Biopolymers in Drug Delivery and Regenerative Medicine

Biopolymers in Drug Delivery and Regenerative Medicine

Editors

Carlos A. García-González
Pasquale Del Gaudio
Ricardo Starbird

MDPI • Basel • Beijing • Wuhan • Barcelona • Belgrade • Manchester • Tokyo • Cluj • Tianjin

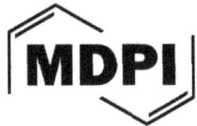

Editors

Carlos A. García-González
University of Santiago de
Compostela
Spain

Pasquale Del Gaudio
University of Salerno
Italy

Ricardo Starbird
Instituto Tecnológico de Costa Rica
Costa Rica

Editorial Office
MDPI
St. Alban-Anlage 66
4052 Basel, Switzerland

This is a reprint of articles from the Special Issue published online in the open access journal *Molecules* (ISSN 1420-3049) (available at: https://www.mdpi.com/journal/molecules/special_issues/Biopolymer_Drug_Delivery_Medicine).

For citation purposes, cite each article independently as indicated on the article page online and as indicated below:

LastName, A.A.; LastName, B.B.; LastName, C.C. Article Title. *Journal Name* **Year**, *Volume Number*, Page Range.

ISBN 978-3-0365-0900-6 (Hbk)
ISBN 978-3-0365-0901-3 (PDF)

Cover image courtesy of Carlos A. García-González.

© 2021 by the authors. Articles in this book are Open Access and distributed under the Creative Commons Attribution (CC BY) license, which allows users to download, copy and build upon published articles, as long as the author and publisher are properly credited, which ensures maximum dissemination and a wider impact of our publications.

The book as a whole is distributed by MDPI under the terms and conditions of the Creative Commons license CC BY-NC-ND.

Contents

About the Editors vii

Ricardo Starbird-Perez, Pasquale Del Gaudio and Carlos A. García-González
Special Issue: Biopolymers in Drug Delivery and Regenerative Medicine
Reprinted from: *Machines* 2021, 26, 568, doi:10.3390/molecules26030568 1

Marlon Osorio, Estefanía Martinez, Tonny Naranjo and Cristina Castro
Recent Advances in Polymer Nanomaterials for Drug Delivery of Adjuvants in Colorectal Cancer Treatment: A Scientific-Technological Analysis and Review
Reprinted from: *Machines* 2020, 25, 2270, doi:10.3390/molecules25102270 5

Emily Goel, Megan Erwin, Claire V. Cawthon, Carson Schaff, Nathaniel Fedor, Trevor Rayl, Onree Wilson, Uwe Christians, Thomas C. Register, Randolph L. Geary, Justin Saul and Saami K. Yazdani
Pre-Clinical Investigation of Keratose as an Excipient of Drug Coated Balloons
Reprinted from: *Machines* 2020, 25, 1596, doi:10.3390/molecules25071596 41

Clara López-Iglesias, Enriqueta R. López, Josefa Fernández, Mariana Landin and Carlos A. García-González
Modeling of the Production of Lipid Microparticles Using PGSS® Technique
Reprinted from: *Machines* 2020, 25, 4927, doi:10.3390/molecules25214927 53

Giulia Auriemma, Paola Russo, Pasquale Del Gaudio, Carlos A. García-González, Mariana Landín and Rita Patrizia Aquino
Technologies and Formulation Design of Polysaccharide-Based Hydrogels for Drug Delivery
Reprinted from: *Machines* 2020, 25, 3156, doi:10.3390/molecules25143156 67

Antonella Caterina Boccia, Guido Scavia, Ilaria Schizzi and Lucia Conzatti
Biobased Cryogels from Enzymatically Oxidized Starch: Functionalized Materials as Carriers of Active Molecules
Reprinted from: *Machines* 2020, 25, 2557, doi:10.3390/molecules25112557 103

Milica Pantić, Gabrijela Horvat, Željko Knez and Zoran Novak
Preparation and Characterization of Chitosan-Coated Pectin Aerogels: *Curcumin* Case Study
Reprinted from: *Machines* 2020, 25, 1187, doi:10.3390/molecules25051187 115

Fernando Alvarado-Hidalgo, Karla Ramírez-Sánchez and Ricardo Starbird-Perez
Smart Porous Multi-Stimulus Polysaccharide-Based Biomaterials for Tissue Engineering
Reprinted from: *Machines* 2020, 25, 5286, doi:10.3390/molecules25225286 129

Karla Ramírez Sánchez, Aura Ledezma-Espinoza, Andrés Sánchez-Kopper, Esteban Avendaño-Soto, Mónica Prado and Ricardo Starbird Perez
Polysaccharide κ-Carrageenan as Doping Agent in Conductive Coatings for Electrochemical Controlled Release of Dexamethasone at Therapeutic Doses
Reprinted from: *Machines* 2020, 25, 2139, doi:10.3390/molecules25092139 151

Christian B. Schimper, Paul S. Pachschwoell, Hubert Hettegger, Marie-Alexandra Neouze, Jean-Marie Nedelec, Martin Wendland, Thomas Rosenau and Falk Liebner
Aerogels from Cellulose Phosphates of Low Degree of Substitution: A TBAF·H$_2$O/DMSO Based Approach
Reprinted from: *Machines* 2020, 25, 1695, doi:10.3390/molecules25071695 165

About the Editors

Carlos A. García-González Department of Pharmacology, Pharmacy and Pharmaceutical Technology, University of Santiago de Compostela. Interests: aerogels; supercritical fluids; regenerative medicine; pharmaceutical technology; 3D-bioprinting; porous materials; scaffolds; biomedical applications.

Pasquale Del Gaudio Università di Salerno, Salerno, Italy. Interests: Polysaccharides; Controlled drug delivery; Wound healing; Aerogels; Personalized therapies; Pulmonary delivery; Micro-Nanoencapsulation.

Ricardo Starbird Escuela de Química, Instituto Tecnológico de Costa Rica, 30102 Cartago, Costa Rica. Interests: polymer science; structuration of biomass and conductive polymers; composites and electrochemical sensors.

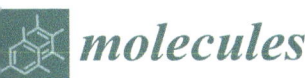

Editorial

Special Issue: Biopolymers in Drug Delivery and Regenerative Medicine

Ricardo Starbird-Perez [1,2,*], Pasquale Del Gaudio [3,*] and Carlos A. García-González [4,*]

1. Centro de Investigación y de Servicios Químicos y Microbiológicos (CEQIATEC), School of Chemistry, Instituto Tecnológico de Costa Rica, 159-7050 Cartago, Costa Rica
2. Centro de Investigación en Ciencia e Ingeniería de Materiales (CICIMA), Universidad de Costa Rica, 11501-2060 San José, Costa Rica
3. Department of Pharmacy, University of Salerno, Via Giovanni Paolo II 132, I-84084 Fisciano, Italy
4. Department of Pharmacology, Pharmacy and Pharmaceutical Technology, I+D Farma Group (GI-1645), Faculty of Pharmacy and Health Research Institute of Santiago de Compostela (IDIS), Universidade de Santiago de Compostela, E-15782 Santiago de Compostela, Spain
* Correspondence: rstarbird@itcr.ac.cr (R.S.-P.); pdelgaudio@unisa.it (P.D.G.); carlos.garcia@usc.es (C.A.G.-G.)

Citation: Starbird-Perez, R.; Del Gaudio, P.; García-González, C.A. Special Issue: Biopolymers in Drug Delivery and Regenerative Medicine. *Molecules* **2021**, *26*, 568. https://doi.org/10.3390/molecules26030568

Academic Editor: Farid Chemat
Received: 15 January 2021
Accepted: 18 January 2021
Published: 22 January 2021

Publisher's Note: MDPI stays neutral with regard to jurisdictional claims in published maps and institutional affiliations.

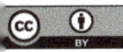

Copyright: © 2021 by the authors. Licensee MDPI, Basel, Switzerland. This article is an open access article distributed under the terms and conditions of the Creative Commons Attribution (CC BY) license (https://creativecommons.org/licenses/by/4.0/).

Biopolymers and biocomposites have emerged as promising pathways to develop novel materials and substrates for biomedical applications. Moreover, the availability, processability, and low toxicity of biopolymers encourage their use in drug delivery and regenerative medicine. The engineering of biopolymer-based materials for their structuration at the nano- and microscale along with their chemical properties allows the design of advanced formulations used as carriers for drug products and as cell scaffolding materials. Finally, combination products including—or based on—biopolymers for controlled drug release offer a powerful solution to improve the tissue integration and biological response of these materials.

In this Special Issue, original research and review articles ranging from the chemical synthesis and characterization of modified biopolymers to their processing in different morphologies and hierarchical structures and in vitro and in vivo evaluation have been gathered together with the aim of contributing to the progress in the biomedicine field.

Recent findings on the applications and processing of biopolymers in the drug delivery area are presented. In a review article, Osorio et al. [1] described different polymer-based drug delivery systems, including polysaccharides and derived polysaccharides, used for the specific case of colorectal cancer treatments. In another biomedical application, Goel et al. carried out a preclinical study (New Zealand White rabbits model) to test the use of keratose, an oxidized form of keratin, as a drug excipient to control the release of paclitaxel, an anti-proliferative drug, from coated biomedical devices (angioplasty balloons) for the treatment of peripheral arterial disease [2]. The benefits of the presence of this biopolymer, in terms of minimizing the adverse impact of peripheral vascular motion on drug retention and reaching a favorable biological response, were assessed. From the processing point of view, López-Iglesias and coworkers [3] introduced a novel production strategy of solid lipid microparticles using a solvent-free technique, the so-called Particles from Gas-Saturated Solutions (PGSS®) process. Artificial neural networks and fuzzy logic tools were used to model the process in terms of temperature, pressure and nozzle diameter to obtain optimized microparticulate systems. The obtained lipid microparticles can be of a potential interest in several biomedical, food and environmental applications. In an alternative processing approach, a comprehensive review by Auriemma et al. presents a description of the theoretical and practical aspects behind the production of different polysaccharide-based hydrogel particles with a special focus on the prilling technology in tandem with several ageing and drying techniques [4]. The value of these techniques is related to its versatility and scalability. Moreover, the gel drying method is a critical step that makes it possible to obtain carriers with specific morphology and inner structure, which may have effects on the release properties. Particularly, the processing of dry polysaccharide-based gels, in the form of cryogels and aerogels, is an emerging field for drug delivery, and European initiatives (e.g., the European Commission-funded AERoGELS CA18125 COST Action) are currently ongoing, with the aim of displaying the full potential of these nanostructured materials for biomedical purposes [5,6]. In this regard, an alternative approach based on the synthesis starch cryogels from enzymatically modified starch combined with lyophilization has been reported by Boccia and coworkers [7]. The chemical nature plays a crucial role in the ability of the prepared cryogels from modified starch to act as drug carriers with promising applications for wound healing and for certain specific administration routes. Additionally, in an experimental application from Pantić et al. [8], tablet-shaped pectin aerogels and pectin aerogels coated with an external layer of chitosan were tested as carriers for oral administration of curcumin, being able to modify the release profile of this drug. Results showed that uncoated pectin aerogel provided a prompt curcumin release, whereas the multilayer biopolymer-based aerogel resulted in a carrier providing a prolonged release of the drug during 24 h.

Advantageous uses of biopolymers as cell scaffolds or for extracellular stimulation were presented in this Special Issue for the development of diverse strategies and implant systems in the regenerative medicine field. In a review article by Alvarado-Hidalgo et al. [9], the recent uses and fabrication methods of biopolymers for extracellular biochemical stimulation of cells as biomimetic 3D scaffold systems were presented. The potential modulation of the extracellular environment through mechanical, electrical, and biochemical stimulation was introduced, with a particular focus on biophysical and biochemical cues of cells that drive their molecular reprogramming. An example of this concept was presented in the research article from Ramírez Sánchez et al. [10]. A smart conductive composite material was processed using κ-carrageenan as a doping agent to improve its electrical properties. The obtained material was electroactive and allowed the release of dexamethasone by electrochemical stimulation, providing a stable system to be used in bioelectronic applications. Finally, cellulose phosphate aerogels for biomedical uses were developed by Schimper et al. [11] through an environmentally friendly methodology based on the conversion of biomass into functional materials. The obtained derivatized cellulose aerogels can be beneficial for the design of dual-porous cell scaffolding materials with interconnected mesopores and micron-size pores.

Therefore, the objective of the Special Issue on "Biopolymers in Drug Delivery and Regenerative Medicine"—to provide the most recent advances on biopolymer research for biomedical applications, particularly in regenerative medicine and drug delivery—has been extensively achieved.

Funding: This research received no external funding.

Acknowledgments: The Guest Editors wish to thank all the authors for their contributions to this Special Issue, all the Reviewers for their work in evaluating the submitted articles, and the editorial staff of Molecules for their kind assistance.

Conflicts of Interest: The authors declare no conflict of interest.

References

1. Osorio, M.; Martinez, E.; Naranjo, T.W.; Castro-Herazo, C. Recent Advances in Polymer Nanomaterials for Drug Delivery of Adjuvants in Colorectal Cancer Treatment: A Scientific-Technological Analysis and Review. *Molecules* **2020**, *25*, 2270. [CrossRef] [PubMed]
2. Goel, E.; Erwin, M.; Cawthon, C.V.; Schaff, C.; Fedor, N.; Rayl, T.; Wilson, O.; Christians, U.; Register, T.C.; Geary, R.L.; et al. Pre-Clinical Investigation of Keratose as an Excipient of Drug Coated Balloons. *Molecules* **2020**, *25*, 1596. [CrossRef] [PubMed]
3. López-Iglesias, C.; López, E.R.; Fernández, J.; Landin, M.; García-González, C.A. Modeling of the Production of Lipid Microparticles Using PGSS®Technique. *Molecules* **2020**, *25*, 4927. [CrossRef] [PubMed]
4. Auriemma, G.; Russo, P.; Del Gaudio, P.; García-González, C.A.; Landin, M.; Aquino, R.P. Technologies and Formulation Design of Polysaccharide-Based Hydrogels for Drug Delivery. *Molecules* **2020**, *25*, 3156. [CrossRef] [PubMed]
5. AERoGELS CA18125 COST Action Website. Available online: https://cost-aerogels.eu/ (accessed on 20 January 2021).

7. García-González, C.A.; Budtova, T.; Durães, L.; Erkey, C.; Del Gaudio, P.; Gurikov, P.; Koebel, M.M.; Liebner, F.; Neagu, M.; Smirnova, I. An Opinion Paper on Aerogels for Biomedical and Environmental Applications. *Molecules* **2019**, *24*, 1815. [CrossRef] [PubMed]
8. Boccia, A.C.; Scavia, G.; Schizzi, I.; Conzatti, L. Biobased Cryogels from Enzymatically Oxidized Starch: Functionalized Materials as Carriers of Active Molecules. *Molecules* **2020**, *25*, 2557. [CrossRef] [PubMed]
9. Pantić, M.; Horvat, G.; Knez, Ž.; Novak, Z. Preparation and Characterization of Chitosan-Coated Pectin Aerogels: Curcumin Case Study. *Molecules* **2020**, *25*, 1187. [CrossRef] [PubMed]
10. Alvarado-Hidalgo, F.; Ramírez-Sánchez, K.; Starbird-Perez, R. Smart Porous Multi-Stimulus Polysaccharide-Based Biomaterials for Tissue Engineering. *Molecules* **2020**, *25*, 5286. [CrossRef] [PubMed]
11. Ramírez-Sánchez, K.; Ledezma-Espinoza, A.; Sánchez-Kopper, A.; Avendaño-Soto, E.; Prado, M.; Starbird-Perez, R. Polysaccharide κ-Carrageenan as Doping Agent in Conductive Coatings for Electrochemical Controlled Release of Dexamethasone at Therapeutic Doses. *Molecules* **2020**, *25*, 2139. [CrossRef] [PubMed]
12. Schimper, C.B.; Pachschwoell, P.S.; Hettegger, H.; Neouze, M.-A.; Nedelec, J.-M.; Wendland, M.; Rosenau, T.; Liebner, F. Aerogels from Cellulose Phosphates of Low Degree of Substitution: A TBAF·H2O/DMSO Based Approach. *Molecules* **2020**, *25*, 1695. [CrossRef] [PubMed]

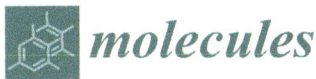

Review

Recent Advances in Polymer Nanomaterials for Drug Delivery of Adjuvants in Colorectal Cancer Treatment: A Scientific-Technological Analysis and Review

Marlon Osorio [1], Estefanía Martinez [1], Tonny Naranjo [2,3] and Cristina Castro [1,*]

[1] School of Engineering, Universidad Pontificia Bolivariana, Circular 1 # 70-01, Medellín 050031, Colombia; marlonandres.osorio@upb.edu.co (M.O.); estefania.martinezc@upb.edu.co (E.M.)
[2] School of Health Sciences, Universidad Pontificia Bolivariana, Calle 78 B # 72 A-109, Medellín 050034, Colombia; tonny.naranjo@upb.edu.co
[3] Medical and Experimental Mycology Group, Corporación para Investigaciones Biológicas, Carrera 72 A # 78 B-141, Medellín 050034, Colombia
* Correspondence: cristina.castro@upb.edu.co; Tel.: +57-448-8388 (ext. 13288)

Academic Editors: Carlos A. García-González, Pasquale Del Gaudio and Ricardo Starbird
Received: 19 April 2020; Accepted: 1 May 2020; Published: 12 May 2020

Abstract: Colorectal cancer (CRC) is the type with the second highest morbidity. Recently, a great number of bioactive compounds and encapsulation techniques have been developed. Thus, this paper aims to review the drug delivery strategies for chemotherapy adjuvant treatments for CRC, including an initial scientific-technological analysis of the papers and patents related to cancer, CRC, and adjuvant treatments. For 2018, a total of 167,366 cancer-related papers and 306,240 patents were found. Adjuvant treatments represented 39.3% of the total CRC patents, indicating the importance of adjuvants in the prognosis of patients. Chemotherapy adjuvants can be divided into two groups, natural and synthetic (5-fluorouracil and derivatives). Both groups can be encapsulated using polymers. Polymer-based drug delivery systems can be classified according to polymer nature. From those, anionic polymers have garnered the most attention, because they are pH responsive. The use of polymers tailors the desorption profile, improving drug bioavailability and enhancing the local treatment of CRC via oral administration. Finally, it can be concluded that antioxidants are emerging compounds that can complement today's chemotherapy treatments. In the long term, encapsulated antioxidants will replace synthetic drugs and will play an important role in curing CRC.

Keywords: colorectal cancer; antioxidants; 5-fluorouracil; polymer nanomaterials; nanocapsules; chemotherapy

1. Introduction

Every sixth death in the world is due to cancer, making it the second leading cause of death [1,2], and despite survival rates increasing, according to the Institute for Health Metrics and Evaluation of the University of Seattle, more than a million people died because of cancer globally in 2017 [3]. In 2016, more than 8.15 million people suffered from breast cancer, which was the type with the most morbidity, followed by colorectal cancer (CRC) and prostate cancer with 6.32 million and 5.7 million cases, respectively [1]. Of these three cancer types, CRC represents the highest number of deaths [3]. Several factors increase the risk of cancer; however, advancing age is the most important for cancer overall, and for CRC, specifically, a diet rich in meat cooked at high temperatures is associated with an increased risk of CRC [4].

Moreover, moderate-to-heavy alcohol consumption is associated with a 1.2- to 1.5-fold increased risk of CRC [5]. Others factors include African American ethnicity, male sex, inflammatory bowel disease, obesity, a sedentary lifestyle, red meat and processed meat intake, tobacco use, a history of abdominal radiation, acromegaly, renal transplant with use of immunosuppressive medications, diabetes mellitus and insulin resistance, androgen deprivation therapy, cholecystectomy, coronary artery disease, and ureterocolic anastomosis [6].

All of the above have led to a huge interest in cancer research. Today, cancer research is focused on identifying the causes and developing strategies for the prevention, diagnosis, treatment, and cure of cancer [7]. Cancer is one of the most investigated subjects; for instance, the proportion of cancer-related entries in PubMed rose from 6% in 1950 to 16% in 2016 [8], being even higher than for other diseases such as various infections (malaria, AIDS, tuberculosis, among others) and diabetes [8].

Accordingly, there is huge scientific research interest in treating and curing CRC, and several strategies have arisen to improve the therapeutic effects and reduce the side effects of actual chemotherapy for CRC treatment. Most of them include polymer drug delivery systems. Thus, this paper aims to review polymer drug delivery systems for adjuvant treatments for CRC, including an initial scientific-technological analysis of the papers and patents related to cancer, CRC, and adjuvant treatments using polymer approaches. The novelty of this paper lies in its broad overview of polymer families and the interaction of them with adjuvants. Moreover, it is explained how the behavior of those emerging drug delivery strategies is related to the superficial charge and chemical groups of the used polymers, information that, to the knowledge of the authors, is not reviewed in the literature for CRC.

2. Scientific-Technological Analysis

In Scopus, the total of cancer-related papers in 2018 was 2,857,590 (see Figure 1a), and CRC-related papers numbered 167,366 (see Figure 1b); both subjects presented an exponential rise from 1970. The first documents indexed in Scopus related to CRC were report cases of medical interventions; for instance, Mr. Luke (1860) reported the surgery of an intestinal obstruction resulting from CRC [9]. Similarly, Dunphy (1947) reported four cases of CRC and included a gross pathological evaluation of the tumors [10].

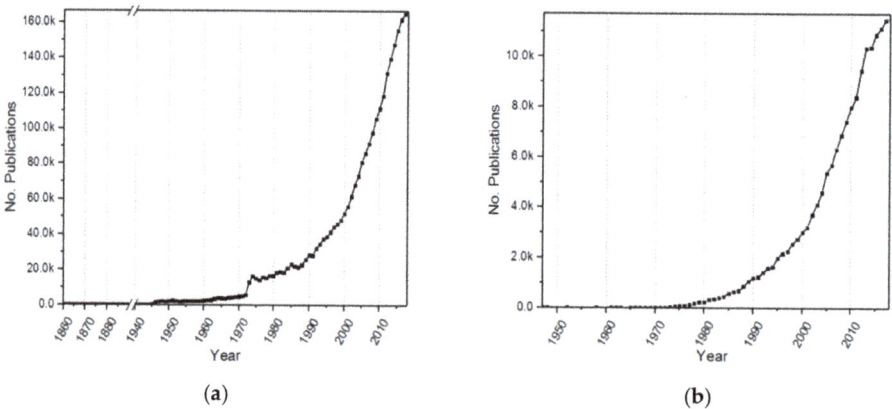

Figure 1. Number of publications of cancer in Scopus; (**a**) total number of cancer-related publications from 1860 to 2018 using the search string "TITLE-ABS-KEY (cancer)"; (**b**) total number of colorectal cancer-related publications from 1947 to 2018 using the search string "TITLE-ABS-KEY (colorectal and cancer)".

In 1970, the first paper that reported the use of adjuvants was published by Adams et al. (1970), in which they compared the use of intralymphatic 5-fluorouracil (5-FU) and radioactive gold as adjuvants to surgical operations for colorectal carcinoma [11]. The next year, another two papers were published, and today, more than 550 papers have been published on this matter per year (Scopus, search string "TITLE-ABS-KEY (colorectal and cancer and adjuvants)"), representing more than 7% (about 11,700 research papers) of the overall CRC research.

Patents related to cancer represented around 2,356,397 entries from 1898 to 2018. The number of patents related to CRC is about 306,240. The pattern of the number of patents per year is presented in Figure 2. It was interesting to find that that the number of patents related to cancer is lower than the number of scientific papers; this behavior can be related to the number of documents of clinical study cases that count for the papers.

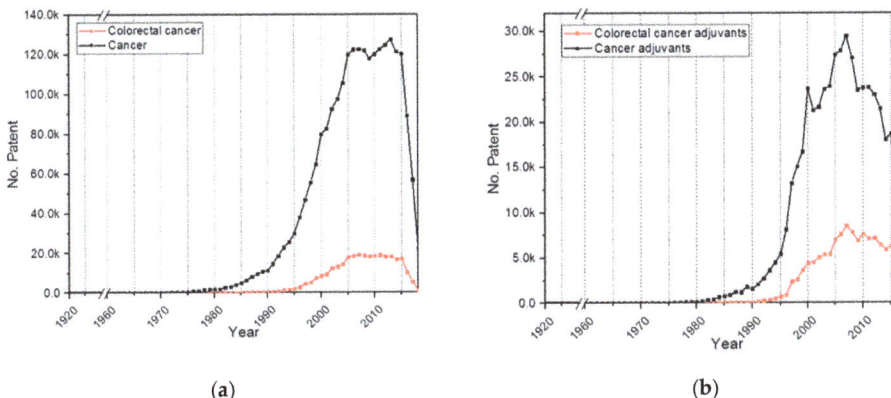

Figure 2. Number of patents per year in (**a**) cancer and colorectal cancer (CRC) (data found in AcclaimIP)—the words "cancer" and "colorectal cancer" were examined in the title, abstract and claims, separately; (**b**) cancer adjuvants and colorectal cancer adjuvants (data found in AcclaimIP)—the words "cancer adjuvant" and "colorectal cancer adjuvant" were searched for in the title, abstract and claims, separately.

Regarding adjuvant therapies, it was found that adjuvants represent 20.0% of the overall cancer patents, and for CRC, adjuvants represent 39.3%. Thus, the number of patents related to adjuvants is proportionally higher for CRC (approximately two-fold) than for overall cancers, which can be explained by the motivation of scientists to cure the most deadly cancer type.

By comparing Figures 1 and 2, it can be seen that adjuvants are more likely to be patented than to be scientifically published (12.6 K vs. 478.9 K) because scientists and companies prefer to protect their intellectual property that can be economically exploited. For instance, the global adjuvant market size was valued at USD 308.99 million in 2016 and is anticipated to grow with a compound annual growth rate (CAGR) of 10.6% [12]. Furthermore, it can be observed that while scientific papers grew rapidly, the number of patents grew until 2010 and then dropped. This behavior can be attributed to the recent difficulty of patenting because applicants' claims should be new and clearly different to previous work [13], which is vast in cancer research, meaning that only 50% of patent applications are adjudicated. This is also discouraging new applications, since authors and companies do not see an attractive cost–benefit ratio for the patenting process [13].

By analyzing the keywords in the latest 2000 papers in Scopus and the title phrases in 1000 patents in the Derwent software (Clarivate Analytics, PA, USA) and then grouping the main subjects (see Figure 3), it was found that adjuvants are the second group for cancer and CRC, with 28.5% and 23.0% of entries, respectively, showing the importance of adjuvant therapy for improving the success of cancer treatments. Emerging strategies such as immunotherapy and biomarkers for treating and classifying cancer were also found.

Regarding the group of adjuvants, it was found that the terms "drug" and "chemotherapy" are more important for CRC than for cancer overall (see Table 1), again exposing the importance of drug delivery strategies for CRC. The drugs with more studies in recent papers (organized per decreasing number of entries) for CRC treatment are 5-fluoraucil, bevacizumab, capecitabine, metformin, aspirin, and irinotecan. Aspirin and metformin drew attention because they are drugs that are used for other purposes. For instance, aspirin and acetyl-salicylates, are used for treating fever, inflammation and pain [14]; however, Garcia et al. (2012) concluded that daily aspirin use at any dose was associated with a 21% lower risk of all-cancer death [15], and Chang et al. (2009) reported that aspirin reduces the risk of colorectal neoplasia in randomized trials and inhibits tumor growth and metastases in animal models, especially in tumors that overexpress cyclooxygenase-2, whereas aspirin can reduce that expression [16].

Table 1. Comparison of keyword groups in scientific papers for cancer adjuvants and colorectal cancer adjuvants. Two thousand papers were extracted from Scopus and examined in their keywords and the documents up to 31/12/2018; the keywords were grouped using VantagePoint.

Keyword Groups	Percentage	
	Cancer Adjuvants	Colorectal Cancer Adjuvants
Chemotherapy	41.2	45.3
Others adjuvant therapies	23.8	13.9
Drugs	10.4	28.0
Radiotherapy	19.9	9.2
Others	4.8	3.6

By analyzing the patents, it was found that the title phrases were more difficult to group and that the topics, in general, were more disperse (see Figure 3c,d); however, adjuvants and pharmaceutical compositions represent more than the 15% of the entries, coming in second place after cancer types, which includes the entries of all cancer names. Likewise, the drugs grouped in pharmaceutical composition for CRC are more diverse, but include indazoles derivatives, heteroaryl derivatives, heterocyclic compounds, quinoline compounds, and tumorigenic inhibitors, among others. These compounds are anticancer agents that have shown antiproliferative activity against cancer cells [17,18].

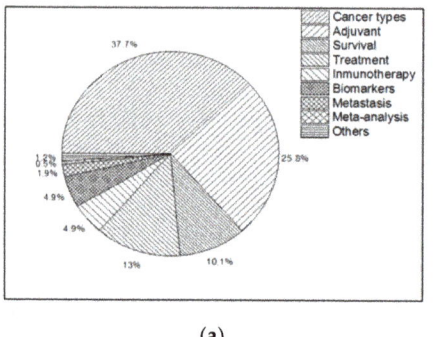 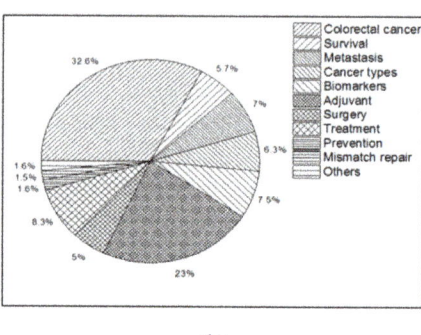

(a) (b)

Figure 3. *Cont.*

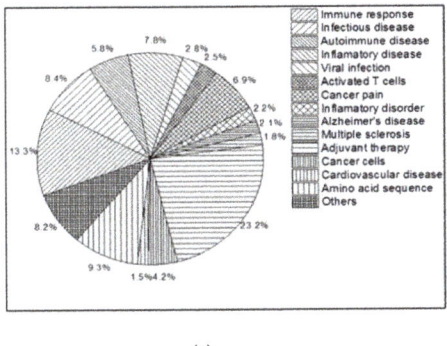
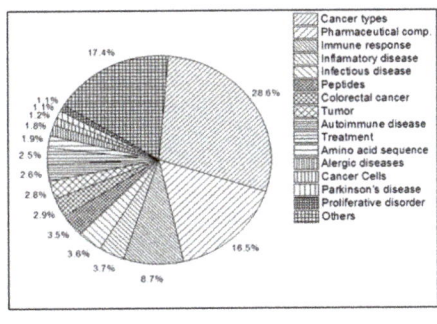

(c)   (d)

Figure 3. Keyword and title phrase groups in the latest papers and patents up to 31/12/2018; (**a**) grouped keywords of cancer adjuvants in scientific papers; (**b**) grouped keywords of colorectal cancer adjuvants in scientific papers; (**c**) grouped title phrases of cancer adjuvants in patents; (**d**) grouped title phrases of colorectal cancer adjuvants in patents. Authors' keywords were extracted from 2000 scientific papers in Scopus and analyzed using VantagePoint. Title patent phrases were extracted from 1000 patents of Derwent and analyzed using VantagePoint.

3. Cancer

According to the World Health Organization, "cancer is a generic term for a large group of diseases characterized by the growth of abnormal cells beyond their usual boundaries that can then invade adjoining parts of the body and/or spread to other organs" [19]. Cancer involves carcinogenesis, which means cancer development; more accuracy, carcinogenesis was first defined by Hecker in 1976 as the "generation of neoplasia" [20]. Neoplasia is an abnormal growth not coordinated with the surrounding tissue [21].

Cancer is initiated via carcinogens in the environment that induce mutations in critical genes, and these mutations direct the cell in which they occur, as well as all of its progeny cells, to grow abnormally. The result of this abnormal growth appears years later as a tumor [21].

Cancer has been traditionally classified in three ways: by the type of tissue in which cancer originates (histological type), by the primary body site, and by the staging (see Figure 4) [19,21].

Histologically, cancer is classified as carcinoma, sarcoma, myeloma, leukemia, and lymphoma [22,23]. Carcinoma refers to a malignant neoplasm of epithelial origin, skin, and tissues that line or cover internal organs. There are two subtypes, adenocarcinoma, which develops in an organ or gland, and squamous cell carcinoma, which originates in the squamous epithelium [23].

Sarcoma refers to cancer that originates in supportive and connective tissues such as the bones, tendons, cartilage, muscle, and fat [22]. Myeloma is cancer that originates in the plasma cells of the bone marrow. Leukemias are also presented in the bone marrow, but this cancer type is associated with the overproduction of immature white blood cells. Leukemia also affects red blood cells and can cause poor blood clotting and fatigue due to anemia [23].

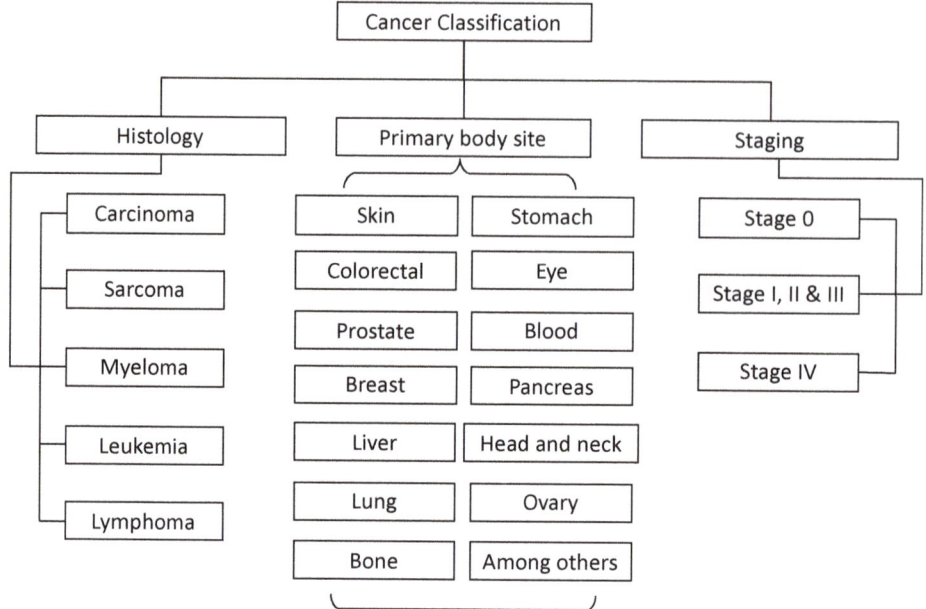

Figure 4. Traditionally cancer classification, histology, primary body site and staging.

Lymphomas develop in the glands or nodes of the lymphatic system—a network of vessels, nodes, and organs (specifically the spleen, tonsils, and thymus) that purify bodily fluids and produce infection-fighting white blood cells, or lymphocytes [22,23].

The body site classification is more familiar to patients, and it refers to the anatomical site at which the cancer appears, for instance, the brain, colorectal tissues, skin, or breast, among others. Finally, staging refers to the process of determining the size of cancer in the body and its localization [23]. To assess the staging of cancer, several diagnostic tests are required (X-rays, biopsies, and ultrasound, among others). In Stage 0, abnormal cells are present but have not spread to nearby tissue [24]; in Stages I, II, and III, cancer is present (the higher stage number, the larger the tumor and the more it has spread into surrounding tissues); and in stage IV, cancer has spread to distant parts of the body (metastasis) [23].

There are also other systems more precise from the medical point of view, for instance, the tumor-node-metastasis (TNM) system that is suggested by The American Joint Committee on Cancer. The TNM is updated periodically, based on advances in the understanding of cancer prognosis, to remain current and relevant for clinical practice; this manual is also described for every anatomical site [23,25].

Recently, there have been other efforts to generate an integrated system to classify cancer [26]. Cancer cells are classified using the cell morphology, leaving behind the functional attributes of these cancer cells. Using techniques in biology based on genomics, transcriptomics, and proteomics, scientists can model the attributes of cancer stem cells and their potential contribution to treatment responses and metastases [26–30].

4. Colorectal Cancer

The name "colorectal cancer" is used to describe bowel cancer that starts in the colon or the rectum. CRC almost always develops from growths called colorectal polyps that form in the lining of the colon (adenocarcinoma in more than 95% of cases) [22,31]. After the diagnosis, the treatment depends on various factors, including the stage of cancer. In the early stages of CRC, the tumor just needs to be surgically removed, but in advanced stages, additional treatments may be considered, such as chemotherapy and radiation therapy, among other adjuvant therapies [31].

5. Colorectal Cancer Treatments

As mentioned above, CRC treatment depends on cancer staging, but it is classified into two groups, surgery and adjuvant therapy.

5.1. Surgery

Colorectal cancers may be cured by surgery (hemicolectomy) [2], but only if the entire tumor is localized and no cells have spread to other sites (adenocarcinoma in situ) [22,32]. Moreover, in most of the cases, complementary therapies (adjuvants) are needed before or after surgery and vary from traditional to novel. Traditional chemotherapies are based on 5-FU, which inhibits cancer cell division. Nobody doubts that traditional adjuvant treatments have improved the prognosis of patients; however, they are not beneficial for all cases. For instance, not all women with breast cancer derive benefit from 5-FU-based adjuvant chemotherapy. Many older women (age > 70) with hormone receptor-positive early stage breast cancer treated with adjuvant chemotherapy will not accrue a survival advantage [33]. For CRC, it was demonstrated that extra cycles of traditional chemotherapy, either before or after chemoradiotherapy, have been shown not to improve survival compared with chemoradiotherapy alone. An argument for less chemotherapy is also presented by results from trials investigating neoadjuvant or preoperative therapy in esophageal and gastric cancers. In randomized trials, which enrolled patients with esophageal and gastro-esophageal junction adenocarcinoma, no survival benefit with four cycles of the ECX regimen (epirubicin, cisplatin, and capecitabine) were reported beyond that achieved with two cycles of fluorouracil and cisplatin. These results support the use of a shorter duration of preoperative chemotherapy [34].

5-FU can cause local and systematic toxicity (DNA damage) to healthy cells, generating undesired side effects, and favor the mutation of them to malignant cells. These problems can be overcome by using novel approaches such as targeting specific cancer-relevant proteins (such as oncogenic tyrosine kinases), immunotherapy, and reactive oxygen species (ROS)-modulated therapies, which are more specific in generating cancer cell apoptosis and reducing the side effects associated with traditional chemotherapy [35,36].

5.2. Adjuvant Therapy

Adjuvant therapy is defined by the United States National Cancer Institute (NCI) as "additional cancer treatment given after the primary treatment (surgery) to lower the risk that cancer will come back" [2], eliminating any residual microscopic cancer cells. Neoadjuvant therapy is an adjuvant therapy given before the primary treatment to make it more effective or easier [37]. Adjuvant therapies for CRC can be divided into five groups, i.e., radiation, hormones, targeted therapy, immunotherapy, and chemotherapy.

5.2.1. Radiation Therapy

Radiation therapy (RT) is the application of ionizing radiation to treat cancer. Cancer cells are more sensitive to DNA damage than normal tissue cells; this characteristic provides the therapeutic effect [38]. It is estimated than 50% of the population with cancer can benefit from this therapy [38]. For colorectal cancer, RT is used as a neoadjuvant treatment to improve patient prognosis, heightening the overall survival rate, diminishing the local recurrence rate, and improving the quality of the surgical procedures [39].

Besides some side effects—such as incontinence of the anal sphincter or urinary tract problems, vaginal dryness, and sexual dysfunction, among others—related to neoadjuvant RT, new techniques have focused efforts on modulating the beam intensity and improving the beam precision and development of delivery systems for encapsulated radionuclides (brachytherapy) [39,40].

5.2.2. Hormone Therapy

Bowel health largely depend on hormones; for instance, Jhonson et al. (2009) found that sex hormones such as estrogen and progestin are related to protective effects against CRC in menopausal women [41]. Similar results were found by Rennert et al. (2009) in 5214 women in perimenopausal/postmenopausal stages with CRC, where the use of estrogen/progestin replacement therapy reduced the risk of CRC by 63% [41]. For men, Lin et al. (2014) found that higher levels of testosterone are related to lower risks of CRC [42]. Hormone therapy is a systemic approach with several side effects such as abdominal pain, headache, depression, acne, nausea, leg cramps, and stroke, among others [43,44]. The use of drug delivery systems can help in reducing the needed doses, which can lower the undesired side effects of the treatment [45].

5.2.3. Targeted Therapy

Targeted therapy is a type of treatment that uses drugs or other substances to identify and attack specific types of cancer cell with less harm to healthy cells. Targeted therapy may have fewer side effects than other types of cancer treatment. Targeted therapies are either small molecule drugs or monoclonal antibodies [23]. The most investigated monoclonal antibodies are bevacizumab, cetuximab, and panitumumab [46,47].

Bevacizumab is a recombinant humanized monoclonal IgG antibody that selectively binds to vascular endothelial growth factor A (VEGF-A), and it demonstrates anti-tumor activity by blocking vascular endothelial growth factor receptor 2 (VEGFR2). Furthermore, patients treated with cetuximab and panitumumab showed a survival benefit in metastatic CRC [46]. Cetuximab is an anti-epithelial grow factor (EGFR) monoclonal antibody of the IgG1 class targeted against the extracellular domain of the EGFR. By binding to the EGFR, cetuximab blocks intracellular EGFR signaling and modulates tumor cell growth by inhibiting proliferation, angiogenesis, and differentiation; stimulating apoptosis; and preventing metastasis. Panitumumab is a fully human, monoclonal antibody targeting the EGFR with high affinity. Its mechanism of inhibiting the EGFR signaling pathway is similar to that of cetuximab, as described above [46]. Nevertheless, to improve the efficacy of the treatment, the therapy should be complemented with cytotoxic chemotherapy using 5-FU [48,49].

5.2.4. Immunotherapy

Immunotherapy was first proposed in 1909 by Nobel Prize winner Paul Ehrlich. The idea behind it is that immune cells can control malignant cells and eradicate cancers before they manifest clinically [35]. However, in spite of several mechanisms active in the immune system to recognize and eliminate tumor cells, some variants of these cells selectively acquire increased resistance against immune responses. Thereafter, resistant cells continue to grow, evading the immune responses, and tumor cells develop resistance against both innate and adaptive immune mechanisms (cancer immunoediting) [35]. To avoid cancer immunoediting, patients can be vaccinated (monoclonal antibodies, adaptive T cells, DNA viral vectors, heat shock proteins, and dendritic cells, among others [35,50–54]) to raise specific immune responses. Moreover, this therapy is followed in parallel with another adjuvant therapy to potentiate the immune system [35].

5.2.5. Chemotherapy

Chemotherapy for cancer treatment uses drugs (plant-derived or synthetic) called cytostatic drugs (cytotoxic chemotherapy), which aim to stop cancer cells from continuing to divide uncontrollably [55].

It is estimated that 20–30% of newly diagnosed patients with CRC present with unresectable metastatic disease. In addition, a considerable proportion of patients (40–50%) experience disease recurrence after surgical resection or develop metastatic disease, typically in the liver or lungs [56]. To improve the life prognosis of those patients, several drugs have been developed, such as 5-FU, which is considered the gold standard for CRC chemotherapy [56].

5-FU was developed in 1957 by Charles Heidelberger and colleagues at the University of Wisconsin, who observed that tumor tissues preferentially used uracil-type molecules for nucleic acid biosynthesis and postulated that a fluorouracil analog would be easily taken up by cancer cells. Likewise, it would inhibit tumor cell division by blocking the conversion of deoxyuridine monophosphate (dUMP) to deoxythymidine monophosphate (thymidylate) [56].

From 1957 to date, 5-FU has been complemented with other adjuvants to improve the overall survival of patients. For instance, Petrelli et al. (1987) found that mixing 5-FU with leucovorin at 500 mg/m^2 in metastatic patients improved overall survival [57]. Goldberg et al. (2004) studied the efficacy in metastatic CRC patients of 5-FU plus leucovorin, irinotecan, and oxaliplatin combinations (FOLFOX) in 795 patients, finding a median survival rate of 19.5 months, which is 35% higher compared with that with other treatments [58], and recently, Magne et al. (2012) investigated the efficacy of cetuximab with continuous or intermittent 5-FU, leucovorin, and oxaliplatin (Nordic FLOX) treatment versus FLOX alone in the first-line treatment of metastatic CRC, finding an overall survival of up to 20.4 months [59].

Today, there is a growing interest in researching natural drugs as adjuvants for CRC; most of them act against reactive oxygen species (ROS). Reactive oxygen species (ROS) include oxygen molecules, superoxide anion radicals, hydroxyl free radicals, and hydrogen peroxide. ROS are generated in the mitochondrial respiratory pathway. Although an increase in the level of intracellular ROS leads to oxidative stress and DNA damage, the effects of ROS are normally balanced by antioxidants, such as reduced glutathione (GSH), ascorbic acid, and uric acid [60]. Disruption of the oxidant–antioxidant balance through alterations to cellular homeostasis or the defective repair of ROS-induced damage is involved in carcinogenesis. Furthermore, it is known that anticancer drugs induce oxidative stress in patients with cancer being treated with chemotherapy [60]. To reduce oxidative stress, investigations are focusing on natural antioxidants. In Table 2, the latest studies for CRC using natural antioxidants are presented. Natural antioxidants are presented as extracts (fruits, plants, and coffee, among others) or polyphenol fractions from those extracts [61].

Table 2. Natural antioxidants for the prevention and treatment of colorectal cancer; recent reports from 2015 to 2019.

Natural Antioxidant	Authors	Main Findings	Reference
Ginseng extracts	Jin et al. (2016)	Meta-analysis indicated a significant 16% lower risk of developing cancer in patients who consumed ginseng.	[62]
	Wong et al. (2015)	Carcinogenic modulation. Cancer cells do not generate resistance to ginseng extracts. Kill cancer cells while exerting low toxicity toward healthy cells.	[63]
	Chong-Zin et al. (2016)	Ginseng extract enhanced the antiproliferative effect of 5-FU on human colorectal cancer cells.	[64]
	Tang et al. (2018) Kim et al. (2018)	Inhibits metastasis and reduces the invasion of CRC in vitro and in vivo.	[65,66]
Ginger (Zerumbone)	Sithara et al. (2018) Girisa et al. (2019)	Inhibits the proliferation of CRC cells (SW480) and thereby induced apoptosis, which might be due to mitochondria transmembrane dysfunction, translocation of phosphatidylserine, and chromatin condensation. Oral administration of zerumbone at more than 100 ppm for 17 weeks to mice significantly inhibited the multiplicity of and inflammation in colonic adenocarcinomas.	[67,68]

Table 2. Cont.

Natural Antioxidant	Authors	Main Findings	Reference
Garlic	Kim et al. (2019)	Diallyl disulfide from garlic increased tumor necrosis factor-related apoptosis in CRC cell lines and in vivo.	[69]
	Roy et al. (2018)	S-allyl-L-cysteine-sulfoxide (SACS)/alliin compounds from garlic showed higher affinity towards EGFR in silico, and in vitro, showed anticancer activity modulating the EGFR in CRC cells.	[70]
Lactoferrin	Li et al. (2017)	Lactoferrin inhibited cell viability, with the 50% concentration of inhibition at 81.3 ± 16.7 mg/mL and 101 ± 23.8 mg/mL for HT29 and HCT8 cells, respectively. Moreover, lactoferrin reduces the relative tumor volume in mouse models compared with negative control.	[71]
	Sugihara et al. (2017)	Rats given 500 and 1000 mg/kg/day of lactoferrin harbored significantly fewer colon aberrant crypt foci, adenomas, and adenocarcinomas than the rats from the control group, due to lactoferrin inhibiting cell growth and TNF-α mRNA expression.	[72]
Polyphenols	Yang et al. (2016)	Polyphenol (−)-epigallocatechin-3-gallate from green tea inhibited growth and the activation of the VEGF/VEGFR axis in human colorectal cancer cells.	[73]
	Gómez-Juaristi et al. (2017)	Yerba mate tea flavonoids are highly adsorbed and metabolized by the human body, especially in the colon microbiota.	[74]
	Amigo-Benavent et al. (2017)	Yerma mate, its phenolic components, and metabolites decrease cancer cell viability and proliferation; evaluated in vitro in Caco-2 colon cells.	[75]
	Schmit et al. (2016)	Coffee consumption was associated with 26% lower odds of developing colorectal cancer.	[76]
	Amigo-Benavent et al. (2017)	Green coffee bean, its phenolic components, and metabolites decrease cancer cell viability and proliferation; evaluated in vitro in Caco-2 colon cells.	[75]
	Scafuri et al. (2016)	Apple phenolic compounds interfere with the activity of nucleotide metabolism and methylation enzymes, similarly to some classes of anticancer drug.	[77]
	Darband et al. (2018)	The polyphenol quercetin poses anticancer effects in colon cancer; it inhibits cell proliferation, angiogenesis, and tumor metastasis, along with promoting apoptosis and autophagy and reducing the drug resistance.	[78]
	Huang et al. (2017)	Curcumin enhances the effects of irinotecan on CRC cells through the generation of reactive oxygen species and activation of the endoplasmic reticulum stress pathway.	[79]
	Ravindranathan et al. (2018)	Curcumin and oligomeric proanthocyanidins offer superior anti-tumorigenic properties in CRC, affecting DNA replication, the cell cycle, and mismatch repair in CRC cells.	[80]
	Marjaneh et al. (2018)	Combination of curcumin with 5-FU dramatically reduced the tumor number and tumor size in both the distal and middle parts of colon in colitis-associated CRC. Additionally, curcumin suppressed colonic inflammation and notably recovered the levels of antioxidant activity.	[81]
	Agudelo et al. (2017)	Polyphenols in *Vaccinium meridionale Swartz* juices showed an apoptotic effect on SW480. The caspase 3 activity was increased in a time-dependent manner in SW480-treated cells; the proapoptotic proteins were increased by 1.6- to 2.0-fold. In addition, SW480 cells significantly increased the production of intracellular ROS, parallel with a reduction in the intracellular content of glutathione (GSH) and consequently a decrease in the GSH/oxidized glutathione (GSSG) ratio.	[82]
	Buhrmann et al. (2018) Buhrmann et al. (2019)	Resveratrol suppressed the formation of cancer-like stem cells in two different CRC lines, and this was accompanied with a significant increase in apoptosis. Moreover, resveratrol suppresses the tumor necrosis factor B, which is a pro-carcinogenic compound.	[83,84]

Table 2. *Cont.*

Natural Antioxidant	Authors	Main Findings	Reference
Fermented skim milk	Chang et al. (2019)	*Lactobacillus paracasei* subsp. *paracasei* NTU 101-fermented skim milk in combination with chemotherapy for CRC in vivo significantly suppressed tumor growth and metastasis compared to chemotherapy alone via regulating vascular endothelial growth factor, matrix metalloprotein-9, and tissue inhibitor of matrix metalloproteinase-1 levels.	[85]
Rosa canina extracts	Turan et al. (2018)	*Rosa canina* extract exhibited a selective cytotoxic effect on CRC cells compared with normal colon cells. The extract induced cell cycle arrest at the S phase and apoptosis via reducing matrix metalloproteinases in CRC cells.	[86]
Vitamin C	Aguilera et al. (2018)	Vitamin C uncouples the Warburg metabolic switch in KRAS mutant colorectal cancer, inducing apoptosis.	[87]
Chlorophyll	Semeraro et al. (2018)	Chlorophyll a is a good candidate for photodynamic therapy due to its intense absorption of red and near-infrared light. In combination with β-cyclodextrins, it was demonstrated that it selectively kills CRC via a necrotic mechanism.	[88]
Piperin	Bantal et al. (2018)	Piperin at 50 mg/kg reduced CRC's effects in vivo (mouse model), i.e., inflammation and focal congestion in sub-mucosa and muscularis layers.	[89]
Manilkara Zapota extract	Tan et al. (2019)	*Manilkara Zapota* extract leaf water extract can inhibit the viability of CRC cells in 72 h, at a concentration ranging from 21 to 84 µg/mL.	[90]

Accordingly, most of the antioxidants in Table 2 are polyphenols, due to most plant-based food naturally containing them. The basic monomer in polyphenols is a phenolic ring, and generally, these are classified as phenolic acids and phenolic alcohols [61]. Polyphenol consumption is strongly associated with a low cancer risk. For instance, the Mediterranean diet (rich in olive oil polyphenols [91]), reduces the risk of CRC by approximately 4% [92]. However, 4% is still modest; thus, polyphenols are extracted to present higher antioxidant activity and consequentially higher anticancer effects. Moreover, the colorectal anticancer effect can be potentiated if the antioxidant is supplied using a drug delivery system [93].

6. Polymer-Based Drug Delivery Systems for Adjuvants for Colorectal Cancer

Ideally, drugs would target the cancer cells with the exact therapeutic concentration. However, drug delivery is not easily controlled. Drug release rates, cell- and tissue-specific targeting, and drug stability are difficult to predict [93]. Furthermore, when targeting colon cells, the drug may avoid degradation and/or be released early, which would reduce its therapeutic effect.

Likewise, natural and synthetic compounds can be easily degraded by air, UV light, and moisture, and lose their antioxidant potential [94]. Thus, encapsulation is important for improving their stability and, overall, generating long-term desorption profiles that improve the CRC adjuvant treatments.

6.1. Nanoencapsulation

Nanoencapsulation is a nanostructured drug delivery system (10–1000 nm [95]) that can be loaded with small molecules or macromolecules, thus acting as a vehicle for chemotherapeutic drugs. Such materials are able to transport chemotherapeutic molecules to the desired area, increasing the drug concentration, to be subsequently released in a controlled manner. A great number of nanoformulations—such as liposomes, micelles, nanoemulsions, and polymeric nanoparticles, among others—have been reported as drug delivery systems to be applied in cancer treatment [96–99].

Nanoencapsulation can be performed to generate two categories of nanodevice (see Figure 5), nanocapsules and matrixial nanomaterials. In the nanocapsules group, the chemotherapeutic drug is surrounded by a wall or shell material to generate spheres or irregular nanocapsules where the chemotherapeutic drug can be mononucleated (a single core) or polynucleated (multicore) [100–102].

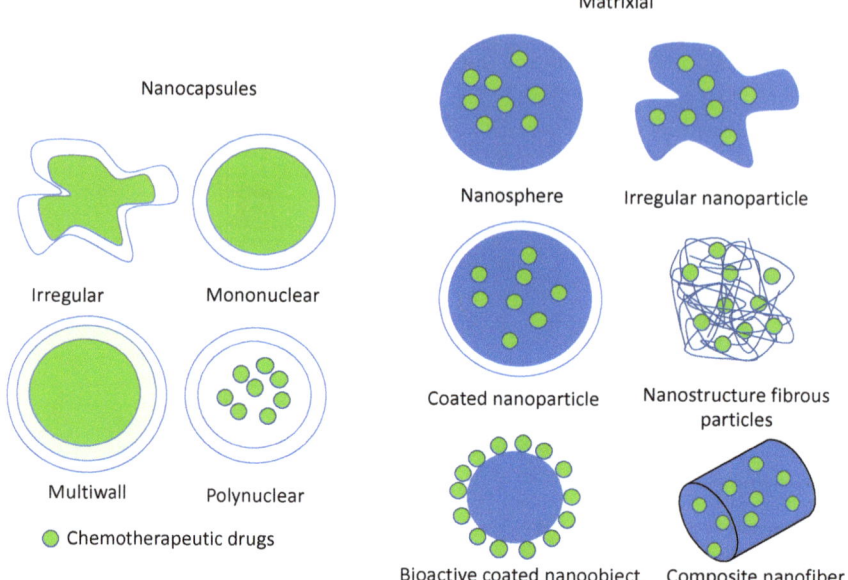

Figure 5. Nanodevices for the encapsulation of chemotherapeutic drugs/antioxidants.

Matrixial nanomaterials are more varied. Generally, the bioactive compound (chemotherapeutic drug) is embedded or superficially adsorbed in a polymer matrix. The polymer matrix can be configured in different forms, nanospheres, irregular nanoparticles, and nanofibers, among others [103–105]. Likewise, the nanoparticle may or not may be coated by another polymer. The nanoparticle can be solid or nanostructured by fibers [106,107].

The techniques used for achieving nanoencapsulation are complex. This is mainly due to the difficulty in attaining the complex morphology of the capsule and core material and the demands of controlling the release rate of the nanocapsules [108]. Various techniques have been developed and used for nanoencapsulation purposes. For instance, emulsification, coacervation, inclusion complexation, solvent evaporation, nanoprecipitation, and supercritical fluid techniques can produce capsules in the nanometer range (10–1000 nm) [95,108]. Most of the documents regarding encapsulation relate to particles between 100 and 1000 nm. However, there also some reports with capsules ranging from 10 to 100 nm.

6.2. Release Mechanism

Nanodevices (nanocapsules and matrixial nanomaterials) can provide several forms of release for the chemotherapeutic drugs (see Figure 6). Drugs can be desorbed from the matrix or core reservoir (nanocapsules) because of a concentration gradient that can be assisted by swelling or material relaxation, facilitating the release of the bioactive component [109].

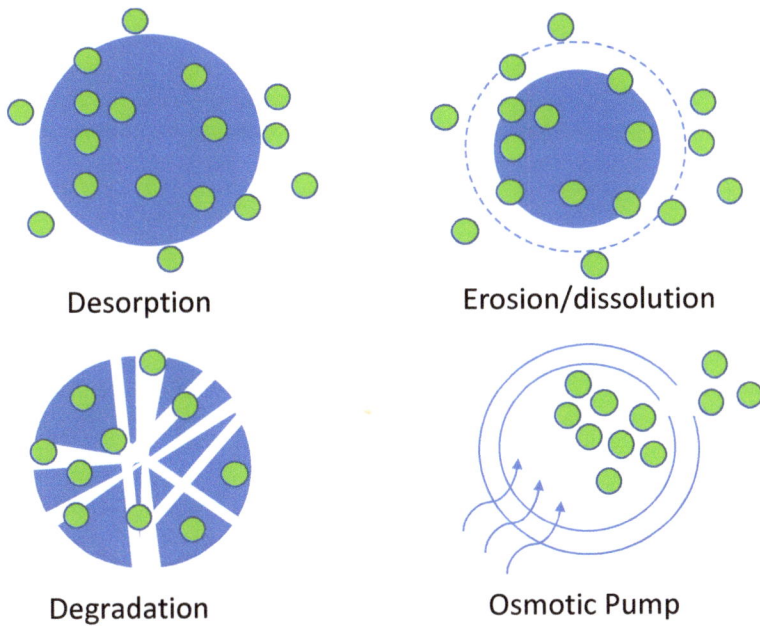

Figure 6. Drug-releasing mechanism of chemotherapeutic drugs.

The erosion/dissolution implies the loss of the shell or matrix integrity to favor the diffusion of the bioactive component. The erosion/dissolution of the nanodevice can be triggered by pH changes and water content, among others. Usually these systems deliver the bioactive compound quickly once the capsule is in contact with the target environment. Otherwise, the degradation mechanism tends to be a slow as it is mediated by enzymatic reactions [110,111].

An osmotically active drug can be delivered using an osmotic pump, in which the bioactive component is pushed away by a fluid that goes into the capsule via a semipermeable membrane and force the drug to pass throughout an orifice [112].

Along with the nanodevice type, the interaction of the biomaterial/bioactive compound modulates the releasing profile. Bioactive components for CRC treatment are complex; for instance, antioxidants poses aromatic rings with hydroxyl lateral groups, conferring to them a hydrophilic nature [113], and hydroxyl groups can easily generate hydrogen bond interactions with biomaterials. Antioxidants of high molecular weight present an amphiphilic nature, with hydrophilic and lipophilic zones such in the case of vitamin E and carotenoids [114], which can interact with either polar or nonpolar polymers.

Plant extracts contains several bioactive compounds (mixtures of hydrophilic and lipophilic compounds). Nevertheless, most CRC adjuvant extracts are, in general, hydrophilic in nature and water-soluble [90,115–117] and thus can interact with hydrophilic polymers. Likewise, synthetic bioactive compounds have an amphiphilic nature; for instance, 5-FU is a pyrimidine with oxygen and flour lateral groups, conferring it with a hydrophilic nature, but 5-FU can present resonance diminishing its water solubility [118]. According to the above, given the diversity of CRC adjuvants, several polymer-based biomaterials have been used for generating nanodevices for drug delivery systems.

6.3. Polymers for Oral Drug Delivery Systems

Biomaterials have improved the delivery and efficacy of a range of pharmaceutical compounds. In particular, polymer- and lipid-based materials have been designed to release therapeutics for extended periods of time and for targeting specific locations within the body, thereby reducing the toxicity to the patient whilst keeping the therapeutic effect [110]. Lipid-based drug delivery systems are beyond of the goals of this paper; these formulations types are reviewed in the following references [119–121]. For polymer drug delivery, the oral route has been proven to be most convenient route for chronic drug therapy [119]. For instance, in studies of CRC patients, it has been proven that the oral administration of adjuvant treatments is most suitable for the patient and cost-saving for health systems [122,123]. However, oral administration is challenging for CRC as the drug needs to be protected during passage through the digestive tract before proper delivery. For this application, polymers are advantageous due to their processability at the nanoscale, their wide range of functional groups, and the possibility of generating mixtures, composites, and copolymers, among others [124], favoring the protection of the drug and its delivery profile.

Drug delivery polymers for colorectal cancer can be classified according to polymer nature, into non-charged polymers and charged polymers (anionic, cationic, and zwitterionic), as presented in Figure 7. Non-charged polymers cannot be charged via dissociation; thus, they are strongly stable at any pH value, and they can interact via hydrogen bonding and Van der Waals interactions. Alternatively, charged polymers can generate anionic, cationic, or zwitterionic charges on their surface and can switch from neutral to charged, depending on the hydrogen potential of the surrounding environment. The switching from neutral to charged will influence the chain polymer organization. For instance, Han et al. (2016) found that the carboxylic lateral groups of polyacrylic acid copolymers induces polymer changes in terms of roughness, thickness, and porosity, from pH 5.5 to 9 [125]. Those systems have the advantage of modulating the drug release by pH, as presented in the gastrointestinal fluids. The interaction with these polymers is more likely to be ionic, which is stronger, but requires at least polar or ionic charges in the bioactive compounds.

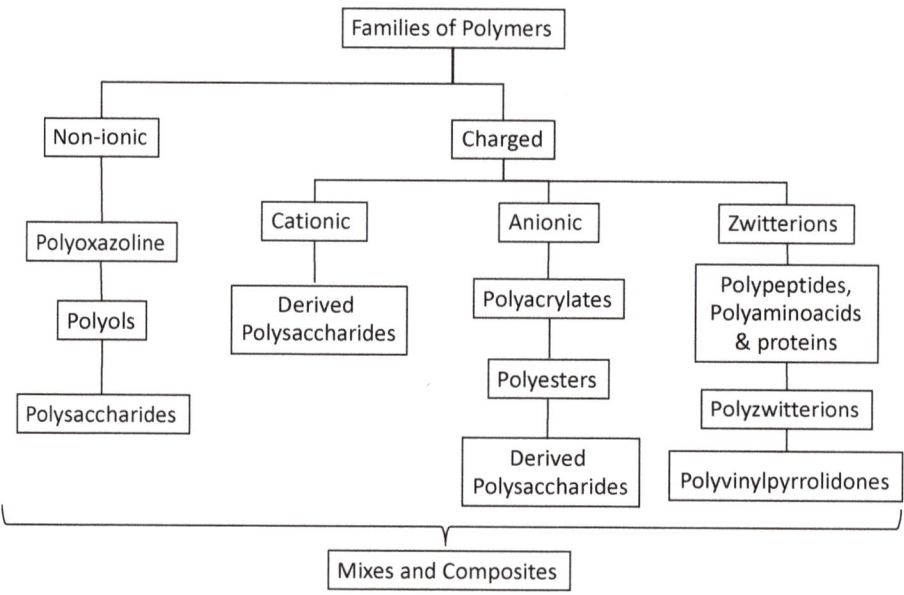

Figure 7. Polymer families for drug delivery systems of antioxidants for CRC.

Mixtures and composites are alternative strategies for creating a synergistic response in the system [126,127]. In the following sections, the strategies for each polymer type in drug delivery systems for CRC are described.

6.4. Polymers for Encapsulating Antioxidants for Colorectal Cancer

Antioxidants for drug delivery have more than 4600 documents indexed in Scopus, with an accelerated growth from 2000 to date. From those, around 44.6% include the word "polymer", which hints at the relevance of creating polymer-based drug delivery systems to protect these compounds. For encapsulating antioxidants, all polymer families have been used for the drug delivery of these compounds.

6.4.1. Polysaccharides and Derived Polysaccharides

Polysaccharides are carbohydrate polymers composed of long chains of monosaccharides, such as glucose, fructose, and galactose, among others [128]. Polysaccharides can respond to pH, colon enzyme degradation, or peristaltic movement. For instance, chitosan can response to pH changes, starches can be degraded by amylase enzymes, and ethyl cellulose can be broken by colon waves [129]. Polysaccharides have garnered attention because, like antioxidants, they come from natural sources, allowing the development of bio-based therapies for CRC. Antioxidants have been successfully encapsulated using polysaccharides for nanocapsules such as cellulose, chitosan, and alginate, among others.

Cellulose is the most abundant polymer on earth; it is composed of β1-4 linked D (+) glucose [124,130,131]. Cellulose and its derivatives have been reported as carriers of antioxidants. For instance, Sunnasee et al. (2019) grafted β-cyclodextrins in cellulose nanocrystals, demonstrating that this system is not immunogenic and does not induce oxidative stress in the cell, thus it is safe for intracellular drug delivery [132]. Li et al. (2019) developed a nanoformulation of quercetin and cellulose nanofibers with sustained antioxidant activity. The nanocellulose fibers were an effective nanocarrier of the antioxidant with a loading capacity of 78.91% and encapsulation efficiency of 88.77%; moreover, the quercetin delivery profile was extended to higher times [133]. Ching et al. (2019) encapsulated curcumin in cellulose nanocrystals (via acid hydrolysis), adding surfactants to improve the loading capacity of the release profile of the antioxidant [134]. Ngwabebhoh et al. (2018) developed a Pickering suspension for encapsulating curcumin using cellulose nanocrystals [106], finding that the capsules were stable for up to 8 days at different pHs [106]. However, the application was directed to antimicrobial properties instead of antioxidants for CRC.

Chitosan is a polysaccharide obtained from chitin deacetylation, composed of β-(1→4)-linked D-glucosamine (deacetylated unit) and *N*-acetyl-D-glucosamine (acetylated unit) [135]. It is a cationic polymer that responds to pH changes and can be converted into hydrogels, making this polymer attractive for the drug delivery of antioxidants. For instance, Kumar et al. (2015) encapsulated naringenin (polyphenol) using chitosan nanocapsules. Their studies proved that encapsulated naringenin has a better anticancer effect than free naringenin [136]. Jeong et al. (2016) crosslinked chitosan with resveratrol modified with phospholipids to improve its oral bioavailability and low water solubility. The researchers found an encapsulation efficiency of up to 85.59%, and an in vitro drug release study suggested a slow and a sustained release governed by diffusion [137].

Shi et al. (2017) encapsulated β-carotene and anthocyanin in (2,2,6,6-Tetramethylpiperidin-1-yl)oxyl (TEMPO)oxidized polysaccharides, specifically Konjac Glucomannan, in which some polysaccharides' hydroxyl lateral groups were converted into carbonyl groups, and then the spheres were coated with chitosan. The advantage of the system was its ability to generate oil–water stable systems and to retain the antioxidants at gastric pH values; moreover, the capsules exhibited anticancer effects [138].

Alginates are salts derived from alginic acid, in which the polymer has a carbonyl lateral group liked to a glucose unit, making the polymer negatively charged [139]. Sookkasem et al. (2015) developed novel alginate beads for encapsulating curcumin for colon target therapy; the capsule was able to prevent release in the upper gastrointestinal tract and immediately release the drug upon the arrival of the beads in the colon [139]. However, the approach of Sookkasem et al. was not at the nanoscale; the alginate beads had a diameter in millimeters (macroscale). Similarly, Wang et al. (2019) developed a macroscale capsule but using ZnO instead of Ca^{2+} as the crosslinking agent to improve the release profile to a longer time [140]. Approaches at the nanoscale for this polymer have been tested using mixtures and composites, especially with chitosan [141,142], as reported in the following sections.

Maltodextrin (α 1–4 D (+) glucose) is a low molecular weight polysaccharide that has been broadly used for the encapsulation of food and pharmaceutical ingredients [143]. Ming et al. (2018) encapsulated red ginseng extract, generating a water/oil emulsion, and then coated it with maltodextrin using spray-drying. The researchers found particles ranging from 58 to 400 nm and optimized the conditions to produce them [143]; however, they did not evaluate the release or anticancer effects of the produced nanocapsules.

Pan et al. (2018) encapsulated curcumin in soybean polysaccharides (mixture of cellulose, xylogalacturonan, and arabinogalactan, among others), polysaccharides that easily link lipophilic compounds. The capsules were stable at a pH ranging from 2.0 to 7.0 [144]. Li et al. (2017) encapsulated phenolic acid antioxidants to prove the effectiveness of producing hollow Arabic gum and short linear glucans from starch templates. Hollow nanocapsules enhanced the antioxidant activity of the phenolic acids and improved the stability of their antioxidant activity in challenging environments with high salt concentrations, and when exposed to UV radiation and high temperatures [145].

Assis et al. (2017) incorporated lycopene nanocapsules in starch films to generate an edible film material, but the application was focused on packaging instead of biomedical efficacy [146]. Amah et al. (2019) encapsulated catechin in starch-based nanoparticles, providing protection to the catechin against the harsh gastric environment and helping to retain its bioactive properties during an in vitro digestion process [147]. Jana et al. (2017) reviewed different strategies for generating three-stimuli-responsive guar gum composites (pH, time, and enzymes) for colon-specific drug delivery [148]. Finally, Saffarzadeh-Matin et al. (2017) prepared an apple pomace polyphenolic extract and encapsulated it in maltodextrin in nanocapsules of 52 nm diameter, optimizing the loading efficiency of the process [149].

6.4.2. Polyacrylates

Polyacrylates are polymers derived from acrylic acid via free radical polymerization. Nevertheless, Garay-Jimenez et al. (2011) reported an alternative method for producing polyacrylate nanoparticles between 40 and 50 nm by emulsion polymerization using a 7:3 mixture of butyl acrylate and styrene in water containing sodium dodecyl sulfate as a surfactant and potassium persulfate as a water-soluble radical initiator. The resulting method seemed promising for the encapsulation of bioactive agents of interest in the biomedical field [150].

Polyacrylates are anionic polymers that present maximum swelling at pH neutral to alkaline, and minimum under acidic conditions, making them ideal for colon-specific drug delivery systems [151].

Feuser et al. (2016) modified with folic acid polymethyl meta acrylate and ferrous sulfate to produce superparamagnetic nanoparticles with excellent colloidal stability and high efficacy in encapsulating lauryl gallate (antioxidant). The release profile of lauryl gallate showed an initial burst effect followed by a slow and sustained release, indicating a biphasic release system. The lauryl gallate loaded in superparamagnetic polymethyl methacrylate (PMMA) nanoparticles did not have any cytotoxic effects on non-tumoral cells. Moreover, the folic acid promoted folate receptor-mediated endocytosis in tumoral cells, enhancing the anticancer effect of lauryl gallate [152].

Ramalingam et al. (2018) loaded curcumin in electrospun fibers to generate a dressing for the treatment of skin cancer. The dressing induced cell proliferation and free radical scavenging activity and up-regulated the expression of CDKN2A in A375 melanoma cells. The cell death of A375 melanoma cells was dose- and time-dependent, which indicates that treatment with curcumin loaded in the nanofibers inhibited the growth and induced the cell death of the skin cancer cells [151].

Ballestri et al. (2018) developed a synthetic antioxidant (porphyrin) and encapsulated it in polymethyl methacrylate (PMMA) core-shell nanoparticle (70 nm diameter) for photodynamic cancer therapy. Photodynamic cancer therapy uses a light to activate an antioxidant compound. The capsule protected porphyrin against unwanted bleaching while preserving the anticancer activity, which was similar to that of free porphyrin under in vitro testing [153].

Recently, Sobh et al. (2019) synthesized a multi-walled carbon nanotube (MWCNT)/Poly(methyl methacrylate-co-2-hydroxyethyl methacrylate) P(MMA-co-HEMA) nanocomposite loaded with either curcumin or its water-soluble derivative via an in situ microemulsion polymerization technique by using different ratios of multi-walled carbon nanotube MWCNT to drug. Curcumin could be loaded in higher amounts with high entrapment efficiency values with improved thermal stability with an increased MWCNT ratio. The in vitro drug release studies of the nanocomposite showed a prolonged controlled release in the intestinal fluid at pH 7.4 and that $\leq 8\%$ of the drug was lost in the stomach fluid at pH 1.2 [154].

Sunoqrot et al. (2019) developed a pH-sensitive polymeric nanoparticle of quercetin as a potential colon cancer-targeted nanomedicine. Quercetin is an abundant plant polyphenol with demonstrated efficacy in CRC. The researcher developed polymeric nanoparticles of quercetin based on the pH-sensitive polymer methacrylic acid and copolymers (Eudragit® S100) to achieve colon pH-specific drug release. The researchers found nanoparticles with a mean diameter of 66.8 nm and a partially negative surface charge of -5.2 mV. In vitro release testing showed a delay in drug release in acidic pH but complete release within 24 h at pH 7.2. A cytotoxicity assay on CT26 murine colon carcinoma cells displayed a significantly higher potency of encapsulated quercetin (IC50 = 0.8 µM) than free quercetin (IC50 = 65.1 µM) [155].

6.4.3. Polyols

Polyols are polymers with hydroxyl groups [156]. A representative polymer of this family is the polyvinyl alcohol (PVA), which is synthesized by the hydrolysis of polyvinyl acetate [157,158]. PVA is a water-soluble polymer that can generate hydrogels by chemical or physical crosslinking [159]. Recent advances are presented below.

Li et al. (2019) improved the solubility of curcumin using D-α-Tocopherol polyethylene glycol 1000 succinate (TPGS), a water-soluble derivative of vitamin E that acts as a surfactant with the ability to form micellar nanoparticles in water. More importantly, TPGS acts as a potent antioxidant. The complex TPGS/curcumin was encapsulated using PVA, in which were obtained stable nanoparticles of 12 nm diameter. The nanoparticle satisfactorily released curcumin in simulated colonic and gastric fluids; furthermore, the nanoparticles decreased intracellular ROS levels and apoptosis and inhibited the migration of HT-29 human colon cancer cells more potently than free curcumin. The pharmacokinetic analysis demonstrated that the nanocapsules were more bioavailable than free curcumin after oral administration to rats [160].

Wen et al. (2019) developed a core-shell electrospun nanofiber, core (PVA and phycocyanin), and shell (Polyoxyethylene) for the targeted therapy of CRC. Phycocyanin (PC), a water-soluble biliprotein (antioxidant), exhibits potent anti-colon cancer properties. The PC-loaded electrospun fiber mat inhibited HCT116 cell growth in a dose-dependent and time-dependent manner. In particular, the PC-loaded mat exerted its anticancer activity by blocking the cell cycle at the G0/G1 phase and inducing cell apoptosis, involving a decrease in Bcl-2/Bax, the activation of caspase 3, and the release of cytochrome c [161].

Golkar et al. (2019) fabricated via electrospinning, *Plantago major Mucilage* (PMM) blended with PVA, in order to produce an electrospun nanofiber. The researchers optimized the electrospinning parameters (voltage, tip-to-collector distance, feed rate, and PMM/PVA ratio) to obtain nanofibers with an average diameter of 250 nm. The viscosity, electrical conductivity, and surface tension of the PMM/PVA solution were 550 Cp, 575 µS/cm, and 47.044 mN/m, respectively [162]. The systems seem promising for biomedical applications. However, the researchers did not evaluate the effects of the fibers for CRC treatment.

6.4.4. Polyzwitterions

Polyzwitterions are a class of polymers consisting of zwitterionic moieties (anionic and cationic groups) as monomers. Poly(sulfobetaines), poly(carbobetaines), and poly(phosphobetaines) are representatives of a special class of polyzwitterions [163]. Gromadzki et al. (2017) developed a core-shell nanocapsule consisting of a dimer fatty acid-based aliphatic polyester core and zwitterionic poly(sulfobetaine) shell for the controlled delivery of curcumin, obtaining nanoparticles of <100 nm in size with an encapsulation efficiency of 98%. The researchers evaluated free and encapsulated curcumin for cytotoxicity and antioxidant activity in a panel of human cell lines and rat liver microsomes, respectively. Encapsulated curcumin had superior cytotoxic and antioxidant activity versus the free drug. In addition, cell viability experiments with non-loaded nanoparticles, both coated and noncoated, demonstrated that the developed nanoparticles are nontoxic, making them potentially suitable candidates for systemic passive targeting in cancer therapy, namely for the treatment of solid tumors exhibiting a high tumor accumulation of the capsules due to enhanced permeability and retention effects [164].

6.4.5. Polyoxazoline

Poly (2-oxazoline) (POZ) is a class of polymers formed by cationic ring-opening that were first identified and synthesized over 50 years ago. These polymers are nonionic, biostable, and water-soluble, and some are polar organic solvents. POZ can be synthesized from readily available non-toxic materials. The interest in using POZ in medical devices and drug delivery is very recent, and their application in multiple platforms is now being recognized by drug delivery scientists [165]. Although there is limited literature about the use of POZ for cancer treatment, some formulations for the treatment of skin cancer are reported. For instance, Simon et al. (2019) developed ointments with quercetin (core) encapsulated in POZ (shell). The POZ produced a stable formulation of spherical nanocapsules of 18 nm in size. Moreover, a good quercetin encapsulation (94% ± 4%) efficiency was observed with these nanosystems, allowing its homogeneous distribution in the nanocapsule.Therefore, Q-MM can be used as a reservoir of quercetin. Once loaded, quercetin's impact on cancer cell viability was doubled while its antioxidant efficacy was preserved [166]. Accordingly, POZ are an alternative for the encapsulation of antioxidants; hopefully, some new advances in oral drug formulations will be presented in the following years that can be used for CRC.

6.4.6. Polypeptides and Polyaminoacids

Polyaminoacids (PAA) and polypeptides (PPD) are polydisperse structures formed by the condensation of amino acid monomers through amide bonds that, contrary to proteins, cannot fold into globular or fibrillar structures [167]. In addition, they can carry versatile reactive functional groups on their side chains (carboxylic acid, hydroxyl, amino, and thiol groups) that allow for a variety of chemical modifications and compatibility with a wide range of bioactive compounds. Some outstanding nanocapsules of polyaminoacids have been developed for cancer treatment. For instance, Choi et al. (2018) encapsulated Celastrol (antioxidant) in PEGylated polyaminoacid-capped mesoporous silica nanoparticles for mitochondria-targeted delivery in solid tumors [107], and Patsula et al. (2019) modified maghemite nanoparticles with poly (L) poly(L-lysine) to protect the iron dioxide core from reaction with the encapsulated antioxidant (epigallocatechin-3-gallate from tea) and to promote the internalization of the nanoparticle of the system into the cancer cell [168].

PPD are special polymers that exhibit antioxidant properties themselves; in Table 3, some recent studies are presented.

Table 3. Recent advances in polypeptides (PPD) with antioxidant effects for CRC.

Polypeptide	Authors	Main Findings	Reference
Arca subcrenata Polypeptides	Hu et al. (2019)	Arca subcrenata polypeptides (PAS) inhibited the growth of HT-29 cells with an LC50 value of 117 µg/mL after 48h treatment, and significantly suppressed the tumor growth in nude mice bearing xenografted HT-29 cells at a dosage of 63mg/kg, with little influence on normal colon cells and normal colonic mucosa. PAS were then inspiringly found to induce apoptosis and G2/M phase arrest in HT-29 cells. The effect's mechanism involved in the inhibition of IGF-1/IGF-1R signaling activation, which was responsible for inactivating the downstream Akt/mTOR pathway. PAS significantly inhibited the ATP production of HT-29 cells both in vitro and in vivo.	[169]
Legume Seed Polypeptides	Lima et al. (2016)	Albumin and globulin fractions from legume seeds were screened for MMP-9 inhibitors (enzymes related to cancer growth and metastasis). Lupin seeds contain the most efficient MMP-9 inhibitors of all legume seeds analyzed, inhibiting both gelatinases and HT29 migration and growth, while pea seeds showed no effect. Results reveal legume protein MMPIs as novel metalloproteinase inhibitors of possible pharmacological interest.	[170]
Black Soybean Peptides	Chen et al. (2019)	The peptide fractions that were collected in each step were tested for their antioxidant capacity and anticancer activities against cancer cell lines. The most active fraction with a molecular weight of 455.0 Da showed the highest free radical scavenging and hydroxyl radical scavenging activity with LC50 values of 0.12 and 0.037 µM, respectively. Moreover, it showed high cytotoxic potential against cancer cells. The amino acid sequence was identified as Leu/Ile-Val-Pro-Lys (L/I-VPK).	[171]
Polypeptides from Intestinal Digestion of Germinated Soybean	González-montoya et al. (2018)	The protein concentrate from germinated soybean was hydrolyzed with pepsin/pancreatin and fractionated by ultrafiltration. Whole digest and fractions > 10, 5–10, and < 5 kDa caused cytotoxicity to Caco-2, HT-29, and HCT-116 human colon cancer cells, and reduced inflammatory responses caused by lipopolysaccharide in macrophages RAW 264.7. Antiproliferative and anti-inflammatory effects were generally higher in 5–10 kDa fractions. The most potent fraction was mainly composed of β-conglycinin and glycinin fragments rich in glutamine.	[172]
Sweet Potato Protein Hydrolysates	Zhang et al. (2018)	Six sweet potato protein hydrolysates (SPPH) showed certain antiproliferative effects on HT-29 cells. Specifically, Alcalase exhibited the highest antiproliferative effect with the lowest LC50 value of 119.72 µg/mL. SPPH by Alcalase were further separated into four fractions (> 10, 5–10, 3–5 and < 3 kDa). Fractions < 3kDa showed the strongest antiproliferative effects, which were 43.87% at 100 µg/mL ($p < 0.05$). The <3 kDa fractions could cause G2/M cell cycle arrest with increased p21 expression and induce apoptosis via decreasing Bcl-2 expression, increasing Bax expression, and inducing caspase-3 activation in HT-29 cells. In addition, <3 kDa fractions could significantly inhibit the cell migration of HT-29 cells.	[173]

Regarding proteins, there are reports of silk proteins that are able to stabilize polar and non-polar antioxidants, due to the amphiphilic properties of fibroin. For example, Lou et al. (2016) used fibroin to stabilize vitamin C, curcumin, and epigallocatechin gallate. The results indicated that these antioxidants presented improved environmental stabilities of up to 14 days due to the binding of antioxidant molecules to the hydrophobic or the hydrophilic/hydrophilic boundary regions of silk [174]. Despite this work not being directly focused on CRC, it is highly relevant because antioxidants can easily react with air and other environmental conditions, losing their ROS-scavenging properties, prior to be consumed by the patient; without stabilization, the antioxidant simply will have little or no effect in the patient. Lerdchai et al. (2016) designed a mixture of Thai silk fibroin/gelatin (denaturalized protein) sponges for the dual controlled release of curcumin and docosahexaenoic acid for localized cancer treatment. The sponges were fabricated by freeze-drying and glutaraldehyde cross-linking techniques. The highly cross-linked and slowly degrading silk fibroin/gelatin (50/50) sponge released curcumin and/or DHA at the slowest rate (for 24 days). Sponges were not toxic to L929 mouse fibroblasts, but a ratio of 1:4 (curcumin/docosahexaenoic acid) had the highest inhibitory effect on the growth of cancer cells [175]. Finally, Lozano-Pérez et al. (2017) encapsulated quercetin in silk fibroin nanoparticles (175 nm diameter). The nanoparticles had a negative surface charge that allowed the sustained release of the antioxidant that occurred throughout the experiment in both phosphate buffer saline (pH 7.4) and simulated intestinal fluid (pH 6.8) [176].

6.4.7. Polyesters

Polyesters are polymers that contain the ester functional group in their main chain [156]. Polyesters are produced via condensation or ring-opening reactions. Due to the strong presence of oxygen groups, this polymer can poses a negative charge that can respond to pH changes [177]. Moreover, some polyesters can be enzymatically degraded such as in the case of polycaprolactone (PCL), polylactic acid (PLA), and polyhydroxyalkanoates (PHA), among others [178–181]. Lipases are an important group of esterases for the biodegradation of aliphatic polyesters. They are produced in the pancreas, liver, and digestive system to break down fat [180]. Fat and polyesters have the same functional groups (esters), which leads the enzyme to degrade these polymers. For CRC, antioxidants have been successfully encapsulated in PLA and in Poly (DL-lactic-co-glycolic) acid (PLGA). PCL and PHA have been employed via mixtures and copolymers, as described in Section 6.4.9.

Alippilakkotte et al. (2018) encapsulated curcumin in polylactic acid (PLA) using an eco-friendly emulsification-solvent evaporation strategy. The method resulted in an efficiency of around 90%. The in vitro release studies showed a sustained curcumin release, after a burst release, in the initial 12 h. The curcumin-loaded PLA nanocapsules could easily penetrate into the cancer cells and can cause a sustained drug release for effective cancer treatment [177].

Pereira et al. (2018) encapsulated Guabiroba phenolic extract in Poly (DL-lactic-co-glycolic) acid (PLGA) nanoparticles to improve the stability, bioavailability, and bioactivity of the extract. The encapsulated extract proved to present a higher antioxidant capacity compared to free extract. Moreover, a reduction in ROS generation in non-cancer cells was achieved with lower extract concentrations ($p < 0.05$) after encapsulation [181].

6.4.8. Poly(vinylpyrrolidones)

Polyvinylpyrrolidone (PVP), commonly called polyvidone or povidone, is a water-soluble polymer made from the monomer N-vinylpyrrolidone by free-radical polymerization in the presence of AIBN as an initiator [182]. Dry PVP is a hygroscopic powder and readily absorbs up to 40% of water by its weight [182]. Nanofibers, particles, and films have been loaded with antioxidant extracts for drug delivery systems.

Sriyanti et al. (2017) and Andjani et al. (2017) developed electrospun nanofiber mats of polyvinyl(pyrrolidone) (PVP) with *Garcinia mangostana* extract (GME). The researchers found strong interactions of the PVP with the extract, which was molecularly dispersed in the electrospun PVP nanofiber matrix. The composite nanofiber mats exhibited very high antioxidant activities despite having been exposed to a high voltage during electrospinning [183,184]. A similar strategy was adopted by Andjani et al. (2017) and Zahra et al. (2019) using rotatory force spinning for encapsulating GME and Garlic (*Allium sativum*) extract; however, the obtained fibers were at the microscale [185,186].

Kamaruddin et al. (2018) developed sub-micron particles by the electrospraying of PVP and green tea extract. The researchers optimized the processes for obtaining the particles and saw the potential for drug delivery systems [186]. However, the particles were not tested for drug delivery applications for colorectal cancer. Similarly, Guamán-Balcázar et al. (2019) generated sub-micron particles of PVP with mango leaf extract, finding a relationship between the mango leaf extract/PVP ratio, temperature, and pressure of the supercritical antisolvent extraction process with the particle size (some of the particles were at the nanoscale). The in vitro desorption test showed a release profile of the extract components lasting up to 8 h under simulated intestinal fluids at pH 6.8 [187].

Contardi et al. (2019) produced a new material of PVP plasticized with p-coumaric acid for the encapsulation of bioactive compounds of interest in the pharmaceutical industry. An initial model of the encapsulation of carminic acid was evaluated, finding that by varying the ratio of PVP to p-coumaric acid, the release profile can be adjusted from minutes to hours; for instance, a ratio of 2:1 (PVP/p-coumaric acid) has a release profile lasting up to 70 h to obtain 100% release [188].

6.4.9. Composites, Copolymers, and Mixtures

Composites and polymer mixtures take advantage of the synergystic effects of two polymers. For instance, one polymer may be highly compatible with the bioactive compound but not pH sensitive, thus the combination with another shell polymer will tailor the release profile. Some recent advances are presented below.

Thanyacharoen et al. (2018) developed a composite material of polyvinyl alcohol with chitosan to deliver gallic acid (antioxidant). The results seem promising as the gallic acid was released for periods longer than 16 h and its antioxidant properties were conserved [189].

Al-Ogaidi (2018) mixed two polysaccharides, alginate, and chitosan, to load vitamin C into nanoparticles of 25–30 nm in size. Moreover, Al-Ogaidi evaluated the effect of the pH on the overall size of the system, finding higher release at a pH of 6. Furthermore, it was found that entrapping vitamin C within the nanoparticle enhanced its anticancer activity [142]. Similar studies were carried out by Aluani et al. (2017) using quercetin instead of vitamin C [190]. Rahaiee et al. (2017) developed alginate–chitosan nanoparticles to stabilize crocin, an antioxidant with anticancer effects; crocin is highly sensitive to pH, heat, and oxidative stress, making its effectiveness reduced. The alginate–chitosan nanoparticles showed a controlled release profile in simulated gastrointestinal fluids and effectively protected crocin from the environment prior to being released [191].

Huang et al. (2016) improved the water dispersibility of curcumin, using core-shell nanoparticles of zein (core) and alginate–pectin (shell). The researcher found that curcumin-loaded core-shell nanoparticles were shown to have superior antioxidant and radical scavenging activities compared to curcumin solubilized in ethanol [192]. Likewise, Wei et al. (2019) developed zein–propylene glycol alginate–rhamnolipid composite nanoparticles to overcome the limitations of resveratrol such as water insolubility and chemical instability; the nanoparticles controlled the release for up to 2 h [193].

Arunkumar created nanocapsules of 100 nm using poly (lactic-co-glycolic acid)-polyethylene glycol to improve the solubility and stability of lutein (an antioxidant with poor solubility). The capsules showed higher stability and improved the bioability of the lutein, enhancing the antiproliferative effect of the antioxidant, evidenced by the lower lethal concentration (LC50) of 10.9 µM for the nanocapsules and 25 µM for free lutein [194].

Jaiswal et al. (2019) synthesized methyl methacrylate (MMA)-modified chitosan (CS) by a green method via a Michael addition reaction between CS and MMA in ethanol. The nanoparticles of approximately 100 nm had, in an in vitro drug release study, a maximal curcumin entrapment efficiency up to 68% with a high release at a pH of 5.0 and a lower one at physiological pH [195]. Positive charges on chitosan will generate maximum delivery at acid pH (stomach) rather than neutral (colon). Consequently, this strategy is not recommended for CRC treatment, since curcumin would be delivered before arriving at the desired area.

Eatemadi et al. (2016) developed a nanoparticle of PCL-PEG-PCL to encapsulate chrysin (antioxidant). The researcher investigated the effect of chrysin-loaded PCL-PEG-PCL on the T47D breast cancer cell line. The cell viability assay showed that chrysin has a time-dependent cytotoxic effect on the T47D cell line. Furthermore, the conducted studies showed that encapsulated chrysin has a higher antitumor effect on the gene expression of FTO, BRCA1, and hTERT than free chrysin [196]. This study was not focused on CRC, but these systems can be easily extrapolated to gastrointestinal drug delivery.

Wu et al. (2016) evaluated the structural, mechanical, antioxidant, and cytocompatibility properties of membranes prepared from PHA and arrowroot (*Maranta arundinacea*) starch powder (ASP). Furthermore, the researchers grafted acrylic acid to PHA (PHA-g-AA). The PHA-g-AA/ASP membranes had better mechanical properties than the PHA/ASP membrane. This effect was attributed to greater compatibility between the grafted PHA and ASP. The water-resistance of the PHA-g-AA/ASP membranes was greater than that of the PHA/ASP membranes, and a cytocompatibility evaluation with human foreskin fibroblasts indicated that both materials were nontoxic. Moreover, ASP enhanced the polyphenol content and antioxidant properties when they were encapsulated [197].

6.5. Polymers for Encapsulating Synthetics and Hybrid Adjuvants for CRC

Synthetics and hybrid adjuvants are based on 5-FU. As explained previously, 5-FU is the gold standard for cancer and CRC adjuvant treatment. However, along with the growing interest in natural antioxidants, new hybrid compounds derived from 5-FU conjugated with natural or synthetic molecules have been developed; for example curcumin, has been conjugated with 5-FU to act synergistically by enhancing cellular uptake and accumulation, by inducing the destabilization of the cytoskeleton and loss of mitochondrial membrane potential, initiating early and late apoptosis in cancer cells [198]. Furthermore, synthetic drugs can be mixed with other natural or synthetic compounds to potentiate them or reduce the side effects. An example of this strategy is the mixing of 5-FU with resveratrol to reduce the toxicity of 5-FU against healthy cells [199]. Examples of other hybrids and mixtures were reviewed by Carrillo et al. (2015); the paper can be consulted in the following reference: [200].

The first attempts at looking at polymer encapsulation techniques for 5-FU and its derivatives are limited, mainly due to 5-FU being first patented in 1957 and then the research into encapsulating the molecule being governed by pharmaceutical companies. However, today, most of the patents have expired, making these compounds attractive for developing drug delivery systems. According to Scopus, there are more than 2800 documents related to 5-FU drug delivery systems. In 2018, more than 180 papers were published, and among them, 114 include the word "polymer". In the Table 4, some representative work from 2015 to 2019 is presented.

Table 4. Recent advances in using 5-fluorouracil (5-FU) and its derivatives in polymer encapsulation strategies for CRC.

Compounds	Polymers	Highlights	References
5-FU Mixed with Doxorubicin (Dox)	Dendritic nanomicelle of poly lactic acid (core) and polyamidoamine dendron (shell)	The nanocapsule has a diameter of 68.6 ± 3.3 nm and shows a pH-sensitive drug release behavior. The parallel activity of 5-FU and Dox shows synergistic anticancer efficacy.	[201]
	Core-shell nanocapsules; core: mesoporous silica; shell: chitosan/PEG	Drug loading (0.15–0.18 mg of 5FU/mg capsule). Controlled release profiles (15–65%) over 72 h. Cell specific cytotoxicity in cancer cells.	[202]
	Nanoparticles of PLGA conjugated with folic acid	Lower LC50 for encapsulated 5-FU against HT-29 cancer cells compared with free 5-FU. Folic acid on the surface of the nanoparticles induces a rapid intake of the nanoparticle into the cell.	[203]

Table 4. Cont.

Compounds	Polymers	Highlights	References
5-FU	Complex of casein-coated iron oxide nanoparticles and folic acid-conjugated chitosan-graft-poly (2-dimethylaminoethyl methacrylate)	Lower toxicity to normal cells. pH-sensitive nanoparticles. Magnetic-sensitive nanoparticles.	[204,205]
	Loaded β-cyclodextrin-carrying polymeric poly(methylmethacrylate)-coated samarium ferrite nanoparticles		
	Zirconium metal organic nanoparticles (5-FU encapsulated in the crystal structure of Zirconium) coated with PEG	The encapsulation system is photosensitive, releasing the drug in response to the light	[206,207]
	5FU conjugated with chitosan		
	Non-coated and chitosan-coated alginate beads in a 3D printed tablet of polyacrilates	Controlled release of 5-FU from the alginate beads encapsulated within the hollow pH-sensitive tablet matrix at pH values corresponding to the colonic environment.	[208]
	Electrospum nanofibers of PCL/chitosan	High chitosan ratios led to increasing the drug release period. The release mechanism for all nanofibers was Fickian diffusion according to Korsmeyer–Peppas model.	[208]
	Crosslinked Sesbaniam gum (polyssacharide)	pH-responsive encapsulation system for colon-specific release.	[209–213]
	Carboxymethyl chitosan-grafted-poly (Acrylic Acid)-based		
	5-FU poly (L-lactide) composite by supercritical CO_2 antisolvent		
	ZnO/carboxymethyl cellulose/chitosan nanocomposite beads		
	Azo hydrogels consisting in acryloyl chloride copolymerized with polyacrylates		
	Carboxylic curdlan and chitosan	Spherical morphology with an average size of about 180 nm and a zeta potential of around 41 mV. Encapsulation efficiency (86.47%) and loading content (10.81%).	[214]
5-FU and Metformin (ME)	Injectable hydrogels of PEG-b-poly(L-lysine)	In vitro degradation and drug release studies demonstrated that both ME and 5FU were released through hydrogels in a controlled and pH-dependent manner. The hydrogels had synergistic inhibitory effects on the cell cycle progression and cell proliferation in colon cancer cells, resulted from a combination of p53-mediated G1 arrest and apoptosis in C26 cells.	[215]
5-fluorouracil and Oxaliplatin	Poly (3-hydroxybutyrate-co-3-hydroxyvalerate acid)/poly (lactic-co-glycolic acid)	Higher anticancer activity using encapsulated drugs over free drugs. The nanoparticles are hemocompatible. Platform for co-delivery of anticancer compounds.	[210]
Doxorubicin	Lycium barbarum polysaccharides	The doxorubicin release from the nanoparticles was pH-dependent and was accelerated by decreasing pH. Cytotoxicity study showed that the loaded nanoparticles have significantly enhanced cytotoxicity in vitro, especially for human cancer cell lines.	[216]
5-FU and Curcumin	Chitosan/reduced graphene oxide nanocomposites	Higher encapsulationn efficiency (>90%). The synergistic cytotoxicity was observed upon addition of 5-FU and curcumin loaded in the nanocomposite, which shows the effectiveness of the system toward the inhibition of growth of HT-29 colon cancer cells. Better cytotoxicity with an LC50 of 23.8 µg/mL was observed for the dual-drug-loaded nanocomposite.	[217]

According to the above table, recent advances in synthetic adjuvants have been focused on improving the bioavailability of 5-FU. For example, for a pH-sensitive polymer that will deliver the 5-FU in the colonic area, the modification of the polymer surface with folic acid makes it selective for receptors that are more active in cancer cells, for targeted therapy. Moreover, the blending of polymers and bioactive compounds is a new approach to reducing the toxic side effects of 5-FU and enhancing its therapeutic effects.

7. Conclusions

Actual cancer treatment is helping to increase the survival rates and prognosis and, in some cases, to cure cancer in patients. Nevertheless, the fight against cancer is not over, especially for CRC, which is one of the most aggressive cancer types. Consequently, cancer is and will remain a hot topic in research.

Among the different adjuvant therapies for complementing or avoiding the surgical removal of the affected area, oral chemotherapy is the most convenient for patients and health professionals. Chemotherapy treatment is continuously evolving to reduce side effects and enhance the therapeutic effects of natural and synthetics drugs, using strategies involving the encapsulation of bioactive compounds. Furthermore, thanks to molecular biology and chemistry, researchers can quickly check the anticancer properties of bioactive compounds in vitro and in vivo in order to compare treatments.

Polymers are versatile biomaterials that can be loaded with CRC-targeting compounds and processed to tailor the desorption kinetics to respond to pH, enzymes, cellular receptors, and time, among others. Despite none of the studies aiming to compare response types (pH, enzymes, time, or cellular receptors), pH-responsive polymers are seemingly the most promising, so new research should be focused on studying polymer families with other ways of responding to stimuli. In vivo pharmacokinetics are a useful tool to compare polymers and bioactive compounds in order to optimize the therapeutic effects of such compounds.

Finally, it can be concluded that antioxidants are emerging compounds that, in the short term, will complement current chemotherapy treatments, and in the long term, these natural drugs will replace 5-FU and will play an important role in curing colorectal cancer.

Author Contributions: Conceptualization, M.O.; data acquisition, M.O.; writing—original draft preparation, M.O.; writing—review and editing, M.O., E.M., T.N. and C.C.; project administration, C.C.; All authors have read and agreed to the published version of the manuscript.

Funding: This research was funded by MINCIENCIAS, Colombia under the project Nanobiocáncer grand number FP44842-211-2018.

Acknowledgments: Authors wants to thanks to Ana Colorado from the VIGILA Department of the Universidad Pontificia Bolivariana for the valuable help in the use of Vantage, AcclaimIP and Derwent.

Conflicts of Interest: The authors declare no conflict of interest.

References

1. Roser, M.; Ritchie, H. Cancer. Available online: https://ourworldindata.org/cancer (accessed on 25 February 2019).
2. Becker, D.; Hershman, D.L. Adjuvant Therapy for Elderly Patients with Breast, Colon, and Lung Cancer. In *Management of Cancer in the Older Patient*; Elsevier: Philadelphia, PA, USA, 2012; pp. 79–88.
3. Institute for Health Metrics and Evaluation (IHME) Global Burden of Disease Collaborative Network. Available online: http://ghdx.healthdata.org/gbd-results-tool.%0D%0A (accessed on 25 February 2019).
4. Chiavarini, M.; Bertarelli, G.; Minelli, L.; Fabiani, R. Dietary intake of meat cooking-related mutagens (HCAs) and risk of colorectal adenoma and cancer: A systematic review and meta-analysis. *Nutrients* **2017**, *9*, 514. [CrossRef] [PubMed]
5. Romieu, I.; Bagnardi, V.; Scotti, L.; Negri, E.; La Vecchia, C.; Tramacere, I.; Rota, M.; Fedirko, V.; Straif, K.; Jenab, M.; et al. Alcohol drinking and colorectal cancer risk: An overall and dose-response meta-analysis of published studies. *Ann. Oncol.* **2011**, *22*, 1958–1972. [CrossRef]

6. Lewis, R.; Burden, S. Colorectal cancer and nutrition. *Adv. Nutr. Diet. Gastroenterol.* **2014**, 255–262. [CrossRef]
7. Ornitz, D.M.; Itoh, N. Protein family review Fibroblast growth factors Gene organization and evolutionary history. *Genome Biol.* **2001**, *2*, 1–12. [CrossRef] [PubMed]
8. Reyes-Aldasoro, C.C. The proportion of cancer-related entries in PubMed has increased considerably; Is cancer truly "the Emperor of All Maladies"? *PLoS ONE* **2017**, *12*, 1–15. [CrossRef]
9. Luke, M. Intestinal obstruction from cancer of the rectum, operation for artificial anus in the left groin; death in six hours. *Lancet* **1860**, *6*, 243. [CrossRef]
10. Dunphy, J.E. Recurrent Cancer of the Colon and Rectum. *N. Engl. J. Med.* **2010**, *237*, 1–3. [CrossRef]
11. Adams, J.T.; Schwartz, S.I.; Rubin, P.; Rob, C.G. Intralymphatic 5-Fluorouracil and radioactive gold as an adjuvant to surgical operation for colorectal carcinoma. *Dis. Colon Rectum* **1970**, *13*, 201–206. [CrossRef]
12. Grand View Research Vaccine Adjuvants Market sie and Analysis. Available online: https://www.grandviewresearch.com/industry-analysis/vaccine-adjuvants-market (accessed on 17 March 2019).
13. Gaudry, B.K.; Rothwell, R. The Unpredictable Prospects of Patenting Cancer Innovation. Available online: https://www.ipwatchdog.com/2018/03/01/unpredictable-patenting-cancer-innovation/id=94280/ (accessed on 17 March 2019).
14. Vainio, H.; Morgan, G. Aspirin for the second hundred years: New uses for an old drug. *Pharmacol. Toxicol.* **1997**, *81*, 151–152. [CrossRef]
15. X. Garcia-Albeniz, A.T.C. Aspirin for the prevention of colorectal cancer. *Best Pr. Res Clin Gastroenterol.* **2012**, 1–18. [CrossRef]
16. Chan, A.T. Aspirin Use and Survival After Diagnosis of Colorectal Cancer. *Jama* **2009**, *302*, 649–659. [CrossRef] [PubMed]
17. Solomon, V.R.; Lee, H. Anti-breast cancer activity of heteroaryl chalcone derivatives. *Biomed. Pharmacother.* **2012**, *66*, 213–220. [CrossRef] [PubMed]
18. R. Solomon, V.; Lee, H. Quinoline as a Privileged Scaffold in Cancer Drug Discovery. *Curr. Med. Chem.* **2011**, *18*, 1488–1508. [CrossRef] [PubMed]
19. World Health Organization Cancer. Available online: https://www.who.int/cancer/en/ (accessed on 5 March 2019).
20. Hecker, E. Definitions and terminology in cancer (tumor) etiology. *Bull. World Health Organ.* **1976**, *54*, 463. [CrossRef]
21. National Institutes of Health (US); Biological Sciences Curriculum Study. Understanding Cancer. *NIH Curric. Suppl. Ser.* **2007**.
22. Pelengaris, S.; Khan, M. *The Molecular Biology of Cancer: A Bridge from Bench to Bedside*, 2nd ed.; Pelengaris, S., Khan, M., Eds.; Wiley: West Sussex, UK, 2013; Volume 28.
23. NIH National Cancer Institutes Cancer Classification. Available online: https://training.seer.cancer.gov/disease/categories/classification.html (accessed on 11 March 2019).
24. Gajdos, C.; Tartter, P.I.; Bodian, C.; Brower, S.T.; Bleiweiss, I.J. Stage 0 to stage III breast cancer in young women. *J. Am. Coll. Surg.* **2003**, *190*, 523–529. [CrossRef]
25. Edge, S.B.; Compton, C.C. The american joint committee on cancer: The 7th edition of the AJCC cancer staging manual and the future of TNM. *Ann. Surg. Oncol.* **2010**, *17*, 1471–1474. [CrossRef] [PubMed]
26. Idikio, H.A. Human cancer classification: A systems biology-based model integrating morphology, cancer stem cells, proteomics, and genomics. *J. Cancer* **2011**, *2*, 107–115. [CrossRef] [PubMed]
27. Ali, H.R.; Rueda, O.M.; Aparicio, S.A.; Caldas, C.; Dunning, M.J.; Curtis, C. Genome-driven integrated classification of breast cancer validated in over 7,500 samples. *Genome Biol.* **2014**, *15*, 1–14. [CrossRef]
28. Hoadley, K.A.; Yau, C.; Hinoue, T.; Wolf, D.M.; Lazar, A.J.; Drill, E.; Shen, R.; Taylor, A.M.; Cherniack, A.D.; Thorsson, V.S.; et al. Cell-of-Origin Patterns Dominate the Molecular Classification of 10,000 Tumors from 33 Types of Cancer. *Cell* **2018**, *173*, 291–304. [CrossRef]
29. Lee, Z.J. An integrated algorithm for gene selection and classification applied to microarray data of ovarian cancer. *Artif. Intell. Med.* **2008**, *42*, 81–93. [CrossRef] [PubMed]
30. Shen, L.; Toyota, M.; Kondo, Y.; Lin, E.; Zhang, L.; Guo, Y.; Hernandez, N.S.; Chen, X.; Ahmed, S.; Konishi, K.; et al. Integrated genetic and epigenetic analysis identifies three different subclasses of colon cancer. *Proc. Natl. Acad. Sci.* **2007**, *104*, 18654–18659. [CrossRef] [PubMed]
31. Bookshelf, N. Colorectal Cancer: Overview. Available online: https://www.ncbi.nlm.nih.gov/books/NBK279198/?report=printable (accessed on 13 March 2018).

32. Cooper, G.M.; Hausman, R. *The Cell: A Molecular Approach*, 6th ed.; Cooper, G.M., Hausman, R., Eds.; ASM Press: Boston, MA, USA, 2013; ISBN 978-0878939640.
33. Jolly, T.A.; Williams, G.R.; Bushan, S.; Pergolotti, M.; Nyrop, K.A.; Jones, E.L.; Muss, H.B. Adjuvant treatment for older women with invasive breast cancer. *Women's Heal.* **2016**, *12*, 129–146. [CrossRef]
34. Ilson, D.H. Adjuvant therapy in colon cancer: Less is more. *Lancet Oncol.* **2018**, *19*, 442–443. [CrossRef]
35. Kazemi, T.; Younesi, V.; Jadidi-Niaragh, F.; Yousefi, M. Immunotherapeutic approaches for cancer therapy: An updated review. *Artif. Cells, Nanomedicine Biotechnol.* **2016**, *44*, 769–779. [CrossRef] [PubMed]
36. Kumari, S.; Badana, A.K.; Murali Mohan, G.; Shailender, G.; Malla, R.R. Reactive Oxygen Species: A Key Constituent in Cancer Survival. *Biomark. Insights* **2018**, *13*. [CrossRef]
37. Shi, J.; Fang, G.; Sheng, Y. Neo-adjuvant chemotherapy for breast cancer. *Zhonghua Zhong Liu Za Zhi* **2001**, *23*, 423–425. [CrossRef]
38. Jaffray, D.; Gospodarowicz, M. Radiation Therapy for Cancer. In *Cancer: Disease Control Priorities*; Gelband, H., Jha, P., Sankaranarayanan, R., Eds.; The International Bank for Reconstruction and Development: Washington, DC, USA, 2015; p. 10.
39. Häfner, M.F.; Debus, J. Radiotherapy for colorectal cancer: Current standards and future perspectives. *Visc. Med.* **2016**, *32*, 172–177. [CrossRef]
40. Skowronek, J. Current status of brachytherapy in cancer treatment-short overview. *J. Contemp. Brachytherapy* **2017**, *9*, 581–589. [CrossRef]
41. Johnson, J.R.; Lacey, J.V., Jr.; Lazovich, D.; Geller, M.A.; Schairer, C.; Schatzkin, A.; Flood, A. Menopausal Hormone Therapy and Risk of Colorectal Cancer. *Cancer Epidemiol Biomarkers Prev.* **2009**, *18*, 196–203. [CrossRef]
42. Lin, J.H.; Zhang, S.M.; Rexrode, K.M.; Manson, J.E.; Chan, A.T.; Wu, K.; Tworoger, S.S.; Hankinson, S.E.; Fuchs, C.; Gaziano, J.M.; et al. Association between sex hormones and colorectal cancer risk in men and women. *Clin. Gastroenterol. Hepatol.* **2014**, *11*, 419–424.e1. [CrossRef] [PubMed]
43. Rennert, G.; Rennert, H.S.; Pinchev, M.; Lavie, O.; Gruber, S.B. Use of hormone replacement therapy and the risk of colorectal cancer. *J. Clin. Oncol.* **2009**, *27*, 4542–4547. [CrossRef] [PubMed]
44. Venning, G.; Lange, S. Hormone Replacement Therapy. Available online: https://www.ncbi.nlm.nih.gov/books/NBK493191/?report=printable (accessed on 2 July 2019).
45. Machluf, M.; Orsola, A.; Atala, A. Controlled release of therapeutic agents: Slow delivery and cell encapsulation. *World J. Urol.* **2000**, *18*, 80–83. [CrossRef]
46. Ohhara, Y.; Fukuda, N.; Takeuchi, S.; Honma, R.; Shimizu, Y.; Kinoshita, I.; Dosaka-Akita, H. Role of targeted therapy in metastatic colorectal cancer. *World J. Gastrointest. Oncol.* **2016**, *8*, 642. [CrossRef]
47. Hainsworth, J.; Heim, W.; Berlin, J.; Baron, A.; Griffing, S.; Holmgren, E.; Ph, D.; Ferrara, N.; Fyfe, G.; Rogers, B.; et al. Bevacizumab plus Irinotecan, Fluorouracil, and Leucovorin for Metastatic Colorectal Cancer. *N. Engl. J. Med.* **2004**, *350*, 2335–2342.
48. Longley, D.B.; Harkin, D.P.; Johnston, P.G. 5-Fluorouracil: Mechanisms of Action and Clinical Strategies. *Nat. Rev. Cancer* **2003**, *3*, 330–338. [CrossRef]
49. Zouhairi, M.E.; Charabaty, A.; Pishvaian, M.J. Molecularly targeted therapy for metastatic colon cancer: Proven treatments and promising new agents. *Gastrointest. Cancer Res.* **2011**, *4*, 15–21.
50. Pitt, J.M.; Kroemer, G.; Zitvogel, L.; Pitt, J.M.; André, F.; Amigorena, S.; Soria, J.; Eggermont, A. Dendritic cell–derived exosomes for cancer therapy Find the latest version: Dendritic cell–derived exosomes for cancer therapy. *J. Clin. Investig.* **2016**, *126*, 1224–1232. [CrossRef]
51. Adams, G.P.; Weiner, L.M. Monoclonal antibody therapy of cancer. *Nat. Biotechnol.* **2005**, *23*, 1147–1157. [CrossRef]
52. Anderson, R.J.; Schneider, J. Plasmid DNA and viral vector-based vaccines for the treatment of cancer. *Vaccine* **2007**, *25*, 24–34. [CrossRef]
53. Diakos, C.I.; Charles, K.A.; McMillan, D.C.; Clarke, S.J. Cancer-related inflammation and treatment effectiveness. *Lancet Oncol.* **2014**, *15*, e493–e503. [CrossRef]
54. Lianos, G.D.; Alexiou, G.A.; Mangano, A.; Mangano, A.; Rausei, S.; Boni, L.; Dionigi, G.; Roukos, D.H. The role of heat shock proteins in cancer. *Cancer Lett.* **2015**, *360*, 114–118. [CrossRef] [PubMed]
55. Institue for Quality and Efficiency in Health Care How Does Chemotherapy Work? Available online: http://www.ncbi.nlm.nih.gov/pubmedhealth/PMH0041062/ (accessed on 2 July 2019).

56. Gustavsson, B.; Carlsson, G.; MacHover, D.; Petrelli, N.; Roth, A.; Schmoll, H.J.; Tveit, K.M.; Gibson, F. A review of the evolution of systemic chemotherapy in the management of colorectal cancer. *Clin. Colorectal Cancer* **2015**, *14*, 1–10. [CrossRef] [PubMed]
57. Petrelli, N.; Herrera, L.; Rustum, Y.; Burke, P.; Creaven, P.; Stulc, J.; Emrich, L.J.; Mittelman, A. A prospective randomized trial of 5-fluorouracil versus 5-fluorouracil and high-dose leucovorin versus 5-fluorouracil and methotrexate in previously untreated patients with advanced colorectal carcinoma. *J. Clin. Oncol.* **1987**, *5*, 1559–1565. [CrossRef]
58. Goldberg, R.M.; Sargent, D.J.; Morton, R.F.; Fuchs, C.S.; Ramanathan, R.K.; Williamson, S.K.; Findlay, B.P.; Pitot, H.C.; Alberts, S.R. A Randomized Controlled Trial of Fluorouracil Plus Leucovorin, Irinotecan, and Oxaliplatin Combinations in Patients With Previously Untreated Metastatic Colorectal Cancer. *J. Clin. Oncol.* **2004**, *22*, 23–30. [CrossRef]
59. Tveit, K.M.; Guren, T.; Glimelius, B.; Pfeiffer, P.; Sorbye, H.; Pyrhonen, S.; Sigurdsson, F.; Kure, E.; Ikdahl, T.; Skovlund, E.; et al. Phase III Trial of Cetuximab With Continuous or Intermittent Fluorouracil, Leucovorin, and Oxaliplatin (Nordic FLOX) Versus FLOX Alone in First-Line Treatment of Metastatic Colorectal Cancer: The NORDIC-VII Study. *J. Clin. Oncol.* **2012**, *30*, 1755–1762. [CrossRef]
60. Yokoyama, C.; Sueyoshi, Y.; Ema, M.; Mori, Y.; Takaishi, K.; Hisatomi, H. Induction of oxidative stress by anticancer drugs in the presence and absence of cells. *Oncol. Lett.* **2017**, *14*, 6066–6070. [CrossRef]
61. Abbas, M.; Saeed, F.; Anjum, F.M.; Afzaal, M.; Tufail, T.; Bashir, M.S.; Ishtiaq, A.; Hussain, S.; Suleria, H.A.R. Natural polyphenols: An overview. *Int. J. Food Prop.* **2017**, *20*, 1689–1699. [CrossRef]
62. Jin, X.; Che, D.B.; Zhang, Z.H.; Yan, H.M.; Jia, Z.Y.; Jia, X. Bin Ginseng consumption and risk of cancer: A meta-analysis. *J. Ginseng Res.* **2016**, *40*, 269–277. [CrossRef]
63. Wong, A.S.T.; Cheb, C.-M.; Leunga, K.-W. Ginseng as cancer therapeutics: Recent advances in functional and mechanistic overview. *Nat. Prod. Rep.* **2015**. [CrossRef]
64. Chong-zhi, W.; Anderson, S.; Wei, D.U.; Tong-chuan, H.E.; Chun-su, Y. Red ginseng and cancer treatment. *Chin. J. Nat. Med.* **2016**, *14*, 7–16. [CrossRef]
65. Tang, Y.C.; Zhang, Y.; Zhou, J.; Zhi, Q.; Wu, M.Y.; Gong, F.R.; Shen, M.; Liu, L.; Tao, M.; Shen, B.; et al. Ginsenoside Rg3 targets cancer stem cells and tumor angiogenesis to inhibit colorectal cancer progression in vivo. *Int. J. Oncol.* **2018**, *52*, 127–138. [CrossRef]
66. Kim, E.J.; Kwon, K.A.; Lee, Y.E.; Kim, J.H.; Kim, S.H.; Kim, J.H. Korean Red Ginseng extract reduces hypoxia-induced epithelial-mesenchymal transition by repressing NF-κB and ERK1/2 pathways in colon cancer. *J. Ginseng Res.* **2018**, *42*, 288–297. [CrossRef] [PubMed]
67. Girisa, S.; Shabnam, B.; Monisha, J.; Fan, L.; Halim, C.E.; Arfuso, F.; Ahn, K.S.; Sethi, G.; Kunnumakkara, A.B. Potential of zerumbone as an anti-cancer agent. *Molecules* **2019**, *24*, 734. [CrossRef] [PubMed]
68. Sithara, T.; Dhanya, B.P.; Arun, K.B.; Sini, S.; Dan, M.; Kokkuvayil Vasu, R.; Nisha, P. Zerumbone, a Cyclic Sesquiterpene from Zingiber zerumbet Induces Apoptosis, Cell Cycle Arrest, and Antimigratory Effects in SW480 Colorectal Cancer Cells. *J. Agric. Food Chem.* **2018**, *66*, 602–612. [CrossRef] [PubMed]
69. Kim, H.J.; Kang, S.; Kim, D.Y.; You, S.; Park, D.; Oh, S.C.; Lee, D.H. Diallyl disulfide (DADS) boosts TRAIL-Mediated apoptosis in colorectal cancer cells by inhibiting Bcl-2. *Food Chem. Toxicol.* **2019**, *125*, 354–360. [CrossRef]
70. Roy, N.; Nazeem, P.A.; Babu, T.D.; Abida, P.S.; Narayanankutty, A.; Valsalan, R.; Valsala, P.A.; Raghavamenon, A.C. EGFR gene regulation in colorectal cancer cells by garlic phytocompounds with special emphasis on S-Allyl-L-Cysteine Sulfoxide. *Interdiscip. Sci. Comput. Life Sci.* **2018**, *10*, 686–693. [CrossRef]
71. Li, H.Y.; Li, M.; Luo, C.C.; Wang, J.Q.; Zheng, N. Lactoferrin Exerts Antitumor Effects by Inhibiting Angiogenesis in a HT29 Human Colon Tumor Model. *J. Agric. Food Chem.* **2017**, *65*, 10464–10472. [CrossRef]
72. Sugihara, Y.; Zuo, X.; Takata, T.; Jin, S.; Miyauti, M.; Isikado, A.; Imanaka, H.; Tatsuka, M.; Qi, G.; Shimamoto, F. Inhibition of DMH-DSS-induced colorectal cancer by liposomal bovine lactoferrin in rats. *Oncol. Lett.* **2017**, *14*, 5688–5694. [CrossRef]
73. Yang, C.S.; Wang, H. Cancer preventive activities of tea catechins. *Molecules* **2016**, *21*, 1679. [CrossRef]
74. Gómez-Juaristi, M.; Martínez-López, S.; Sarria, B.; Bravo, L.; Mateos, R. Absorption and metabolism of yerba mate phenolic compounds in humans. *Food Chem.* **2018**, *240*, 1028–1038. [CrossRef] [PubMed]

75. Amigo-Benavent, M.; Wang, S.; Mateos, R.; Sarriá, B.; Bravo, L. Antiproliferative and cytotoxic effects of green coffee and yerba mate extracts, their main hydroxycinnamic acids, methylxanthine and metabolites in different human cell lines. *Food Chem. Toxicol.* **2017**, *106*, 125–138. [CrossRef] [PubMed]
76. Schmit, S.L.; Rennert, H.S.; Rennert, G.; Gruber, S.B. Coffee consumption and the risk of colorectal cancer. *Cancer Epidemiol. Biomarkers Prev.* **2016**, *25*, 634–639. [CrossRef]
77. Scafuri, B.; Marabotti, A.; Carbone, V.; Minasi, P.; Dotolo, S.; Facchiano, A. A theoretical study on predicted protein targets of apple polyphenols and possible mechanisms of chemoprevention in colorectal cancer. *Sci. Rep.* **2016**, *6*, 1–13. [CrossRef] [PubMed]
78. Darband, S.G.; Kaviani, M.; Yousefi, B.; Sadighparvar, S.; Pakdel, F.G.; Attari, J.A.; Mohebbi, I.; Naderi, S.; Majidinia, M. Quercetin: A functional dietary flavonoid with potential chemo-preventive properties in colorectal cancer. *J. Cell. Physiol.* **2018**, *233*, 6544–6560. [CrossRef] [PubMed]
79. Huang, Y.-F.; Zhu, D.-J.; Chen, X.-W.; Chen, Q.-K.; Luo, Z.-T.; Liu, C.-C.; Wang, G.-X.; Zhang, W.-J.; Liao, N.-Z. Curcumin enhances the effects of irinotecan on colorectal cancer cells through the generation of reactive oxygen species and activation of the endoplasmic reticulum stress pathway. *Oncotarget* **2017**, *8*, 40264–40275. [CrossRef] [PubMed]
80. Ravindranathan, P.; Pasham, D.; Balaji, U.; Cardenas, J.; Gu, J.; Toden, S.; Goel, A. A combination of curcumin and oligomeric proanthocyanidins offer superior anti-tumorigenic properties in colorectal cancer. *Sci. Rep.* **2018**, *8*, 1–12. [CrossRef]
81. Marjaneh, R.M.; Rahmani, F.; Hassanian, S.M.; Rezaei, N.; Hashemzehi, M.; Bahrami, A.; Ariakia, F.; Fiuji, H.; Sahebkar, A.; Avan, A.; et al. Phytosomal curcumin inhibits tumor growth in colitis-associated colorectal cancer. *J. Cell. Physiol.* **2018**, *233*, 6785–6798. [CrossRef]
82. Carlos, D.A.; Sandra, A.; Fabián, C.-M.; Benjamín, R.; Maria, E.M. Antiproliferative and pro-apoptotic effects of Andean berry juice (Vaccinium meridionale Swartz) on human colon adenocarcinoma SW480 cells. *J. Med. Plants Res.* **2017**, *11*, 393–402. [CrossRef]
83. Buhrmann, C.; Yazdi, M.; Popper, B.; Shayan, P.; Goel, A.; Aggarwal, B.B.; Shakibaei, M. Resveratrol chemosensitizes TNF-β-induced survival of 5-FU-treated colorectal cancer cells. *Nutrients* **2018**, *10*, 888. [CrossRef]
84. Buhrmann, C.; Yazdi, M.; Popper, B.; Shayan, P.; Goel, A.; Aggarwal, B.B.; Shakibaei, M. Evidence that TNF-β induces proliferation in colorectal cancer cells and resveratrol can down-modulate it. *Exp. Biol. Med.* **2019**, *244*, 1–12. [CrossRef] [PubMed]
85. Chang, C.Y.; Ho, B.Y.; Pan, T.M. Lactobacillus paracasei subsp. paracasei NTU 101-fermented skim milk as an adjuvant to uracil-tegafur reduces tumor growth and improves chemotherapy side effects in an orthotopic mouse model of colorectal cancer. *J. Funct. Foods* **2019**, *55*, 36–47. [CrossRef]
86. Turan, I.; Demir, S.; Kilinc, K.; Yaman, S.O.; Misir, S.; Kara, H.; Genc, B.; Mentese, A.; Aliyazicioglu, Y.; Deger, O. Cytotoxic effect of Rosa canina extract on human colon cancer cells through repression of telomerase expression. *J. Pharm. Anal.* **2018**, *8*, 394–399. [CrossRef] [PubMed]
87. Aguilera, O.; Muñoz-Sagastibelza, M.; Torrejón, B.; Borrero-Palacios, A.; del Puerto-Nevado, L.; Martínez-Useros, J.; Rodriguez-Remirez, M.; Zazo, S.; García, E.; Fraga, M.; et al. Vitamin C uncouples the Warburg metabolic switch in KRAS mutant colon cancer. *Oncotarget* **2016**, *7*. [CrossRef]
88. Semeraro, P.; Chimienti, G.; Altamura, E.; Fini, P.; Rizzi, V.; Cosma, P. Chlorophyll a in cyclodextrin supramolecular complexes as a natural photosensitizer for photodynamic therapy (PDT) applications. *Mater. Sci. Eng. C* **2018**, *85*, 47–56. [CrossRef]
89. Bantal, V.; Ghanta, P.; Tejasvi, P. Piperine Presents Chemo-preventive Property Against 1, 2-Dimethyl Hydrazine Induced Colon Cancer in Mice: Biochemical and Physiological Evidences. *Pharmacologia* **2018**. [CrossRef]
90. Tan, B.L.; Norhaizan, M.E. Manilkara zapota (L.) P. Royen leaf water extract triggered apoptosis and activated caspase-dependent pathway in HT-29 human colorectal cancer cell line. *Biomed. Pharmacother.* **2019**, *110*, 748–757. [CrossRef]
91. Brglez Mojzer, E.; Knez Hrnčič, M.; Škerget, M.; Knez, Ž.; Bren, U. Polyphenols: Extraction Methods, Antioxidative Action, Bioavailability and Anticarcinogenic Effects. *Molecules* **2016**, *21*, 901. [CrossRef]
92. Bamia, C.; Lagiou, P.; Buckland, G.; Grioni, S.; Agnoli, C.; Taylor, A.J.; Dahm, C.C.; Overvad, K.; Olsen, A.; Tjønneland, A.; et al. Mediterranean diet and colorectal cancer risk: Results from a European cohort. *Eur. J. Epidemiol.* **2013**, *28*, 317–328. [CrossRef]

93. Tibbitt, M.W.; Dahlman, J.E.; Langer, R. Emerging Frontiers in Drug Delivery. *J. Am. Chem. Soc.* **2016**, *138*, 704–717. [CrossRef]
94. Ferreira, I.; Rocha, S.; Coelho, M. Encapsulation of Antioxidants by Spray-Drying. *Mater. Eng.* **2005**, *11*, 713–717.
95. Kothamasu, P.; Kanumur, H.; Ravur, N.; Maddu, C.; Parasuramrajam, R.; Thangavel, S. Nanocapsules: The weapons for novel drug delivery systems. *BioImpacts* **2012**, *2*, 71–81. [CrossRef] [PubMed]
96. Contreras-Cáceres, R.; Cabeza, L.; Perazzoli, G.; Díaz, A.; López-Romero, J.M.; Melguizo, C.; Prados, J. Electrospun Nanofibers: Recent Applications in Drug Delivery and Cancer Therapy. *Nanomaterials* **2019**, *9*, 656. [CrossRef] [PubMed]
97. Suganya, V.; Anuradha, V. Microencapsulation and Nanoencapsulation: A Review. *Int. J. Pharm. Clin. Res.* **2017**, *9*, 233–239. [CrossRef]
98. Trucillo, P.; Campardelli, R.; Reverchon, E. Production of liposomes loaded with antioxidants using a supercritical CO_2 assisted process. *Powder Technol.* **2018**, *323*, 155–162. [CrossRef]
99. Paini, M.; Daly, S.R.; Aliakbarian, B.; Fathi, A.; Tehrany, E.A.; Perego, P.; Dehghani, F.; Valtchev, P. An efficient liposome based method for antioxidants encapsulation. *Colloids Surfaces B Biointerfaces* **2015**, *136*, 1067–1072. [CrossRef]
100. Li, Q.; Cai, T.; Huang, Y.; Xia, X.; Cole, S.P.C.; Cai, Y. A review of the structure, preparation, and application of NLCs, PNPs, and PLNs. *Nanomaterials* **2017**, *7*, 122. [CrossRef]
101. Thakur, R.P.; Rai, K.N. Advances and Implications in Nanotechnology for Lung Cancer Management. *Curr. drug Metab.* **2017**, *18*. [CrossRef]
102. Bazylińska, U.; Wawrzyńczyk, D.; Kulbacka, J.; Frąckowiak, R.; Cichy, B.; Bednarkiewicz, A.; Samoć, M.; Wilk, K.A. Polymeric nanocapsules with up-converting nanocrystals cargo make ideal fluorescent bioprobes. *Sci. Rep.* **2016**, *6*. [CrossRef]
103. Ibrahim, M.M.; El-Zawawy, W.K.; Nassar, M.A. Synthesis and characterization of polyvinyl alcohol/nanospherical cellulose particle films. *Carbohydr. Polym.* **2010**, *79*, 694–699. [CrossRef]
104. Hirai, A.; Inui, O.; Horii, F.; Tsuji, M. Phase separation behavior in aqueous suspensions of bacterial cellulose nanocrystals prepared by sulfuric acid treatment. *Langmuir* **2009**, *25*, 497–502. [CrossRef] [PubMed]
105. Franco, R.A.; Nguyen, T.H.; Lee, B.T. Electro-spinning of PLGA/PCL blends for tissue engineering and their biocompatibility. *J. Mater. Sci. Mater. Med.* **2011**, *22*, 2207–2218. [CrossRef] [PubMed]
106. Asabuwa Ngwabebhoh, F.; Ilkar Erdagi, S.; Yildiz, U. Pickering emulsions stabilized nanocellulosic-based nanoparticles for coumarin and curcumin nanoencapsulations: In vitro release, anticancer and antimicrobial activities. *Carbohydr. Polym.* **2018**, *201*, 317–328. [CrossRef] [PubMed]
107. Choi, J.Y.; Gupta, B.; Ramasamy, T.; Jeong, J.H.; Jin, S.G.; Choi, H.G.; Yong, C.S.; Kim, J.O. PEGylated polyaminoacid-capped mesoporous silica nanoparticles for mitochondria-targeted delivery of celastrol in solid tumors. *Colloids Surfaces B Biointerfaces* **2018**, *165*, 56–66. [CrossRef] [PubMed]
108. Anandharamakrishnan, C. *Techniques for Nanoencapsulation of Food Ingredients*, 1st ed.; Anandharamakrishnan, C., Ed.; Springer: Madison, WI, USA, 2014.
109. Siepmann, J.; Peppas, N.A. Modeling of drug release from delivery systems based on hydroxypropyl methylcellulose (HPMC). *Adv. Drug Deliv. Rev.* **2001**, *48*, 139–157. [CrossRef]
110. Fenton, O.S.; Olafson, K.N.; Pillai, P.S.; Mitchell, M.J.; Langer, R. Advances in Biomaterials for Drug Delivery. *Adv. Mater.* **2018**, *30*, 1–29. [CrossRef]
111. Montagne, L.; Pluske, J.; Hampson, D. A review of interactions between dietary fibre and the intestinal mucosa, and their consequences on digestive health in young non-ruminant animals. *Anim. Feed Sci. Technol.* **2003**, *108*, 95–117. [CrossRef]
112. Tian, Z.; Yu, Q.; Xie, Y.; Li, F.; Lu, Y.; Dong, X.; Zhao, W.; Qi, J.; Wu, W. Controlling Release of Integral Lipid Nanoparticles Based on Osmotic Pump Technology. *Pharm. Res.* **2016**, *33*, 1988–1997. [CrossRef]
113. Quideau, S.; Deffieux, D.; Douat-Casassus, C.; Pouységu, L. Plant polyphenols: Chemical properties, biological activities, and synthesis. *Angew. Chemie - Int. Ed.* **2011**, *50*, 586–621. [CrossRef]
114. Kiokias, S.; Proestos, C.; Varzakas, T. A Review of the Structure, Biosynthesis, Absorption of Carotenoids-Analysis and Properties of their Common Natural Extracts. *Curr. Res. Nutr. Food Sci. J.* **2016**, *4*, 25–37. [CrossRef]
115. Liyana-Pathirana, C.M.; Shahidi, F. Antioxidant activity of commercial soft and hard wheat (Triticum aestivum L.) as affected by gastric pH conditions. *J. Agric. Food Chem.* **2005**, *53*, 2433–2440. [CrossRef]

116. Pettinato, M.; Aliakbarian, B.; Casazza, A.A.; Perego, P. Encapsulation of Antioxidants from Spent Coffee Ground Extracts by Spray Drying. *Chem. Eng. Trans.* **2017**, *57*, 1219–1224. [CrossRef]
117. Yoon, S.H.; Jin, H.-J.; Kook, M.-C.; Pyun, Y.R. Electrically conductive bacterial cellulose by incorporation of carbon nanotubes. *Biomacromolecules* **2006**, *7*, 1280–1284. [CrossRef] [PubMed]
118. McMurry, J. *Quimica Organica*, 6th ed.; Thomson: Mexico City, Mexico, 2004; ISBN 970 686 3545.
119. Kyatanwar, A.U. Self micro-emulsifying drug delivery system (SMEDDS): Review. *J. Pharm. Res.* **2010**, *7*, 9. [CrossRef]
120. Shrestha, H.; Bala, R.; Arora, S. Lipid-Based Drug Delivery Systems. *J. Pharm.* **2014**, *2014*, 1–10. [CrossRef]
121. García-Pinel, B.; Porras-Alcalá, C.; Ortega-Rodríguez, A.; Sarabia, F.; Prados, J.; Melguizo, C.; López-Romero, J.M. Lipid-Based Nanoparticles: Application and Recent Advances in Cancer Treatment. *Nanomaterials* **2019**, *9*, 638. [CrossRef] [PubMed]
122. Aisner, J. Overview of the changing paradigm in cancer treatment: Oral chemotherapy. *Am. J. Heal. Pharm.* **2007**, *64*, 4–7. [CrossRef]
123. Kerz, T.; Paret, G.; Herff, H. Routes of drug administration. *Int. J. Pharm. Stud. Res.* **2007**, *I*, 614–638. [CrossRef]
124. Osorio-Delgado, M.A.; Henao-Tamayo, L.J.; Velásquez-Cock, J.A.; Cañas-Gutierrez, A.I.; Restrepo-Múnera, L.M.; Gañán-Rojo, P.F.; Zuluaga-Gallego, R.O.; Ortiz-Trujillo, I.C.; Castro-Herazo, C.I. Biomedical applications of polymeric biomaterials. *DYNA* **2017**, *84*. [CrossRef]
125. Han, U.; Seo, Y.; Hong, J. Effect of pH on the structure and drug release profiles of layer-by-layer assembled films containing polyelectrolyte, micelles, and graphene oxide. *Sci. Rep.* **2016**, *6*, 1–10. [CrossRef]
126. Guarino, V.; Causa, F.; Taddei, P.; di Foggia, M.; Ciapetti, G.; Martini, D.; Fagnano, C.; Baldini, N.; Ambrosio, L. Polylactic acid fibre-reinforced polycaprolactone scaffolds for bone tissue engineering. *Biomaterials* **2008**, *29*, 3662–3670. [CrossRef]
127. Mathew, A.P.; Oksman, K.; Pierron, D.; Harmad, M.F. Crosslinked fibrous composites based on cellulose nanofibers and collagen with in situ pH induced fibrillation. *Cellulose* **2012**, *19*, 139–150. [CrossRef]
128. Mérillon, K.G.; RamawatJ, J.-M. *Polysaccharides: Bioactivity and Biotechnology*, 1st ed.; Mérillon, K.G., RamawatJ, J.-M., Eds.; Springer: Zug, Switzerland, 2015; ISBN 978-3-319-16297-3.
129. Kosaraju, S.L. Colon targeted delivery systems: Review of polysaccharides for encapsulation and delivery. *Crit. Rev. Food Sci. Nutr.* **2005**, *45*, 251–258. [CrossRef]
130. Osorio, M.A.; Restrepo, D.; Velásquez-Cock, J.A.; Zuluaga, R.O.; Montoya, U.; Rojas, O.; Gañán, P.F.; Marin, D.; Castro, C.I. Synthesis of thermoplastic starch-bacterial cellulose nanocomposites via in situ fermentation. *J. Braz. Chem. Soc.* **2014**, *25*. [CrossRef]
131. Velásquez-Cock, J.; Castro, C.; Gañán, P.; Osorio, M.; Putaux, J.L.; Serpa, A.; Zuluaga, R. Influence of the maturation time on the physico-chemical properties of nanocellulose and associated constituents isolated from pseudostems of banana plant c.v. Valery. *Ind. Crops Prod.* **2016**, *83*, 551–560. [CrossRef]
132. Sunasee, R.; Despres, H.W.; Nunez, K.D.; Ckless, K.; Pacherille, A.; Carson, M. Analysis of the Immune and Antioxidant Response of Cellulose Nanocrystals Grafted with β-Cyclodextrin in Myeloid Cell Lines. *J. Nanomater.* **2019**, *2019*, 1–9. [CrossRef]
133. Li, X.; Liu, Y.; Yu, Y.; Chen, W.; Liu, Y.; Yu, H. Nanoformulations of quercetin and cellulose nanofibers as healthcare supplements with sustained antioxidant activity. *Carbohydr. Polym.* **2019**, *207*, 160–168. [CrossRef]
134. Ching, Y.C.; Gunathilake, T.M.S.U.; Chuah, C.H.; Ching, K.Y.; Singh, R.; Liou, N.S. Curcumin/Tween 20-incorporated cellulose nanoparticles with enhanced curcumin solubility for nano-drug delivery: Characterization and in vitro evaluation. *Cellulose* **2019**, *26*, 5467–5481. [CrossRef]
135. Elieh-Ali-Komi, D.; Hamblin, M.R. Chitin and Chitosan: Production and Application of Versatile Biomedical Nanomaterials. *Int. J. Adv. Res.* **2016**, *4*, 411–427. [CrossRef]
136. Kumar, S.P.; Birundha, K.; Kaveri, K.; Devi, K.T.R. Antioxidant studies of chitosan nanoparticles containing naringenin and their cytotoxicity effects in lung cancer cells. *Int. J. Biol. Macromol.* **2015**, *78*, 87–95. [CrossRef]
137. Jeong, H.; Samdani, K.J.; Yoo, D.H.; Lee, D.W.; Kim, N.H.; Yoo, I.S.; Lee, J.H. Resveratrol cross-linked chitosan loaded with phospholipid for controlled release and antioxidant activity. *Int. J. Biol. Macromol.* **2016**, *93*, 757–766. [CrossRef] [PubMed]
138. Shi, M.; Bai, J.; Zhao, L.; Yu, X.; Liang, J.; Liu, Y.; Nord, W.; Li, Y. Co-loading and intestine-specific delivery of multiple antioxidants in pH-responsive microspheres based on TEMPO-oxidized polysaccharides. *Carbohydr. Polym.* **2017**, *157*, 858–865. [CrossRef]

139. Sookkasem, A.; Chatpun, S.; Yuenyongsawad, S.; Wiwattanapatapee, R. Alginate beads for colon specific delivery of self-emulsifying curcumin. *J. Drug Deliv. Sci. Technol.* **2015**, *29*, 159–166. [CrossRef]
140. Wang, H.; Gong, X.; Guo, X.; Liu, C.; Fan, Y.Y.; Zhang, J.; Niu, B.; Li, W. Characterization, release, and antioxidant activity of curcumin-loaded sodium alginate/ZnO hydrogel beads. *Int. J. Biol. Macromol.* **2019**, *121*, 1118–1125. [CrossRef]
141. Elgegren, M.; Kim, S.; Cordova, D.; Silva, C.; Noro, J.; Cavaco-paulo, A.; Nakamatsu, J. Ultrasound-Assisted Encapsulation of Sacha Inchi (Plukenetia volubilis Linneo.) Oil in Alginate-Chitosan Nanoparticles Mariela. *Polymers (Basel).* **2019**, *11*, 1245. [CrossRef]
142. Al-Ogaidi, I. Evaluation of the Antioxidant and Anticancer Effects of Biodegradable / Biocompatible Chitosan – Alginate Nanoparticles Loaded with. *Int. J. Pharm. Res. Allied Sci.* **2018**, *7*, 189–197.
143. Min, J.-Y.; Ahn, S.-I.; Lee, Y.-K.; Kwak, H.-S.; Chang, Y.H. Optimized conditions to produce water-in-oil-in-water nanoemulsion and spray-dried nanocapsule of red ginseng extract. *Food Sci. Technol.* **2018**, *38*, 485–492. [CrossRef]
144. Pan, K.; Chen, H.; Seung Joon, B.; Zhong, Q. Self-assembled curcumin-soluble soybean polysaccharide nanoparticles: Physicochemical properties and in vitro anti- proliferation activity against cancer cells Kang. *Food Chem.* **2019**, *344*, 1173–1178. [CrossRef]
145. Li, X.; Li, M.; Liu, J.; Ji, N.; Liang, C.; Sun, Q.; Xiong, L. Preparation of hollow biopolymer nanospheres employing starch nanoparticle templates for enhancement of phenolic acid antioxidant activities. *J. Agric. Food Chem* **2017**, *48*. [CrossRef]
146. Assis, R.Q.; Lopes, S.M.; Costa, T.M.H.; Flôres, S.H.; Rios, A.d.O. Active biodegradable cassava starch films incorporated lycopene nanocapsules. *Ind. Crops Prod.* **2017**, *109*, 818–827. [CrossRef]
147. Ahmad, M.; Mudgil, P.; Gani, A.; Hamed, F.; Masoodi, F.A.; Maqsood, S. Nano-encapsulation of catechin in starch nanoparticles: Characterization, release behavior and bioactivity retention during simulated in-vitro digestion. *Food Chem.* **2019**, *270*, 95–104. [CrossRef]
148. Jana, S.; Maiti, S.; Jana, S. Stimuli-responsive guar gum composites for colon-specific drug delivery. In *Biopolymer-Based Composites: Drug Delivery and Biomedical Applications*; Sougata, J., Sabyasachi, M., Subrata, J., Eds.; Elsevier Ltd: Cambridge, MA, USA, 2017; pp. 61–79. ISBN 9780081019153.
149. Saffarzadeh-Matin, S.; Shahbazi, M. Maltodextrine nanoparticles loaded with polyphenolic extract from apple industrial waste:Preparation, optimization and characterization. *RSM Optim. S. Saffarzadeh-Matin al. / J. Part. Sci. Technol.* **2017**, *3*, 197–209. [CrossRef]
150. Garay-Jimenez, J.C.; Turos, E. A convenient method to prepare emulsified polyacrylate nanoparticles from for drug delivery applications. *Bioorganic Med. Chem. Lett.* **2011**, *21*, 4589–4591. [CrossRef]
151. Ramalingam, N.; Rajiv, S. Curcumin loaded electrospun poly (2-hydroxyethyl methacrylate) p (HEMA) nanofibers as Antioxidant and Anticancer agents. *J. Adv. Res. Nanosci. Nanotechnol.* **2018**, *1*, 1–9.
152. Feuser, P.E.; Arévalo, J.M.C.; Junior, E.L.; Rossi, G.R.; da Silva Trindade, E.; Rocha, M.E.M.; Jacques, A.V.; Ricci-Júnior, E.; Santos-Silva, M.C.; Sayer, C.; et al. Increased cellular uptake of lauryl gallate loaded in superparamagnetic poly(methyl methacrylate) nanoparticles due to surface modification with folic acid. *J. Mater. Sci. Mater. Med.* **2016**, *27*. [CrossRef]
153. Ballestri, M.; Caruso, E.; Guerrini, A.; Ferroni, C.; Banfi, S.; Gariboldi, M.; Monti, E.; Sotgiu, G.; Varchi, G. Core–shell poly-methyl methacrylate nanoparticles covalently functionalized with a non-symmetric porphyrin for anticancer photodynamic therapy. *J. Photochem. Photobiol. B Biol.* **2018**, *186*, 169–177. [CrossRef]
154. Sobh, R.A.; Nasr, H.E.; Moustafa, A.B.; Mohamed, W.S. Tailoring of anticancer drugs loaded in MWCNT/Poly(MMA-co-HEMA) nanosphere composite by using in situ microemulsion polymerization. *J. Pharm. Investig.* **2019**, *49*, 45–55. [CrossRef]
155. Sunoqrot, S.; Abujamous, L. pH-sensitive polymeric nanoparticles of quercetin as a potential colon cancer-targeted nanomedicine. *J. Drug Deliv. Sci. Technol.* **2019**, *52*, 670–676. [CrossRef]
156. Osorio-delgado, M.A.; Henao-tamayo, L.J.; Velásquez-cock, J.A.; Isabel, A.; Restrepo-múnera, L.M.; Gañán-rojo, P.F.; Zuluaga-, R.O.; Ortiz-trujillo, I.C.; Castro-herazo, C.I. Biomedical applications of polymeric biomaterials Aplicaciones biomédicas de biomateriales poliméricos. *DYNA* **2017**, *84*, 241–252. [CrossRef]
157. Kweon, D.K.; Kang, D.O.O.W. Drug-Release Behavior of Chitosan-g-Poly (vinyl alcohol). *J. Appl. Polym. Sci.* **1999**, *74*, 458–464. [CrossRef]

158. Osorio, M.; Velásquez-Cock, J.; Restrepo, L.M.; Zuluaga, R.; Gañán, P.; Rojas, O.J.; Ortiz-Trujillo, I.; Castro, C. Bioactive 3D-Shaped Wound Dressings Synthesized from Bacterial Cellulose: Effect on Cell Adhesion of Polyvinyl Alcohol Integrated In Situ. *Int. J. Polym. Sci.* **2017**, *2017*. [CrossRef]
159. Millon, L.E.; Guhados, G.; Wan, W.K. Anisotropic polyvinyl alcohol-bacterial cellulose nanocomposite for biomedical applications. *J. Biomed. Mater. Res. Part B Appl. Biomater.* **2008**, *86*, 444–452. [CrossRef] [PubMed]
160. Li, H.; Yan, L.; Tang, E.K.Y.; Zhang, Z.; Chen, W.; Liu, G.; Mo, J. Synthesis of TPGS/Curcumin Nanoparticles by Thin-Film Hydration and Evaluation of Their Anti-Colon Cancer Efficacy In Vitro and In Vivo. *Front. Pharmacol.* **2019**, *10*, 1–12. [CrossRef]
161. Wen, P.; Hu, T.G.; Wen, Y.; Linhardt, R.J.; Zong, M.H.; Zou, Y.X.; Wu, H. Targeted delivery of phycocyanin for the prevention of colon cancer using electrospun fibers. *Food Funct.* **2019**, *10*, 1816–1825. [CrossRef]
162. Golkar, P.; Kalani, S.; Allafchian, A.R.; Mohammadi, H.; Jalali, S.A.H. Fabrication and characterization of electrospun Plantago major seed mucilage/PVA nanofibers. *J. Appl. Polym. Sci.* **2019**, *136*, 1–10. [CrossRef]
163. Singh, M.; Tarannum, N. Polyzwitterions. In *Engineering of Biomaterials for Drug Delivery Systems Beyond Polyethylene Glycol*; Parambath, A.B.T.-E., Ed.; Woodhead Publishing: Cambridge, MA, USA, 2018; pp. 69–101. ISBN 978-0-08-101750-0.
164. Gromadzki, D.; Tzankova, V.; Kondeva, M.; Gorinova, C.; Rychter, P.; Libera, M.; Momekov, G.; Marić, M.; Momekova, D. Amphiphilic core-shell nanoparticles with dimer fatty acid-based aliphatic polyester core and zwitterionic poly(sulfobetaine) shell for controlled delivery of curcumin. *Int. J. Polym. Mater. Polym. Biomater.* **2017**, *66*, 915–925. [CrossRef]
165. Viegas, T.X.; Bentley, M.D.; Harris, J.M.; Fang, Z.; Yoon, K.; Dizman, B.; Weimer, R.; Mero, A.; Pasut, G.; Veronese, F.M. Polyoxazoline: Chemistry, properties, and applications in drug delivery. *Bioconjug. Chem.* **2011**, *22*, 976–986. [CrossRef]
166. Simon, L.; Vincent, M.; Le Saux, S.; Lapinte, V.; Marcotte, N.; Morille, M.; Dorandeu, C.; Devoisselle, J.M.; Bégu, S. Polyoxazolines based mixed micelles as PEG free formulations for an effective quercetin antioxidant topical delivery. *Int. J. Pharm.* **2019**, 118516. [CrossRef]
167. González-Aramundiz, J.V.; Lozano, M.V.; Sousa-Herves, A.; Fernandez-Megia, E.; Csaba, N. Polypeptides and polyaminoacids in drug delivery. *Expert Opin. Drug Deliv.* **2012**, *9*, 183–201. [CrossRef]
168. Patsula, V.; Moskvin, M.; Siow, W.X.; Konefal, R.; Ma, Y.H.; Horák, D. Antioxidant polymer-modified maghemite nanoparticles. *J. Magn. Magn. Mater.* **2019**, *473*, 517–526. [CrossRef]
169. Hu, X.; Zheng, W.; Luo, Y.; Ou, X.; Song, L.; Zhang, S.; He, T.; Guo, Z.; Zhu, J.; Shi, H.; et al. Arca subcrenata Polypeptides Inhibit Human Colorectal Cancer HT-29 Cells Growth via Suppression of IGF-1R/Akt/mTOR Signaling and ATP Production. *Nutr. Cancer* **2019**, *0*, 1–13. [CrossRef] [PubMed]
170. Lima, A.I.G.; Mota, J.; Monteiro, S.A.V.S.; Ferreira, R.M.S.B. Legume seeds and colorectal cancer revisited: Protease inhibitors reduce MMP-9 activity and colon cancer cell migration. *Food Chem.* **2016**, *197*, 30–38. [CrossRef] [PubMed]
171. Chen, Z.; Li, W.; Santhanam, R.K.; Wang, C.; Gao, X.; Chen, Y.; Wang, C.; Xu, L.; Chen, H. Bioactive peptide with antioxidant and anticancer activities from black soybean [Glycine max (L.) Merr.] byproduct: Isolation, identification and molecular docking study. *Eur. Food Res. Technol.* **2019**, *245*, 677–689. [CrossRef]
172. González-Montoya, M.; Hernández-Ledesma, B.; Silván, J.M.; Mora-Escobedo, R.; Martínez-Villaluenga, C. Peptides derived from in vitro gastrointestinal digestion of germinated soybean proteins inhibit human colon cancer cells proliferation and inflammation. *Food Chem.* **2018**, *242*, 75–82. [CrossRef] [PubMed]
173. Zhang, M.; Mu, T.H. Contribution of different molecular weight fractions to anticancer effect of sweet potato protein hydrolysates by six proteases on HT-29 colon cancer cells. *Int. J. Food Sci. Technol.* **2018**, *53*, 525–532. [CrossRef]
174. Luo, T.; Yang, L.; Wu, J.; Zheng, Z.; Li, G.; Wang, X.; Kaplan, D.L. Stabilization of Natural Antioxidants by Silk Biomaterials. *ACS Appl. Mater. Interfaces* **2016**, *8*, 13573–13582. [CrossRef]
175. Lerdchai, K.; Kitsongsermthon, J.; Ratanavaraporn, J.; Kanokpanont, S.; Damrongsakkul, S. Thai Silk Fibroin/Gelatin Sponges for the Dual Controlled Release of Curcumin and Docosahexaenoic Acid for Anticancer Treatment. *J. Pharm. Sci.* **2016**, *105*, 221–230. [CrossRef]
176. Lozano-Pérez, A.A.; Rivero, H.C.; Pérez Hernández, M.d.C.; Pagán, A.; Montalbán, M.G.; Víllora, G.; Cénis, J.L. Silk fibroin nanoparticles: Efficient vehicles for the natural antioxidant quercetin. *Int. J. Pharm.* **2017**, *518*, 11–19. [CrossRef]

177. Alippilakkotte, S.; Sreejith, L. Pectin mediated synthesis of curcumin loaded poly(lactic acid) nanocapsules for cancer treatment. *J. Drug Deliv. Sci. Technol.* **2018**, *48*, 66–74. [CrossRef]
178. Grobelski, B.; Wach, R.A.; Adamus, A.; Olejnik, A.K.; Kowalska-Ludwicka, K.; Kolodziejczyk, M.; Bielecki, S.; Rosiak, J.M.; Pasieka, Z. Biocompatibility of Modified Bionanocellulose and Porous Poly(ε-caprolactone) Biomaterials. *Int. J. Polym. Mater. Polym. Biomater.* **2014**, *63*, 518–526. [CrossRef]
179. Seyednejad, H.; Gawlitta, D.; Kuiper, R.V.; De Bruin, A.; Van Nostrum, C.F.; Vermonden, T.; Dhert, W.J.A.; Hennink, W.E. In vivo biocompatibility and biodegradation of 3D-printed porous scaffolds based on a hydroxyl-functionalized poly(ε-caprolactone). *Biomaterials* **2012**, *33*, 4309–4318. [CrossRef] [PubMed]
180. Stoyko, F. *Biodegradable Polyesters*, 1st ed.; Stoyko, F., Ed.; Wiley: Singapore, 2015; ISBN 9781118837252.
181. Pereira, M.C.; Oliveira, D.A.; Hill, L.E.; Zambiazi, R.C.; Borges, C.D.; Vizzotto, M.; Mertens-Talcott, S.; Talcott, S.; Gomes, C.L. Effect of nanoencapsulation using PLGA on antioxidant and antimicrobial activities of guabiroba fruit phenolic extract. *Food Chem.* **2018**, *240*, 396–404. [CrossRef] [PubMed]
182. Kariduraganavar, M.Y.; Kittur, A.A.; Kamble, R.R. Polymer Synthesis and Processing. In *Handbook of Polymer Synthesis*; Kumbar, S.G., Laurencin, C.T., Deng, M.B.T.-N.S.B.P., Eds.; Elsevier: Oxford, UK, 2014; pp. 1–31. ISBN 978-0-12-396983-5.
183. Sriyanti, I.; Edikresnha, D.; Rahma, A.; Munir, M.M.; Rachmawati, H.; Khairurrijal, K. Correlation between Structures and Antioxidant Activities of Polyvinylpyrrolidone/Garcinia mangostana L. Extract Composite Nanofiber Mats Prepared Using Electrospinnin. *J. Nanomater.* **2017**, *2017*. [CrossRef]
184. Andjani, D.; Sriyanti, I.; Fauzi, A.; Edikresnha, D.; Munir, M.M.; Rachmawati, H. Khairurrijal Rotary Forcespun Polyvinylpyrrolidone (PVP) Fibers as a Mangosteen Pericarp Extracts Carrier. *Procedia Eng.* **2017**, *170*, 14–18. [CrossRef]
185. Zahra, F.; Fauzi, A.; Miftahul Munir, M.; Khairurrijal, K. Synthesis and Characterization of Rotary Forcespun Polyvinylpyrrolidone Fibers Loaded by Garlic (Allium sativum) Extract. *IOP Conf. Ser. Mater. Sci. Eng.* **2019**, *515*. [CrossRef]
186. Kamaruddin; Sriyanti, I.; Edikresnha, D.; Munir, M.M.; Khairurrijal, K. Electrosprayed polyvinylpyrrolidone (PVP) submicron particles loaded by green tea extracts. *IOP Conf. Ser. Mater. Sci. Eng.* **2018**, *367*. [CrossRef]
187. Guamán-Balcázar, M.C.; Montes, A.; Pereyra, C.; Martínez de la Ossa, E. Production of submicron particles of the antioxidants of mango leaves/PVP by supercritical antisolvent extraction process. *J. Supercrit. Fluids* **2019**, *143*, 294–304. [CrossRef]
188. Contardi, M.; Heredia-Guerrero, J.A.; Guzman-Puyol, S.; Summa, M.; Benítez, J.J.; Goldoni, L.; Caputo, G.; Cusimano, G.; Picone, P.; Di Carlo, M.; et al. Combining dietary phenolic antioxidants with polyvinylpyrrolidone: Transparent biopolymer films based on: P-coumaric acid for controlled release. *J. Mater. Chem. B* **2019**, *7*, 1384–1396. [CrossRef]
189. Thanyacharoen, T.; Chuysinuan, P.; Techasakul, S.; Nooeaid, P.; Ummartyotin, S. Development of a gallic acid-loaded chitosan and polyvinyl alcohol hydrogel composite: Release characteristics and antioxidant activity. *Int. J. Biol. Macromol.* **2018**, *107*, 363–370. [CrossRef]
190. Aluani, D.; Tzankova, V.; Kondeva-Burdina, M.; Yordanov, Y.; Nikolova, E.; Odzhakov, F.; Apostolov, A.; Markova, T.; Yoncheva, K. Evaluation of biocompatibility and antioxidant efficiency of chitosan-alginate nanoparticles loaded with quercetin. *Int. J. Biol. Macromol.* **2017**, *103*, 771–782. [CrossRef]
191. Rahaiee, S.; Hashemi, M.; Shojaosadati, S.A.; Moini, S.; Razavi, S.H. Nanoparticles based on crocin loaded chitosan-alginate biopolymers: Antioxidant activities, bioavailability and anticancer properties. *Int. J. Biol. Macromol.* **2017**, *99*, 401–408. [CrossRef] [PubMed]
192. Huang, X.; Huang, X.; Gong, Y.; Xiao, H.; McClements, D.J.; Hu, K. Enhancement of curcumin water dispersibility and antioxidant activity using core-shell protein-polysaccharide nanoparticles. *Food Res. Int.* **2016**, *87*, 1–9. [CrossRef] [PubMed]
193. Wei, Y.; Yu, Z.; Lin, K.; Sun, C.; Dai, L.; Yang, S.; Mao, L.; Yuan, F.; Gao, Y. Fabrication and characterization of resveratrol loaded zein-propylene glycol alginate-rhamnolipid composite nanoparticles: Physicochemical stability, formation mechanism and in vitro digestion. *Food Hydrocoll.* **2019**, *95*, 336–348. [CrossRef]
194. Arunkumar, R.; Prashanth, K.V.H.; Manabe, Y.; Hirata, T.; Sugawara, T.; Dharmesh, S.M.; Baskaran, V. Biodegradable poly (lactic-co-glycolic acid)-polyethylene glycol nanocapsules: An efficient carrier for improved solubility, bioavailability, and anticancer property of lutein. *J. Pharm. Sci.* **2015**, *104*, 2085–2093. [CrossRef] [PubMed]

195. Jaiswal, S.; Dutta, P.K.; Kumar, S.; Koh, J.; Pandey, S. Methyl methacrylate modified chitosan: Synthesis, characterization and application in drug and gene delivery. *Carbohydr. Polym.* **2019**, *211*, 109–117. [CrossRef]
196. Eatemadi, A.; Daraee, H.; Aiyelabegan, H.T.; Negahdari, B.; Rajeian, B.; Zarghami, N. Synthesis and Characterization of Chrysin-loaded PCL-PEG-PCL nanoparticle and its effect on breast cancer cell line. *Biomed. Pharmacother.* **2016**, *84*, 1915–1922. [CrossRef]
197. Wu, C.S.; Liao, H.T. Interface design and reinforced features of arrowroot (Maranta arundinacea) starch/polyester-based membranes: Preparation, antioxidant activity, and cytocompatibility. *Mater. Sci. Eng. C* **2016**, *70*, 54–61. [CrossRef]
198. Teiten, M.H.; Dicato, M.; Diederich, M. Hybrid curcumin compounds: A new strategy for cancer treatment. *Molecules* **2014**, *19*, 20839–20863. [CrossRef]
199. Abdel Latif, Y.; El-Bana, M.; Hussein, J.; El-Khayat, Z.; Farrag, A.R. Effects of resveratrol in combination with 5-fluorouracil on N-methylnitrosourea-induced colon cancer in rats. *Comp. Clin. Path.* **2019**. [CrossRef]
200. Carrillo, E.; Navarro, S.A.; Ramírez, A.; García, M.Á.; Griñán-Lisón, C.; Perán, M.; Marchal, J.A. 5-fluorouracil derivatives: A patent review (2012–2014). *Expert Opin. Ther. Pat.* **2015**, *25*, 1131–1144. [CrossRef]
201. Han, R.; Sun, Y.; Kang, C.; Sun, H.; Wei, W. Amphiphilic dendritic nanomicelle-mediated co-delivery of 5-fluorouracil and doxorubicin for enhanced therapeutic efficacy. *J. Drug Target.* **2017**, *25*, 140–148. [CrossRef] [PubMed]
202. Moodley, T.; Singh, M. Polymeric mesoporous silica nanoparticles for enhanced delivery of 5-fluorouracil in vitro. *Pharmaceutics* **2019**, *11*, 288. [CrossRef] [PubMed]
203. Wang, Y.; Li, P.; Chen, L.; Gao, W.; Zeng, F.; Kong, L.X. Targeted delivery of 5-fluorouracil to HT-29 cells using high efficient folic acid-conjugated nanoparticles. *Drug Deliv.* **2015**, *22*, 191–198. [CrossRef]
204. Anirudhan, T.S.; Christa, J. Binusreejayan pH and magnetic field sensitive folic acid conjugated protein–polyelectrolyte complex for the controlled and targeted delivery of 5-fluorouracil. *J. Ind. Eng. Chem.* **2018**, *57*, 199–207. [CrossRef]
205. Hariharan, M.S.; Sivaraj, R.; Ponsubha, S.; Jagadeesh, R.; Enoch, I.V.M.V. 5-Fluorouracil-loaded β-cyclodextrin-carrying polymeric poly(methylmethacrylate)-coated samarium ferrite nanoparticles and their anticancer activity. *J. Mater. Sci.* **2019**, *54*, 4942–4951. [CrossRef]
206. Roth Stefaniak, K.; Epley, C.C.; Novak, J.J.; McAndrew, M.L.; Cornell, H.D.; Zhu, J.; McDaniel, D.K.; Davis, J.L.; Allen, I.C.; Morris, A.J.; et al. Photo-triggered release of 5-fluorouracil from a MOF drug delivery vehicle. *Chem. Commun.* **2018**, *54*, 7617–7620. [CrossRef] [PubMed]
207. Hadjianfar, M.; Semnani, D.; Varshosaz, J. Polycaprolactone/chitosan blend nanofibers loaded by 5-fluorouracil: An approach to anticancer drug delivery system. *Polym. Adv. Technol.* **2018**, *29*, 2972–2981. [CrossRef]
208. Gioumouxouzis, C.I.; Chatzitaki, A.-T.; Karavasili, C.; Katsamenis, O.L.; Tzetzis, D.; Mystiridou, E.; Bouropoulos, N.; Fatouros, D.G. Controlled Release of 5-Fluorouracil from Alginate Beads Encapsulated in 3D Printed pH-Responsive Solid Dosage Forms. *AAPS PharmSciTech.* **2018**, *19*, 3362–3375. [CrossRef]
209. Pal, P.; Pandey, J.P.; Sen, G. Sesbania gum based hydrogel as platform for sustained drug delivery: An 'in vitro' study of 5-Fu release. *Int. J. Biol. Macromol.* **2018**, *113*, 1116–1124. [CrossRef]
210. Ma, Z.; Ma, R.; Wang, X.; Gao, J.; Zheng, Y.; Sun, Z. Enzyme and PH responsive 5-flurouracil (5-FU)loaded hydrogels based on olsalazine derivatives for colon-specific drug delivery. *Eur. Polym. J.* **2019**, *118*, 64–70. [CrossRef]
211. Sun, X.; Liu, C.; Omer, A.M.; Lu, W.; Zhang, S.; Jiang, X.; Wu, H.; Yu, D.; Ouyang, X. kun pH-sensitive ZnO/carboxymethyl cellulose/chitosan bio-nanocomposite beads for colon-specific release of 5-fluorouracil. *Int. J. Biol. Macromol.* **2019**, *128*, 468–479. [CrossRef] [PubMed]
212. Cuadra, I.A.; Zahran, F.; Martín, D.; Cabañas, A.; Pando, C. Preparation of 5-fluorouracil microparticles and 5-fluorouracil/poly(L-lactide) composites by a supercritical CO2 antisolvent process. *J. Supercrit. Fluids* **2019**, *143*, 64–71. [CrossRef]
213. Khan, S.; Anwar, N. Highly Porous pH-Responsive Carboxymethyl Chitosan- Grafted -Poly (Acrylic Acid) Based Smart Hydrogels for 5-Fluorouracil Controlled Delivery and Colon Targeting. *Int. J. Polym. Sci.* **2019**, *2019*. [CrossRef]
214. Yan, J.K.; Qiu, W.Y.; Wang, Y.Y.; Wu, L.X.; Cheung, P.C.K. Formation and characterization of polyelectrolyte complex synthesized by chitosan and carboxylic curdlan for 5-fluorouracil delivery. *Int. J. Biol. Macromol.* **2018**, *107*, 397–405. [CrossRef]

215. Wu, X.; He, C.; Wu, Y.; Chen, X. Synergistic therapeutic effects of Schiff's base cross-linked injectable hydrogels for local co-delivery of metformin and 5-fluorouracil in a mouse colon carcinoma model. *Biomaterials* **2016**, *75*, 148–162. [CrossRef]
216. Wang, Y.; Bai, F.; Luo, Q.; Wu, M.; Song, G.; Zhang, H.; Cao, J.; Wang, Y. Lycium barbarum polysaccharides grafted with doxorubicin: An efficient pH-responsive anticancer drug delivery system. *Int. J. Biol. Macromol.* **2019**, *121*, 964–970. [CrossRef]
217. Dhanavel, S.; Revathy, T.A.; Sivaranjani, T.; Sivakumar, K.; Palani, P.; Narayanan, V.; Stephen, A. 5-Fluorouracil and curcumin co-encapsulated chitosan/reduced graphene oxide nanocomposites against human colon cancer cell lines. *Polym. Bull.* **2019**. [CrossRef]

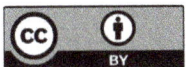

© 2020 by the authors. Licensee MDPI, Basel, Switzerland. This article is an open access article distributed under the terms and conditions of the Creative Commons Attribution (CC BY) license (http://creativecommons.org/licenses/by/4.0/).

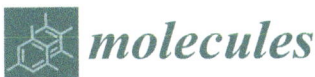

Article

Pre-Clinical Investigation of Keratose as an Excipient of Drug Coated Balloons

Emily Goel [1], Megan Erwin [1], Claire V. Cawthon [1], Carson Schaff [1], Nathaniel Fedor [1], Trevor Rayl [1], Onree Wilson [1], Uwe Christians [2], Thomas C. Register [3], Randolph L. Geary [4], Justin Saul [5] and Saami K. Yazdani [6],*

[1] Department of Mechanical Engineering, University of South Alabama, Mobile, AL 36688, USA; emily.turner.ann@gmail.com (E.G.); megan.m.erwin@vanderbilt.edu (M.E.); clairecawthon@gmail.com (C.V.C.); carson.schaff@gmail.com (C.S.); ntfedor@gmail.com (N.F.); trevorerayl@gmail.com (T.R.); onreewilson@gmail.com (O.W.)
[2] iC42 Clinical Research and Development, Department of Anesthesiology, University of Colorado; Aurora, CO 80045, USA; Uwe.Christians@ucdenver.edu
[3] Department of Vascular Surgery, Wake Forest School of Medicine, Winston-Salem, NC 27157, USA; register@wakehealth.edu
[4] Department of Pathology, Wake Forest School of Medicine, Winston-Salem, NC 27157, USA; rgeary@wakehealth.edu
[5] Department of Chemical, Paper and Biomedical Engineering, Miami University, Oxford, OH 45056, USA; sauljm@miamioh.edu
[6] Department of Engineering, Wake Forest University, Winston-Salem, NC 27101, USA
* Correspondence: yazdanis@wfu.edu; Tel.: +1-336-702-1968

Academic Editors: Carlos A. García-González, Pasquale Del Gaudio and Ricardo Starbird
Received: 13 March 2020; Accepted: 27 March 2020; Published: 31 March 2020

Abstract: Background: Drug-coated balloons (DCBs), which deliver anti-proliferative drugs with the aid of excipients, have emerged as a new endovascular therapy for the treatment of peripheral arterial disease. In this study, we evaluated the use of keratose (KOS) as a novel DCB-coating excipient to deliver and retain paclitaxel. Methods: A custom coating method was developed to deposit KOS and paclitaxel on uncoated angioplasty balloons. The retention of the KOS-paclitaxel coating, in comparison to a commercially available DCB, was evaluated using a novel vascular-motion simulating *ex vivo* flow model at 1 h and 3 days. Additionally, the locoregional biological response of the KOS-paclitaxel coating was evaluated in a rabbit ilio-femoral injury model at 14 days. Results: The KOS coating exhibited greater retention of the paclitaxel at 3 days under pulsatile conditions with vascular motion as compared to the commercially available DCB (14.89 ± 4.12 ng/mg vs. 0.60 ± 0.26 ng/mg, $p = 0.018$). Histological analysis of the KOS–paclitaxel-treated arteries demonstrated a significant reduction in neointimal thickness as compared to the uncoated balloons, KOS-only balloon and paclitaxel-only balloon. Conclusions: The ability to enhance drug delivery and retention in targeted arterial segments can ultimately improve clinical peripheral endovascular outcomes.

Keywords: Keratose; drug-coated balloon; paclitaxel; drug delivery; pre-clinical; peripheral arterial disease; endovascular

1. Introduction

Drug-coated balloons (DCBs) represent a new therapeutic approach to treat peripheral arterial disease (PAD) [1–5]. In the United States, PAD affects more than eight million people, with an annual cost of roughly $21 billion [6]. Traditionally, endovascular treatment of PAD has been performed by balloon angioplasty or the placement of a permanent metallic stent [7,8]. However, results are poor, with 50–85% of patients developing hemodynamically significant restenosis (re-occlusion), and 16–65%

developing occlusions within 2 years post-treatment [9,10]. The use of anti-proliferative drugs in combination with bare metal stents, i.e., drug-eluting stents (DES), was a major breakthrough and highly successful in treating coronary artery disease [11,12]. However, stents have shown very poor clinical outcomes in treating PAD, as they are subjected to biomechanical stress and severe artery deformation (twisting, bending, and shortening), leading to high fracture rates (up to 68%) and restenosis [13].

DCBs, which were FDA-approved for the treatment of PAD in late 2014, provide a new therapeutic approach for interventionalists to practice a 'leave nothing behind' procedure, preserving future treatment options DCBs are angioplasty balloons directly coated with an anti-proliferative therapeutic drug and an excipient (drug carrier) [1,14–18]. The excipient enhances the adhesion of the drug to the balloon surface, increases the stability of the drug coating during handling and delivery, and maximizes drug retention to the targeted arterial segment. [18–24] Current DCBs excipients include polysorbate and sorbitol, urea, polyethylene glycol (PEG) and butyryl-tri-hexyl citrate (BTHC). The rationale for the selection of these various excipients varies. For example, excipients such as polysorbate and PEG are known cosolvents of paclitaxel [25,26], which can alter the vessel interaction of the drug with the DCB device. Conversely, urea acts to increase paclitaxel release at the lesion [18] and PEG has been shown to bind to hydroxylapatite, a primary component of calcified atherosclerotic lesions [17,19,23,24], thereby improving local pharmacodynamics.

However, more recent pre-clinical studies have demonstrated the potential of DCB excipients to embolize and travel downstream to distal tissue post-treatment [27,28]. As peripheral arteries undergo severe mechanical deformation, excipients should aid in maintaining drug residency on the luminal surface, in particular at the early time phase, prior to the buildup of tissue, following delivery onto the luminal surface of the artery. Therefore, novel excipients that are capable of maintaining drug residency while minimizing downstream or off-target effects are needed. Keratins are a class of proteins that can be derived from numerous sources, including from human hair. Keratins have been shown to achieve the sustained release of small-molecule drugs and growth factors [29,30]. Further, keratin films have been reported for use in vascular grafts to reduce thrombosis, suggesting their utility in cardiovascular applications [31]. The goal of this study was thus to examine the ability to use an oxidized form of keratin (known as keratose (KOS)) as a new drug carrier excipient to aid in the delivery and retention of the anti-proliferative drug, paclitaxel. Specifically, the mobility, retention and biological impact of a KOS–paclitaxel-coated DCB was determined using *ex vivo* and *in vivo* models.

2. Results

2.1. Ex Vivo Results

The non-coated angioplasty balloons were successfully coated with the KOS–paclitaxel mixture (Figure 1D,E). To determine the impact of vascular deformation on DCB retention, both the KOS–paclitaxel DCB and the commercially available DCB were tested under only physiological pulsatile conditions (no twisting or shortening) and physiological pulsatile conditions with vascular deformation conditions. The pulsatile flow conditions consisted of pressures ranging from 70 to 120 mmHg with a mean flow rate of 120 mL/min at 60 beats per minute. The vascular deformation conditions consisted of the artery shortening 10% in the axial direction and twisting of the artery at 15°/cm. The frequency of the artery twisting and shortening was 0.05 Hz (3 cycles/min). All DCBs were inserted through a 6 Fr sheath into the closed-circulatory system under the physiological pulsatile conditions. The treated sections of the artery were marked during inflation of the DCBs. It is noted that vascular deformation (twisting and shortening) occurred following 4 h of physiological pulsatile conditions of DCB deployment. At timepoints of 1 h and 3 days, the treated section of the arteries were removed and analyzed for arterial tissue paclitaxel concentration (Figure 2). There was a reduction in arterial paclitaxel levels from 1 h to 3 days post-treatment for both the KOS–paclitaxel and the commercially available DCB under physiological pulsatile conditions (3 days—pulse only: KOS-PXL:

17.56 ± 7.19 ng/mg vs. commercial DCB: 24.44 ± 27.03, $p = 0.96$, Table 1). However, under pulsatile and vascular deformation, paclitaxel was significantly retained within the treated artery (3 days—pulse and vascular deformation: KOS-PXL: 14.89 ± 4.12 ng/mg vs. commercial DCB: 0.60 ± 0.26, $p = 0.018$).

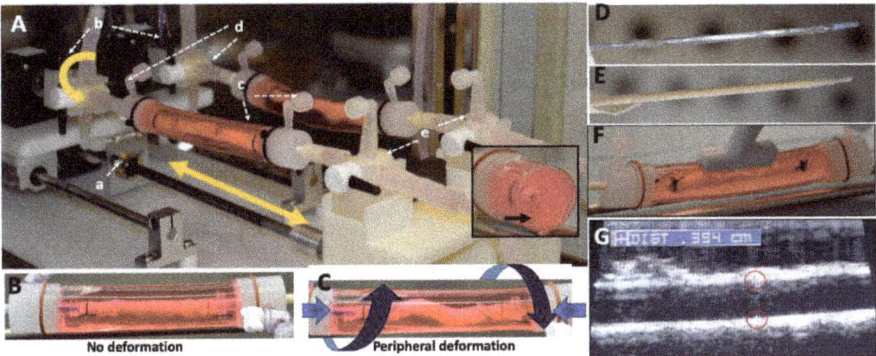

Figure 1. Schematic illustration of the novel peripheral simulating bioreactor system. (**A**) Two servos (a and b) provide axial deformation and twisting, respectively. Servo (a) moves the harvested arteries (c) forward and backward in a linear motion. Servo b rotates the artery by degrees. The three-way values (d and e) are used to introduce flow and pressure to the artery. The artery is surrounded by matrigel, mimicking external tissue, providing support during vascular movement (insert, black arrow). (**B**,**C**) Harvested arteries under pulsatile (no deformation) and pulsatile conditions with peripheral deformation. (**D**,**E**) Gross photos of an uncoated balloon and a keratose–paclitaxel coated balloon. (**F**,**G**) Diameter measurements performed by ultrasound on the harvested artery.

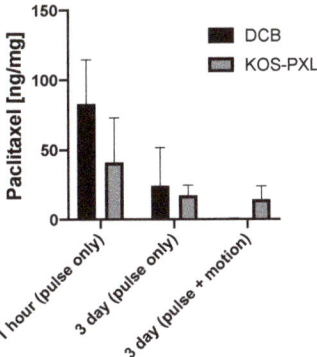

Figure 2. Paclitaxel levels of the drug-coated balloon (DCB) and the keratose–paclitaxel (KOS-PXL)-coated balloon arterial segments undergoing pulsatile flow conditions versus pulsatile flow conditions with vascular motion.

Table 1. *Ex vivo* arterial drug concentration measurements of treated arteries.

Time Points	KOS-PXL ng/mg	Commercial DCB ng/mg	*p* Value
1 h (pulse only)	41.01 ± 32.11	82.88 ± 31.81	0.30
3 day (pulse only)	17.56 ± 7.19	24.44 ± 27.03	0.96
3 day (pulse + vascular motion)	14.89 ± 4.12	0.60 ± 0.26	0.018

2.2. Histomorphometric Results

Following *ex vivo* studies, *in vivo* studies were performed using the rabbit ilio–femoral injury model to determine the impact of the KOS excipients on vascular remodeling. The animals were treated with a KOS-paclitaxel ($n = 4$), KOS-only balloon ($n = 4$), paclitaxel-only balloon ($n = 4$) or an uncoated balloon ($n = 4$). All arteries were treated successfully without any signs of dissection or thrombosis, and all animals survived the duration of the study. At 7 days, morphometric analysis demonstrated similar area measurements, including the EEL, IEL, lumen and media, for all treatment groups (Table 2). Neointimal thickness was significantly different between the varying groups (no coating: 0.10 ± 0.011 mm vs. KOS-only: 0.069 ± 0.022 mm vs. PXL-only: 0.066 ± 0.018 mm vs. KOS-PXL: 0.53 ± 0.003 mm, $p = 0.005$, Figure 3). Although percent area stenosis was the least in the KOS-PXL group, differences between the group were non-significant (no coating: $10.88\% \pm 4.52\%$ vs. KOS-only: $9.99\% \pm 3.78\%$ vs. PXL-only: $7.92\% \pm 3.84\%$ vs. KOS-PXL: $6.80\% \pm 2.74\%$, $p = 0.45$).

Table 2. Summary of the morphometric and histological measurements in the rabbit iliac–femoral injury model.

	No Coating	KOS-only	PXL-only	KTO-PXL	*p* Value
Morphometric Measurements					
EEL, mm^2	1.87 ± 0.33	1.64 ± 0.63	1.98 ± 0.48	1.39 ± 0.39	0.37
IEL, mm^2	1.32 ± 0.24	1.15 ± 0.55	1.58 ± 0.24	0.99 ± 0.45	0.52
Lumen, mm^2	1.18 ± 0.24	1.00 ± 0.55	1.32 ± 0.30	0.92 ± 0.43	0.58
Media, mm^2	0.55 ± 0.10	0.50 ± 0.11	0.59 ± 0.18	0.40 ± 0.08	0.21
Neointimal area, mm^2	0.15 ± 0.06	0.14 ± 0.04	0.11 ± 0.05	0.06 ± 0.02	0.085
Neointimal thickness, mm	0.10 ± 0.011	0.069 ± 0.022	0.066 ± 0.018	0.053 ± 0.003	0.005
Percent area stenosis, %	10.88 ± 4.52	9.99 ± 3.78	7.92 ± 3.84	6.80 ± 2.74	0.45
Histological Analysis					
Injury	1.00 ± 0.41	0.75 ± 1.19	1.13 ± 1.32	0.50 ± 0.41	0.74
EC Score	0.25 ± 0.50	0.00 ± 0.00	0.25 ± 0.50	1.50 ± 0.58	0.013
Inflammation	0.25 ± 0.50	0.00 ± 0.00	0.50 ± 0.58	0.25 ± 0.50	0.86
SMC Loss	0.00 ± 0.00	0.00 ± 0.00	0.25 ± 0.50	1.00 ± 0.82	0.081

Abbreviations: EEL—external elastic lamina, IEL—internal elastic lamina, EC—endothelial cell, SMC—smooth muscle cell.

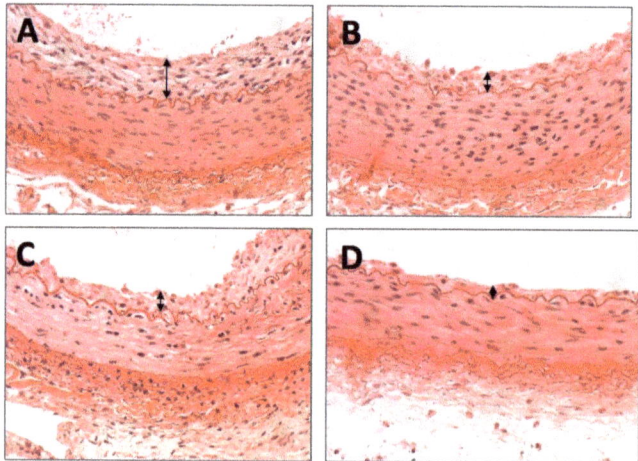

Figure 3. Representative images of the arterial response following the varying treatment groups. H&E staining demonstrated neointimal growth for (**A**) the uncoated balloon group, (**B**) keratose-only coated balloon, (**C**) paclitaxel-only coated balloon and (**D**) keratose–paclitaxel coated balloon at 7 days. Neointimal growth is marked by double-arrow heads.

Histological analysis demonstrated minimal injury for all groups at 7 days with the greatest endothelial cell loss in the KOS–paclitaxel treated arteries (no coating: 0.25 ± 0.50 vs. KOS-only: 0.00 ± 0.00 vs. PXL-only: 0.25 ± 0.58 vs. KOS-PXL: 1.50 ± 0.58, $p = 0.013$). Inflammation was minimal for all groups and there was a trend towards greater SMC loss in the KOS–paclitaxel group (no coating: 0.00 ± 0.00 vs. KOS-only: 0.00 ± 0.00 vs. PXL-only: 0.25 ± 0.50 vs. KOS-PXL: 1.00 ± 0.82, $p = 0.45$). No aneurysmal dilatation or thrombosis was observed in any treated artery.

3. Discussion

This study was designed to evaluate the use of keratose as a novel excipient for peripheral applications and, specifically, to determine the feasibility of the keratose excipient to retain paclitaxel under peripheral vascular mechanical environments. This was accomplished by developing a novel vascular-simulating *ex vivo* flow system and testing in a clinically relevant pre-clinical model. Furthermore, the vascular biological response to the keratose excipient was also investigated in the pre-clinical model. The *ex vivo* model arterial drug concentration results demonstrated that keratose significantly improves the retention of paclitaxel as compared to a commercially available DCB. Histomorphometric results of rabbit arteries treated by keratose demonstrated the safety and efficacy of the excipient in the delivery of paclitaxel. Overall, these results demonstrate the potential of the keratose as a DCB excipient for peripheral applications.

Drug-coated balloons are the next-generation treatment for PAD. Approved in the US since late 2014, DCB represented a shift in the approach to treating peripheral artery disease. While the DES provides a scaffold for long-term drug release, DCBs are limited in the time they can interact with the target lesion (~30 s to 2 min). Therefore, a major goal of any excipient is to support the retention of the therapeutic agent to the arterial wall surface, even under vascular deformation conditions. In two recent studies, the embolization of release particulates from all currently FDA-approved DCB coatings was investigated [27,28]. Twenty-eight days post-delivery, their results also demonstrated evidence of distal embolization, including embolic crystalline material, in downstream tissue. Remarkably, pharmacokinetic analysis of the distal tissue showed similar or higher levels of paclitaxel concentration as compared to the arterial treatment site, in particular for the IN.PACT DCB. These results indicate the mobility of the DCB coating following deployment, although, to date, no studies have directly investigated the impact of vascular deformation on DCB performance.

The vascular-mimicking *ex vivo* system, to our knowledge, is the first system that can evaluate the acute drug-loading of arteries treated by endovascular devices under pulsatile and vascular deformation conditions using explanted pig arteries. Our testing of the KOS coating was performed under vascular deformation conditions of 10% artery shortening, 15°/cm twisting at a frequency of 0.05 Hz (3 cycles/min). These conditions were selected to replicate the human periphery motion of the femoral artery (shortening lengths of 7% and twisting at 11.5°/cm) and the popliteal–tibial artery motion (shortening of 15% and twisting at 19.9°/cm) [32–35]. The frequency of the peripheral movement will be 0.06 Hz (5184 cycles/day or 3.6 cycles/min), which is based upon the average steps per day of adults in the US [36]. Our results indicated that the KOS coating maintained paclitaxel tissue levels under physiological pulsatile and vascular motion conditions 3 days post-delivery.

To further evaluate the DCB coating, we fluorescently tagged (NHS-Fluorescein, Thermo Scientific) the KOS to visualize the presence of the coating acutely (1 h) and three days post-delivery in arteries undergoing vascular deformation. The presence of the KOS was confirmed by confocal microscopy (Figure 4). The mechanism by which this process occurs is not fully elucidated in these studies. In drug-release experiments with small molecule drugs such as ciprofloxacin from hydrogel (rather than coating) forms of KOS, we have demonstrated that the rate of drug release correlates with the degradation rate of the hydrogel material [30]. We note that this degradation process does not refer to the breaking of peptide (amide) bonds in the keratin, but rather the dissolution of the keratin hydrogels. This correlation between drug release and KOS dissolution (or degradation) suggested an interaction between keratin and the drug. In the case of ciprofloxacin, this was found to be associated with electrostatic interactions. While the physiochemical characteristics of paclitaxel are different than ciprofloxacin, such interactions (or others, such as hydrophobic interactions) could be in play and are an area for further study.

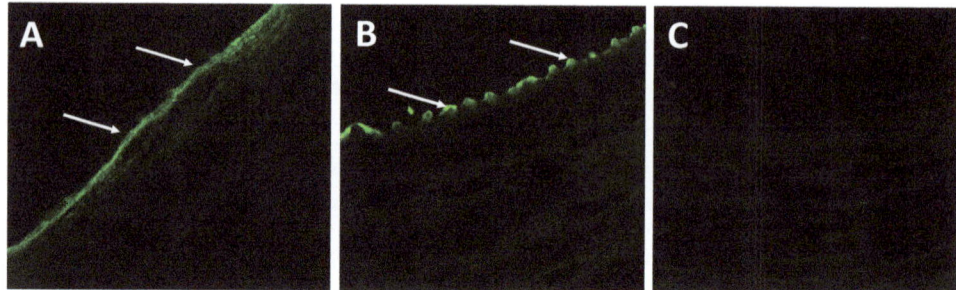

Figure 4. Representative confocal images arterial segments following keratose delivery. Confocal microscopy confirmed the presence of the keratose at (**A**) 1 h and (**B**) 3 days under peripheral deformation conditions. (**C**) Negative control depicts the lack of tissue autofluorescence during confocal imaging.

This previous finding of an interaction between KOS and small molecule drugs is noteworthy due to the findings of paclitaxel retention in the vessel at 3 days with vascular motion compared to DCB (Figure 2) and the presence of (fluorescently labeled) KOS on the vascular walls (Figure 4). That is, it is possible that paclitaxel remains associated with the KOS in a manner not possible with other synthetic polymers (e.g., PEG) or other (e.g., urea) excipients due to the properties of keratin. In particular, KOS has been shown to contain RGD and other integrin-binding sequences which may allow it to bind to the vascular cells [37,38]. Thus, KOS may have a unique ability to associate with the lumen through integrin-binding with vascular cells while simultaneously retaining the paclitaxel through electrostatic or hydrophobic interactions.

While it is well-recognized that arterial repair after balloon injury occurs more rapidly in animals than in humans, animal models still hold a predictive value for the observation of biological effects that may be associated with drug delivery [39]. In this study, histopathologic evaluation of the KOS–paclitaxel DCB, along with uncoated balloons, KOS-only balloons and paclitaxel-only DCBs were performed in a rabbit ilio–femoral injury model, which has been shown to be an appropriate model for the evaluation of endovascular devices [40–43]. Overall, the morphometric results demonstrated minimal neointimal growth, as percent area stenoses were less than eleven percent for all groups at the 7-day time point. These results were expected as, in general, peripheral rabbit arteries appear to be resistant to the development of aggressive neointimal growth with mild balloon to artery ratio (1.1–1.2:1), especially with plain balloon angioplasty [39,43]. Furthermore, as expected, injury scores were mild, ranging from 0.50 to 1.13 in all groups. However, by histologic evaluation, the safety and effectiveness of the KOS–paclitaxel DCB was still evident, based on vascular remodeling and healing. Specifically, neointimal thickness was significantly reduced in the KOS–paclitaxel DCB treatment group (no coating: 0.10 ± 0.011 mm vs. KOS-only: 0.069 ± 0.022 mm vs. PXL-only: 0.066 ± 0.018 mm vs. KOS-PXL: 0.53 ± 0.003 mm, $p = 0.005$). Importantly, the endothelization score was significantly reduced in the KOS–paclitaxel treated arteries, indicative of drug retention (Table 1). Additionally, there was a trend towards a lower neointimal area and higher loss of smooth muscle cells (SMCs) in the KOS–paclitaxel DCB group as compared to all others, indicative of drug effect (no coating: 0.00 ± 0.00 vs. KOS-only: 0.00 ± 0.00 vs. PXL-only: $0.25 \pm 0.0.50$ vs. KOS-PXL: 1.00 ± 0.82, $p = 0.081$). Overall, the *in vivo* data demonstrate the safety of the keratose coating and a reduction in neointimal growth by the keratose–paclitaxel DCB.

While our results support the concept of a keratose coating to deliver anti-proliferative drugs to arterial segments, the study was limited to a healthy animal model and thus did not take into consideration diseased arteries, as observed in patients with PAD. For the *ex vivo* studies, further characteristic testing of paclitaxel delivery via the drug-coated balloon is warranted to quantify the amount of drug remaining on the balloon following delivery and to quantify circulating paclitaxel levels. We also recognize that human lesions are more complex and often include fibrosis, calcification, hemorrhage and, in most cases, require de-bulking using balloons and atherectomy devices, which may alter drug transfer and retention. While preclinical studies involving healthy arteries are the standard model to determine the arterial time drug concentration of cardiac and stent-based intervention devices, further improvement may be found with a KOS-paclitaxel coating in injury models.

4. Materials and Methods

4.1. Keratose-Coated Balloons

The KOS-coated balloons were prepared as previously described [44,45]. Briefly, paclitaxel (LC Laboratories, Woburn, MA, USA) was prepared by dissolving paclitaxel in absolute ethanol followed by sonication at a final concentration of 40 mg/mL. Keratose (KeraNetics LLC, Winston-Salem, NC, USA) solution was prepared by dissolving lyophilized keratose in iohexol (GE Healthcare, Little Chalfont, UK) at a 6% weight-to-volume ratio in. An in-house air spray coating method was used to deposit keratose and paclitaxel in a layered approach on uncoated angioplasty balloons (Abbott Vascular, Abbott Park, IL, USA) [45]. Coated balloons were then sterilized by UV irradiation.

4.2. Peripheral-Simulating Bioreactor

The peripheral-simulating bioreactor was designed to shorten and twist two harvest porcine carotid arteries subjected to pulsatile flow conditions (Figure 1A). The overall system (46 × 19 × 19 cm) was designed to fit inside of a standard CO_2 incubator by arranging the arteries in a parallel configuration. The system utilizes one stepper motor per artery for rotational motion and one stepper motor for the translational motion of both arteries. Custom connectors were machined to mount the arteries to the stepper motors. The motion of the stepper motors was measured using rotary encoders (CUI AMT11, Tualatin, OR, USA) mounted on the shaft of each motor. An Arduino microcontroller with two motor shields was used to control the motors along with an LCD keypad module to provide an intuitive user experience, displaying time and cycles remaining for each test and providing physical inputs to start, stop, input artery length and the duration of testing.

The carotid arteries, positioned within the vascular-simulating bioreactor, were harvested from large pigs (250–350 lbs.) from a local abattoir and transferred in sterile PBS with 1% antibiotic-antimitotic (Gibco, Grand Island, NY, USA). The arteries were then rinsed in sterile PBS in a culture hood and trimmed. Eight-cm-long segments were cut and tied with sutures onto fittings within the *ex vivo* setup. The circulating medium consisted of the system made up of Dulbecco's modified eagle's medium containing 10% fetal bovine serum and 1% antibiotic–antimycotic.

4.3. Ex Vivo DCB Testing and Arterial Time Drug Concentration

Prior to any vascular motion (twisting and shortening), all arteries were subjected to pulsatile flow for 1 h, as defined by a custom LabVIEW program as previously described [42] The pressure was monitored via a pressure catheter transducer (Millar Instruments, Houston, TX). Flow was monitored by an ultrasonic flow meter. Following this pre-conditioning phase, the vessel diameter was measured by ultrasound (Figure 1F,G). Harvested arteries were then treated by either the KOS–paclitaxel-coated balloon or a commercially available DCB (In.PACT Admiral DCB, Medtronic, Santa Rosa, CA, USA). The delivery pressure of the DCB was determined by the manufacturers' specification at a 10–20% overstretch. At timepoints of one hour and three-days, flow was ceased, and the treated portion of the vessel was removed. Excised vessels were flash frozen, stored at −80 °C and shipped on dry ice to iC42 Clinical Research and Development (Aurora, CO, USA) for the quantification of arterial paclitaxel. Quantification of arterial paclitaxel levels was performed using a validated high-performance liquid chromatography (HPLC)-electrospray ionization- tandem mass spectrometry assay (LC-MS/MS) [44–46]. In brief, the LC-MS/MS system was a series 1260 HPLC system (Agilent Technologies, Santa Clara, CA, USA) linked to a Sciex 5000 triple-stage quadrupole mass spectrometer (MS/MS, Sciex, Concord, ON, USA) via a turbo-flow electrospray ionization source. The artery tissue samples were homogenized using an electric wand homogenizer (VWR 200, VWR International, Radnor, PA, USA) after the addition of 1 mL of phosphate buffer. Eight hundred (800) μL of 0.2 M $ZnSO_4$ 30% water/70% methanol v/v protein precipitation solution containing the internal standard (paclitaxel-D_5, 10 ng/mL) was added. Samples were vortexed for 5 min, centrifuged (16,000, 4 °C, 15 min) and transferred into glass HPLC vials. Study samples were diluted as necessary for detector signals to fall within the dynamic MS/MS detector range. One hundred (100) μL of the samples was injected onto a 4.6 × 12.5 mm extraction column (Eclipse XDB C8, 5 μm particle size, Agilent Technologies, Palo Alto, CA, USA). Samples were washed with a mobile phase of 15% methanol and 85% 0.1% formic acid using a flow of 3 mL/min. The temperature for the extraction column was 65 °C. After 1 min, the switching valve was activated and the analytes were eluted in the backflush mode from the extraction column onto a 150 × 4.6 mm analytical column (Zorbax XDB C8, 3.5 μm particle size, Agilent). The analytes were eluted from the analytical column using a gradient of methanol/acetonitrile (1/1 v/v) plus 0.1% formic acid (solvent B) and 0.1% formic acid in HPLC grade water (solvent A). The MS/MS was run in the positive multi-reaction mode and the following ion transitions were monitored: m/z = 876.6 $[M + Na]^+$ → 308.2 (paclitaxel) and m/z = 881.6 $[M + Na]^+$ → 313.1 (the internal standard paclitaxel-D_5). Paclitaxel tissue concentrations were calculated based on paclitaxel/paclitaxel-D_5 peak area ratios using a quadratic regression equation with 1/x weighting. The range of reliable response was 0.5–100 ng/mL tissue homogenate. Inter-day imprecision was less than 15% and accuracy was within 85–115% of the nominal concentrations. There were no significant matrix interferences, carry-over or matrix effects. For more details, please see the aforementioned publications [42,44,45].

4.4. Rabbit Injury Model

This study was approved by the Institutional Animal Care and Use Committee and conformed to the position of the American Heart Association on use of animals in research. The experimental preparation of the animal model has been previously reported [42,46]. Under fluoroscopic guidance, eight anesthetized adult male New Zealand White rabbits underwent endothelial denudation of both iliac arteries using an angioplasty balloon catheter (3.0 × 8 mm). Subsequently, arteries were treated by either KOS–paclitaxel (3.0 × 15 mm), KOS-only balloon (3.0 × 15 mm), paclitaxel-only balloon (3.0 × 15 mm), or an uncoated balloon (3.0 × 15 mm) at a delivery pressure of 8 atm for two minutes. Anti-platelet therapy consisted of aspirin (40 mg/day) given orally 24 h before catheterization, with continued dosing throughout the in-life-phase of the study, while single-dose intra-arterial heparin (150 IU/kg) and lidocaine were administered at the time of catheterization. The animals survived for 7 days and subsequent histological evaluations were performed.

4.5. Arterial Sections

Following the duration of the study, animals were anesthetized and euthanized, and the treated artery segments were removed based on landmarks identified by angiography. The arteries were perfused with saline and formalin-fixed under physiological pressure prior to removal. The segments were stored in 10% formalin at room temperature and then processed to paraffin blocks, sectioned, and stained with Hematoxylin and Eosin (H&E) or Verhoeff's elastin stain (VEG).

4.6. Histomorphometric Analysis

Histological sections were digitized and measurements performed using ImageJ software (NIH). Cross-sectional area measurements included the external elastic lamina (EEL), internal elastic lamina (IEL), and lumen area of each section. Using these measurements, the medial area, neointimal area and percent area stenosis were calculated as previously described [46,47].

Morphological analysis was performed by light microscopy using a grading criterion as previously published [46,47]. The parameters assessed included intimal healing as judged by injury, endothelial cell loss and inflammation. The medial wall was also assessed for drug-induced biological effect, specifically looking at smooth muscle cell loss. These parameters were semi-quantified using a scoring a system of 0 (none), 1 (minimal), 2 (mild), 3 (moderate) and 4 (severe) as previously described [47].

4.7. Statistical Analysis

Results are reported as mean ± standard deviation. Data were compared with analysis of variance (ANOVA) using GrapPad Prism 7 (GraphPad Software, La Jolla, CA, USA). The comparison of quantitative data of multiple groups was performed by Tukey's multiple comparisons post hoc test. Significance is reported as $p < 0.05$.

5. Conclusions

This study provides evidence of the use of keratose as an excipient for peripheral applications. The *ex vivo* results showed a potential benefit of the coating to minimize the adverse impact of vascular motion on drug mobility and favorable biological response in the pre-clinical model. Additional studies are warranted to further demonstrate the safety and efficacy profile of the keratose coating in larger animal models and longer durations. Overall, this approach has the potential to improve interventional outcomes and quality of life of millions of patients suffering with PAD.

Author Contributions: Conceptualization, E.G., M.E, C.V.C., J.S. and S.K.Y.; methodology (*ex vivo*), C.V.C., R.L.G., C.S., N.F., T.R., O.W., U.C., T.C.R., S.K.Y., methodology (*in vivo*), E.G., M.E., S.K.Y., formal analysis, E.G., M.E., C.V.C., U.C., S.K.Y., data curation, E.G., M.E., C.V.C., U.C., S.K.Y.; writing—original draft preparation, E.G., J.S., S.K.Y.; writing—review and editing, all authors. funding acquisition, E.G., S.K.Y. All authors have read and agreed to the published version of the manuscript.

Funding: This research was supported by the American Heart Association [#15SDG25880000] and [#16PRE27350003] and National Institute of Health [#1R15HL127596].

Conflicts of Interest: Saami K. Yazdani serves on the Scientific Advisory Board of Advanced Catheter and has received grant support from Advanced Catheter Therapies, Lutonix, Inc., Alucent Biomedical and Toray Industries and a consultant to Interface Biologics. Other co-authors have no conflict of interest to report.

References

1. Scheinert, D.; Duda, S.; Zeller, T.; Krankenberg, H.; Ricke, J.; Bosiers, M.; Tepe, G.; Naisbitt, S.; Rosenfield, K. The LEVANT I (Lutonix paclitaxel-coated balloon for the prevention of femoropopliteal restenosis) trial for femoropopliteal revascularization: First-in-human randomized trial of low-dose drug-coated balloon versus uncoated balloon angioplasty. *JACC Cardiovasc. Interv.* **2014**, *7*, 10–19. [CrossRef] [PubMed]
2. Tepe, G.; Schnorr, B.; Albrecht, T.; Brechtel, K.; Claussen, C.D.; Scheller, B.; Speck, U.; Zeller, T. Angioplasty of Femoral-Popliteal Arteries With Drug-Coated Balloons: 5-Year Follow-Up of the THUNDER Trial. *JACC Cardiovasc. Interv.* **2015**, *8*, 102–108. [CrossRef] [PubMed]
3. Werk, M.; Albrecht, T.; Meyer, D.R.; Ahmed, M.N.; Behne, A.; Dietz, U.; Eschenbach, G.; Hartmann, H.; Lange, C.; Schnorr, B.; et al. Paclitaxel-coated balloons reduce restenosis after femoro-popliteal angioplasty: Evidence from the randomized PACIFIER trial. *Circ. Cardiovasc. Interv.* **2012**, *5*, 831–840. [CrossRef] [PubMed]
4. Werk, M.; Langner, S.; Reinkensmeier, B.; Boettcher, H.F.; Tepe, G.; Dietz, U.; Hosten, N.; Hamm, B.; Speck, U.; Ricke, J. Inhibition of restenosis in femoropopliteal arteries: Paclitaxel-coated versus uncoated balloon: Femoral paclitaxel randomized pilot trial. *Circulation* **2008**, *118*, 1358–1365. [CrossRef]
5. Tepe, G.; Laird, J.; Schneider, P.; Brodmann, M.; Krishnan, P.; Micari, A.; Metzger, C.; Scheinert, D.; Zeller, T.; Cohen, D.J.; et al. Drug-coated balloon versus standard percutaneous transluminal angioplasty for the treatment of superficial femoral and popliteal peripheral artery disease: 12-month results from the IN.PACT SFA randomized trial. *Circulation* **2015**, *131*, 495–502. [CrossRef]

6. Mahoney, E.M.; Wang, K.; Keo, H.H.; Duval, S.; Smolderen, K.G.; Cohen, D.J.; Steg, G.; Bhatt, D.L.; Hirsch, A.T. Vascular hospitalization rates and costs in patients with peripheral artery disease in the United States. *Circ. Cardiovasc. Qual. Outcomes* **2010**, *3*, 642–651. [CrossRef]
7. Norgren, L.; Hiatt, W.R.; Dormandy, J.A.; Nehler, M.R.; Harris, K.A.; Fowkes, F.G.; Bell, K.; Caporusso, J.; Durand-Zaleski, I.; Komori, K.; et al. Inter-Society Consensus for the Management of Peripheral Arterial Disease (TASC II). *Eur. J. Vasc. Endovasc. Surg. Off. J. Eur. Soc. Vasc. Surg.* **2007**, *33*, S1–S75. [CrossRef]
8. Tsetis, D.; Belli, A.M. Guidelines for stenting in infrainguinal arterial disease. *Cardiovasc. Interv. Radiol.* **2004**, *27*, 198–203. [CrossRef]
9. Schillinger, M.; Sabeti, S.; Dick, P.; Amighi, J.; Mlekusch, W.; Schlager, O.; Loewe, C.; Cejna, M.; Lammer, J.; Minar, E. Sustained benefit at 2 years of primary femoropopliteal stenting compared with balloon angioplasty with optional stenting. *Circulation* **2007**, *115*, 2745–2749. [CrossRef]
10. Tosaka, A.; Soga, Y.; Iida, O.; Ishihara, T.; Hirano, K.; Suzuki, K.; Yokoi, H.; Nanto, S.; Nobuyoshi, M. Classification and clinical impact of restenosis after femoropopliteal stenting. *J. Am. Coll. Cardiol.* **2012**, *59*, 16–23. [CrossRef]
11. Stone, G.W.; Ellis, S.G.; Cox, D.A.; Hermiller, J.; O'Shaughnessy, C.; Mann, J.T.; Turco, M.; Caputo, R.; Bergin, P.; Greenberg, J.; et al. A polymer-based, paclitaxel-eluting stent in patients with coronary artery disease. *N. Engl. J. Med.* **2004**, *350*, 221–231. [CrossRef]
12. Morice, M.C.; Serruys, P.W.; Sousa, J.E.; Fajadet, J.; Ban Hayashi, E.; Perin, M.; Colombo, A.; Schuler, G.; Barragan, P.; Guagliumi, G.; et al. A randomized comparison of a sirolimus-eluting stent with a standard stent for coronary revascularization. *N. Engl. J. Med.* **2002**, *346*, 1773–1780. [CrossRef] [PubMed]
13. Scheinert, D.; Scheinert, S.; Sax, J.; Piorkowski, C.; Braunlich, S.; Ulrich, M.; Biamino, G.; Schmidt, A. Prevalence and clinical impact of stent fractures after femoropopliteal stenting. *J. Am. Coll. Cardiol.* **2005**, *45*, 312–315. [CrossRef] [PubMed]
14. Cortese, B.; Micheli, A.; Picchi, A.; Coppolaro, A.; Bandinelli, L.; Severi, S.; Limbruno, U. Paclitaxel-coated balloon versus drug-eluting stent during PCI of small coronary vessels, a prospective randomized clinical trial. *Heart* **2010**, *96*, 1291–1296. [CrossRef] [PubMed]
15. Scheller, B.; Speck, U.; Romeike, B.; Schmitt, A.; Sovak, M.; Böhm, M.; Stoll, H.P. Contrast media as carriers for local drug delivery: Successful inhibition of neointimal proliferation in the porcine coronary stent model. *Eur. Heart J.* **2003**, *24*, 1462–1467. [CrossRef]
16. Hehrlein, C.; Richardt, G.; Wiemer, M.; Schneider, H.; Naber, C.; Hoffmann, E.; Dietz, U. Description of Pantera Lux paclitaxel-releasing balloon and preliminary quantitative coronary angiography (QCA) results at six months in patients with coronary in-stent restenosis. *EuroIntervention* **2011**, *7*, K119–K1124. [CrossRef] [PubMed]
17. Schroeder, H.; Meyer, D.R.; Lux, B.; Ruecker, F.; Martorana, M.; Duda, S. Two-year results of a low-dose drug-coated balloon for revascularization of the femoropopliteal artery: Outcomes from the ILLUMENATE first-in-human study. *Catheter. Cardiovasc. Interv.* **2015**, *86*, 278–286. [CrossRef]
18. Cremers, B.; Clever, Y.; Schaffner, S.; Speck, U.; Böhm, M.; Scheller, B. Treatment of coronary in-stent restenosis with a novel paclitaxel urea coated balloon. *Minerva Cardioangiol.* **2010**, *58*, 583–588.
19. Lockwood, N. BioInterface. In *Drug Delivery to the Vessel Wall: Coated Balloons and the Role of the Excipient*; Surfaces in Biomaterials Foundation, BioInterface Workshop and Symposium: Scottsdale, AZ, USA, 2015.
20. Seidlitz, A.; Kotzan, N.; Nagel, S.; Reske, T.; Grabow, N.; Harder, C.; Petersen, S.; Sternberg, K.; Weitschies, W. In vitro determination of drug transfer from drug-coated balloons. *PLoS ONE* **2013**, *8*, e83992. [CrossRef]
21. Kempin, W.; Kaule, S.; Reske, T.; Grabow, N.; Petersen, S.; Nagel, S.; Schmitz, K.P.; Weitschies, W.; Seidlitz, A. In vitro evaluation of paclitaxel coatings for delivery via drug-coated balloons. *Eur. J. Pharm. Biopharm. Off. J. Arb. Pharm. Verfahr.* **2015**, *96*, 322–328. [CrossRef]
22. Buszman, P.P.; Tellez, A.; Afari, M.; Cheng, Y.; Conditt, G.B.; McGregor, J.C.; Milewski, K.; Stenoien, M.; Kaluza, G.L.; Granada, J.F. Stent healing response following delivery of paclitaxel via durable polymeric matrix versus iopromide-based balloon coating in the familial hypercholesterolaemic swine model of coronary injury. *EuroIntervention* **2013**, *9*, 510–516. [CrossRef] [PubMed]
23. Spectranetics, Stellarex™ DCB with EnduraCoat Technology. Available online: https://www.usa.philips.com (accessed on 10 February 2020).

24. Venkatasubbu, G.D.; Ramasamy, S.; Avadhani, G.S.; Ramakrishnan, V.; Kumar, J. Surface modification and paclitaxel drug delivery of folic acid modified polyethylene glycol functionalized hydroxyapatite nanoparticles. *Powder Technol.* **2012**, *235*, 437–442. [CrossRef]
25. Tarr, B.D.; Yalkowsky, S.H. A new parenteral vehicle for the administration of some poorly water soluble anti-cancer drugs. *J. Parenteral. Sci. Technol.* **1987**, *41*, 31–33.
26. Adams, J.D.; Flora, K.P.; Goldspiel, B.R.; Wilson, J.W.; Finley, R. Taxol®: A history of pharmaceutical development and current pharmaceutical concerns. *J. Natl. Cancer Inst. Monogr.* **1993**, *15*, 141–147.
27. Torii, S.; Jinnouchi, H.; Sakamoto, A.; Romero, M.E.; Kolodgie, F.D.; Virmani, R.; Finn, A.V. Comparison of Biologic Effect and Particulate Embolization after Femoral Artery Treatment with Three Drug-Coated Balloons in Healthy Swine Model. *J. Vasc. Interv. Radiol.* **2019**, *30*, 103–109. [CrossRef] [PubMed]
28. Kolodgie, F.D.; Pacheco, E.; Yahagi, K.; Mori, H.; Ladich, E.; Virmani, R. Comparison of Particulate Embolization after Femoral Artery Treatment with IN.PACT Admiral versus Lutonix 035 Paclitaxel-Coated Balloons in Healthy Swine. *J. Vasc. Interv. Radiol.* **2016**, *27*, 1676–1685. [CrossRef]
29. Tomblyn, S.; Pettit Kneller, E.L.; Walker, S.J.; Ellenburg, M.D.; Kowalczewski, C.J.; Van Dyke, M.; Burnett, L.; Saul, J.M. Keratin hydrogel carrier system for simultaneous delivery of exogenous growth factors and muscle progenitor cells. *J. Biomed. Mater. Res. Part B Appl. Biomater.* **2016**, *104*, 864–879. [CrossRef]
30. Saul, J.M.; Ellenburg, M.D.; de Guzman, R.C.; Van Dyke, M. Keratin hydrogels support the sustained release of bioactive ciprofloxacin. *J. Biomed. Mater. Res. Part A* **2011**, *98*, 544–553. [CrossRef]
31. Noishiki, Y.; Ito, H.; Hiyamoto, T.; Inagaki, H. Application of Denatured Wool Keratin Derivatives to an Antithrombogenic Biomaterial-Vascular Graft Coated with a Heparinized Keratin Derivative. *Kobunshi Ronbunshu* **1982**, *39*, 221–227. [CrossRef]
32. Klein, A.J.; Chen, S.J.; Messenger, J.C.; Hansgen, A.R.; Plomondon, M.E.; Carroll, J.D.; Casserly, I.P. Quantitative assessment of the conformational change in the femoropopliteal artery with leg movement. *Catheter. Cardiovasc. Interv.* **2009**, *74*, 787–798. [CrossRef]
33. MacTaggart, J.N.; Phillips, N.Y.; Lomneth, C.S.; Pipinos, I.I.; Bowen, R.; Baxter, B.T.; Johanning, J.; Longo, G.M.; Desyatova, A.S.; Moulton, M.J.; et al. Three-dimensional bending, torsion and axial compression of the femoropopliteal artery during limb flexion. *J. Biomech.* **2014**, *47*, 2249–2256. [CrossRef] [PubMed]
34. Young, M.D.; Streicher, M.C.; Beck, R.J.; van den Bogert, A.J.; Tajaddini, A.; Davis, B.L. Simulation of lower limb axial arterial length change during locomotion. *J. Biomech.* **2012**, *45*, 1485–1490. [CrossRef] [PubMed]
35. Desyatova, A.; Poulson, W.; Deegan, P.; Lomneth, C.; Seas, A.; Maleckis, K.; MacTaggart, J.; Kamenskiy, A. Limb flexion-induced twist and associated intramural stresses in the human femoropopliteal artery. *J. R. Soc. Interface* **2017**, *14*, 128. [CrossRef] [PubMed]
36. Bassett, D.R., Jr.; Wyatt, H.R.; Thompson, H.; Peters, J.C.; Hill, J.O. Pedometer-measured physical activity and health behaviors in U.S. adults. *Med. Sci. Sports Exerc.* **2010**, *42*, 1819–1825. [CrossRef] [PubMed]
37. Tachibana, A.; Furuta, Y.; Takeshima, H.; Tanabe, T.; Yamauchi, K. Fabrication of wool keratin sponge scaffolds for long-term cell cultivation. *J. Biotechnol.* **2002**, *93*, 165–170. [CrossRef]
38. Yamauchi, K.; Hojo, H.; Yamamoto, Y.; Tanabe, T. Enhanced cell adhesion on RGDS-carrying keratin film. *Mat. Sci. Eng. C Bio. S.* **2003**, *23*, 467–472. [CrossRef]
39. Schwartz, R.S.; Edelman, E.R.; Carter, A.; Chronos, N.A.; Rogers, C.; Robinson, K.A.; Waksman, R.; Machan, L.; Weinberger, J.; Wilensky, R.L.; et al. Preclinical evaluation of drug-eluting stents for peripheral applications: Recommendations from an expert consensus group. *Circulation* **2004**, *110*, 2498–2505. [CrossRef]
40. Milewski, K.; Tellez, A.; Aboodi, M.S.; Conditt, G.B.; Yi, G.H.; Thim, T.; Stenoien, M.; McGregor, J.C.; Gray, W.A.; Virmani, R.; et al. Paclitaxel-iopromide coated balloon followed by "bail-out" bare metal stent in porcine iliofemoral arteries: First report on biological effects in peripheral circulation. *EuroIntervention* **2011**, *7*, 362–368. [CrossRef]
41. Albrecht, T.; Speck, U.; Baier, C.; Wolf, K.J.; Bohm, M.; Scheller, B. Reduction of stenosis due to intimal hyperplasia after stent supported angioplasty of peripheral arteries by local administration of paclitaxel in swine. *Investig. Radiol.* **2007**, *42*, 579–585. [CrossRef]
42. Atigh, M.K.; Turner, E.A.; Christians, U.; Yazdani, S.K. The use of an occlusion perfusion catheter to deliver paclitaxel to the arterial wall. *Cardiovasc. Ther.* **2017**, *35*, e12269. [CrossRef]
43. Schwartz, R.S.; Chronos, N.A.; Virmani, R. Preclinical restenosis models and drug-eluting stents: Still important, still much to learn. *J. Am. Coll. Cardiol.* **2004**, *44*, 1373–1385.

44. Turner, E.; Erwin, M.; Atigh, M.; Christians, U.; Saul, J.M.; Yazdani, S.K. In vitro and in vivo Assessment of Keratose as a Novel Excipient of Paclitaxel Coated Balloons. *Front. Pharmacol.* **2018**, *9*, 808. [CrossRef] [PubMed]
45. Turner, E.A.; Atigh, M.K.; Erwin, M.M.; Christians, U.; Yazdani, S.K. Coating and Pharmacokinetic Evaluation of Air Spray Coated Drug Coated Balloons. *Cardiovasc. Eng. Technol.* **2018**, *9*, 240–250. [CrossRef] [PubMed]
46. Yazdani, S.K.; Sheehy, A.; Nakano, M.; Nakazawa, G.; Vorpahl, M.; Otsuka, F.; Donn, R.S.; Perkins, L.E.; Simonton, C.A.; Kolodgie, F.D.; et al. Preclinical evaluation of second-generation everolimus- and zotarolimus-eluting coronary stents. *J. Invasive Cardiol.* **2013**, *25*, 383–390. [PubMed]
47. Yazdani, S.K.; Pacheco, E.; Nakano, M.; Otsuka, F.; Naisbitt, S.; Kolodgie, F.D.; Ladich, E.; Rousselle, S.; Virmani, R. Vascular, downstream, and pharmacokinetic responses to treatment with a low dose drug-coated balloon in a swine femoral artery model. *Catheter. Cardiovasc. Interv.* **2014**, *83*, 132–140. [CrossRef] [PubMed]

Sample Availability: Samples of the compounds are not available from the authors.

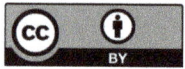

© 2020 by the authors. Licensee MDPI, Basel, Switzerland. This article is an open access article distributed under the terms and conditions of the Creative Commons Attribution (CC BY) license (http://creativecommons.org/licenses/by/4.0/).

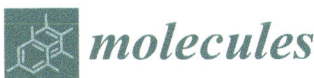

Article

Modeling of the Production of Lipid Microparticles Using PGSS® Technique

Clara López-Iglesias [1,*], Enriqueta R. López [2], Josefa Fernández [2], Mariana Landin [1] and Carlos A. García-González [1,*]

[1] Department of Pharmacology, Pharmacy and Pharmaceutical Technology, I+D Farma group (GI-1645), Faculty of Pharmacy, Agrupación Estratégica de Materiales (AeMAT) and Health Research Institute of Santiago de Compostela (IDIS), Universidade de Santiago de Compostela, 15782 Santiago de Compostela, Spain; m.landin@usc.es

[2] Laboratorio de Propiedades Termofísicas, Grupo NaFoMat, Departamento de Física Aplicada, Facultad de Física, Agrupación Estratégica de Materiales (AeMAT), Universidade de Santiago de Compostela, 15782 Santiago de Compostela, Spain; enriqueta.lopez@usc.es (E.R.L.); josefa.fernandez@usc.es (J.F.)

* Correspondence: clara.lopez.iglesias@rai.usc.es (C.L.-I.); carlos.garcia@usc.es (C.A.G.-G.); Tel.: +34-881-814-882 (C.L.-I. & C.A.G.-G.)

Academic Editor: Rita Cortesi
Received: 25 September 2020; Accepted: 23 October 2020; Published: 24 October 2020

Abstract: Solid lipid microparticles (SLMPs) are attractive carriers as delivery systems as they are stable, easy to manufacture and can provide controlled release of bioactive agents and increase their efficacy and/or safety. Particles from Gas-Saturated Solutions (PGSS®) technique is a solvent-free technology to produce SLMPs, which involves the use of supercritical CO_2 (scCO_2) at mild pressures and temperatures for the melting of lipids and atomization into particles. The determination of the key processing variables is crucial in PGSS® technique to obtain reliable and reproducible microparticles, therefore the modelling of SLMPs production process and variables control are of great interest to obtain quality therapeutic systems. In this work, the melting point depression of a commercial lipid (glyceryl monostearate, GMS) under compressed CO_2 was studied using view cell experiments. Based on an unconstrained D-optimal design for three variables (nozzle diameter, temperature and pressure), SLMPs were produced using the PGSS® technique. The yield of production was registered and the particles characterized in terms of particle size distribution. Variable modeling was carried out using artificial neural networks and fuzzy logic integrated into neurofuzzy software. Modeling results highlight the main effect of temperature to tune the mean diameter SLMPs, whereas the pressure-nozzle diameter interaction is the main responsible in the SLMPs size distribution and in the PGSS® production yield.

Keywords: lipid microparticles; PGSS®; supercritical CO_2; modeling; solvent-free technology

1. Introduction

Particulate systems like microparticles have attracted interest in several biomedical, food and environmental applications [1–5]. Namely, the encapsulation of bioactive agents in these carriers improves their efficacy and safety, since better control of the dosage and release are provided [6,7]. Microparticles also enhance physicochemical stability, protecting the cargo from environmental and physiological factors [8]. The size of microparticles, between 0.1–100 µm [9], can hamper their absorption through biological membranes, increasing their permanence in the application site, thus providing local and sustained drug release and mitigating their toxic effects [10].

Lipids are advantageous matrices for particulate drug delivery systems since they are physiological compounds and therefore well tolerated by living systems [11,12]. For instance, a variety of lipids such as sorbitan esters, phosphatidylcholine, and unsaturated polyglycolized glycerides are widely used as surfactants in lipid-based formulations [13]. Among lipid systems, solid lipid microparticles (SLMPs) are easy to produce on a large scale and sterilize, exhibiting better stability properties than others, such as liposomes [14]. Several SLMP-based formulations have been developed as drug delivery systems for oral, parenteral, pulmonary and topical applications [14,15].

Solvent-free strategies are especially attractive for the manufacturing of SLMPs from the processing, environmental and economical points of view. Namely, supercritical CO_2 (scCO_2) technology has been highlighted as a processing tool for environmentally friendly, safe and cost-efficient techniques at mild conditions—pressure (P) > 73.8 bar and temperature (T) > 31.1 °C [16]. Processes based on supercritical fluid technology (foaming, sterilization) usually avoid or at least mitigate the use of organic solvents thus reducing their carbon footprint. The PGSS® (Particles from Gas-Saturated Solutions) technique is based on the use of compressed CO_2 or scCO_2 for the production of microparticles in an atomization-wise process [17–19]. PGSS® process comprises two main steps: (i) CO_2 sorption in the polymer, and (ii) polymer expansion and particle formation. In the first step, high amounts (5–50 wt.%) of CO_2 dissolve in a molten substance at a moderate pressure in an extent depending on the soaking time and CO_2 affinity to the polymer [20]. Then a rapid expansion to atmospheric pressure of the melt through a nozzle causes an intense cooling effect and CO_2 supersaturation within the melt, resulting in the precipitation of solid particles [21]. scCO_2 used in the PGSS® technique differs from other compressed fluids (e.g., compressed air) used in conventional atomization processes (spray drying) in their chemical interaction with the processed polymers at a molecular level, as scCO_2 can decrease the melting temperature of the polymer thus contributing to costs optimization and energy consumption savings [22]. PGSS® is an adequate technique for the processing of polymeric particles incorporating thermolabile compounds, although its use is limited to polymer matrices with relatively low melting temperatures and with an affinity of CO_2 to the polymer [23]. Compared to other processes for particle production involving the use of scCO_2, such as the gas antisolvent (GAS), supercritical antisolvent (SAS) and supercritical fluid extraction of an emulsion (SFEE) techniques, the PGSS® technique does not use any organic solvents [16,24]. Moreover, the substance to be micronized does not require to be soluble in CO_2 unlike in the rapid expansion of supercritical fluids (RESS) process [25,26]. Overall, PGSS® emerges as an appealing and advantageous technique for the processing of SLMPs at reduced melting temperatures and in the absence of organic solvents.

The morphology and size of the SLMPs produced by the PGSS® process are mainly influenced by the formulation (chemical composition and rheology of the compounds to be precipitated), the technical details of the equipment used (volume of the saturator, precipitator and collector, diameter of the nozzle and length of the tubing) and the operating conditions (pressure, temperature, soaking time) [27,28]. The PGSS® processing variables are numerous, making it difficult to elucidate their influence on the characteristics of the microparticles using conventional statistical methods [29–31]. Despite PGSS® being a simple and versatile method, the lack of knowledge of the effects of the variables on the results of PGSS® technology may entail an obstacle towards the robust SLMPs production and the scaling-up of the process [32]. Approaches based on DoE (design of experiments) and multiple regression have been proposed to manage the number of experiments, to select the critical variables and to optimize the operation conditions, but mainly regarding their influence on the dissolution profile of the drug incorporated in the particles [33]. Some mathematical models were also proposed to simulate the physicochemical processes taking place during the PGSS® processing, such as the behavior of a CO_2-supersaturated solution drop in low-pressure environments [34,35]. In this context, artificial intelligence technologies emerge as tools with great potential for simplifying the study of processes in which many variables are involved, even when a small number of experiments are available. Some of them, such as the neurofuzzylogic systems, allow multiple variables to be modeled and the models expressed through language, which generates in-depth knowledge about the process. Neurofuzzylogic software is a hybrid system that combines artificial neural networks (ANN) and fuzzy logic (FL). ANN are computer programs that simulate how the human brain processes information. They detect patterns and relationship in data, and learn from experience, leading to "black-box" mathematical models [36]. When combined with FL, the models are expressed as simple linguistic IF ... THEN rules together with a membership degree, losing their black-box character and being easily understandable.

Artificial intelligence tools have been previously used in the development and optimization of microparticles [37] and polymeric and lipid nanoparticles [38,39]. To the best of our knowledge, these tools are applied in this work for the first time to model the production of SLMPs by the PGSS® technology. SLMPs consist of a matrix of commercial glyceryl monostearate (GMS), a lipid widely used as an emulsifier in pharmaceutical preparations due to its good biocompatibility and safety [40,41]. First, the melting point depression of commercial GMS in contact with scCO$_2$ was studied to establish the limits of the adequate knowledge space for the processing of PGSS®. Subsequently, an unconstrained D-optimal design for three variables (nozzle diameter, pressure and temperature) at 2, 3 and 3 levels, respectively, was used to prepare SLMPs using the PGSS® technique. The microparticles were characterized in terms of size and shape. The generated database was modeled through a neurofuzzylogic system and the design space was established with respect to the melt GMS processability (fine particle production yield) and the characteristics of the particles.

2. Results and Discussion

2.1. Melting Point Depression of GMS in the Presence of CO_2

Melting pressure-temperature curve of the commercial GMS under compressed CO_2 was measured to determine the feasible operating range of conditions for the PGSS® technique (Figure 1). This step is crucial since it is necessary to establish a set of pressure-temperature conditions (grey region in Figure 1) where the lipid mixture is molten. The melting point of GMS in the presence of CO_2 has been previously studied [42], but these determinations are essential because it is well known that GMS can have inter-batch and inter-manufacturer variability as it is commercially provided as a mixture of components (mono- and diglycerides).

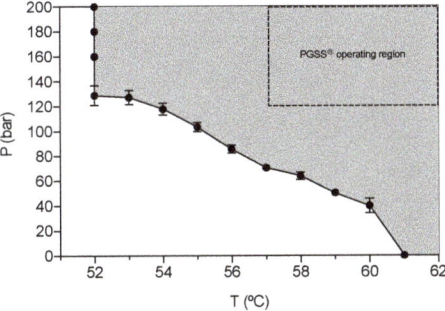

Figure 1. Glyceryl monostearate (GMS) melting points obtained at different pressures of CO_2 using a variable-volume high-pressure view cell. Grey area represents the pressure-temperature region at which GMS will be molten. The area delimited by the dashed line represents the operating region established for solid lipid microparticles (SLMPs) production by PGSS® technique.

The melting point of the commercial GMS without CO_2 was 61 °C at ambient pressure. CO_2 can act as a plasticizer agent, being able to melt other substances, like lipids or polymers, below their normal melting points. Melting point depletion effect of GMS in contact with CO_2 is highly dependent on the working pressure and decreased proportionally up to 52 °C as can be seen in Figure 1. This effect was related to the increase in the amount of CO_2 dissolved in the lipid when the pressure increases [43]. A plateau in temperature was reached at 52 °C and pressures above 120 bar were not able to cause an additional melting point depletion. This second effect was related to the competing mechanism of increased CO_2 solubility in the lipid and the hydrostatic pressure promoting the melting point depletion and increase, respectively, that are counteracting at pressures above 120 bar for GMS [42]. The reduced melting temperature in the presence of compressed CO_2 is advantageous for the energy optimization of the PGSS® particle processing when transferring formulations from lab to pilot scale [44,45].

2.2. Particle Size Distribution (PSD), Morphological and Physichochemical Characterization of GMS Particles

Based on the melting point values obtained in Section 2.1, the range of values of pressure and temperature selected for the experimental study of the PGSS® processing of GMS particles were set at 120–200 bar and 57–67 °C, respectively. In this work, an increment of ca. 5 °C with respect to the melting temperature of GMS at a certain pressure in the presence of compressed CO_2 was established as a rule-of-thumb (dashed and grey rectangle in Figure 1) to ensure the complete melting and to avoid clogging of the nozzle during the PGSS® expansion-spraying step. The selection of the nozzle diameter was based on the technical possibilities of the PGSS® equipment, being 4 and 1 mm the maximum nozzle diameter and the minimum nozzle diameter that did not cause clogging events upon depressurization using the established P-T range in the experimental design, respectively.

PSDs of the SLMPs showed mean diameters between 100 and 190 μm and standard deviations between 30 and 65 μm (Table 1). In general, the PSDs fitted well to a normal distribution (Figure 2) with good correlation levels ($R^2 > 0.95$) in all cases. The yield of particle production was determined from the weight percentage of fine particles with respect to the initial GMS (Table 1). The loss of material during the PGSS® processing was due to GMS remaining in the tubing and the saturator of the equipment, molten material that was not solidified into particles and formed a crust in the walls of the precipitator. Some mass losses were attributed to small particles that remained suspended in the outlet gaseous stream and were vented out during the depressurization step along with the CO_2.

Table 1. Yield of particle production, mean diameter and standard deviation of SLMPs of GMS processed using PGSS® technique. Particles were denoted as GMS-x-y-z, where x is the nozzle diameter (mm), y the processing temperature (degrees Celsius) and z the processing pressure (bar).

SLMPs	Mean Diameter (μm)	Standard Deviation (μm)	% Fine Particles
GMS-4-57-120	138.7	47.0	17.4
GMS-4-57-200	182.6	63.3	43.7
GMS-4-62-120	128.0	41.8	12.8
GMS-4-62-200	147.4	48.3	18.3
GMS-4-67-120	103.5	33.1	11.0
GMS-4-67-200	154.3	52.1	27.5
GMS-1-57-120	171.6	56.8	39.5
GMS-1-57-160	172.3	51.6	34.8
GMS-1-57-200	186.2	57.5	25.7
GMS-1-67-120	131.9	44.4	23.5
GMS-1-67-160	130.3	50.0	27.1
GMS-1-67-200	125.4	43.1	34.8

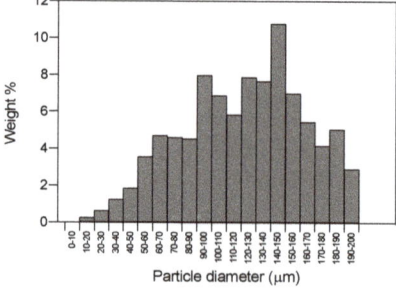

Figure 2. Frequency histogram of GMS-1-67-200 particles (mean particle diameter = 125.4 ± 43.1 μm). The normal distribution of this histogram is representative of all the GMS formulations tested.

The processing using PGSS® technique led to particles with reduced circularity (60.7 ± 18.2%) with respect to the original GMS (round particles, Figure 3A). PGSS®-processed lipid microparticles had a decreased bulk density (0.14 g/cm^3) with respect to the raw material (0.53 g/cm^3). However, skeletal density was similar (0.995 ± 0.017 g/cm^3) to the unprocessed GMS (0.980 ± 0.003 g/cm^3), suggesting that the chemical structure of the GMS was not unaltered during the process, as also confirmed by X-ray diffraction (XRD) and Attenuated Total Reflectance/Fourier Transform infrared spectroscopy (ATR/FT-IR) (Figure A1).

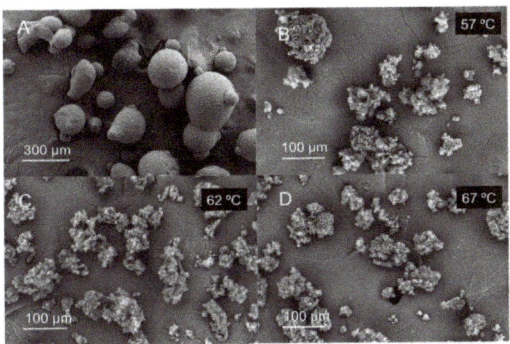

Figure 3. Effect of temperature in the PGSS® processing of GMS particles: (**A**) unprocessed GMS particles and (**B**) GMS-1-57-200, (**C**) GMS-1-62-200 and (**D**) GMS-1-67-200 particles.

2.3. Morphological Characterization and Modeling of GMS Particle Production Using Neurofuzzy Tool

The processing of GMS using the PGSS® technique resulted in porous particles of varied shape and of lower particle diameter than the original material (Figures 3 and 4).

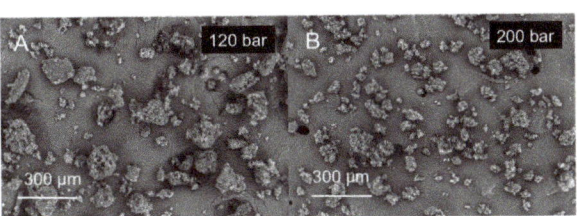

Figure 4. Effect of pressure in the PGSS® processing of GMS particles: (**A**) GMS-1-67-120 and (**B**) GMS-1-67-200 particles.

Neurofuzzylogic software succeeded in modeling the influence of the parameters of pressure, temperature and nozzle diameter (inputs) on the output mean diameter (Table 2) with high predictability ($R^2 > 90\%$) and accuracy ($p < 0.01$). The three parameters help to explain the variations in particle size, with temperature (submodel 1) having the main effect. An interaction between the pressure and the nozzle can be also observed (submodel 2).

Table 2. Inputs selected by FormRules® for the different outputs evaluated in this work, with their respective parameters to evaluate the quality of each model. The most relevant submodels are highlighted in bold.

Output	Submodel	Inputs Selected	R^2	Degrees of Freedom	f Value	Critical f Value
Mean diameter	1	T	91.5012	5 and 6	12.92	4.39
	2	P × Nozzle				
Standard deviation	1	P × Nozzle	58.3925	4 and 7	2.46	4.12
% fine particles	1	P × Nozzle	75.1098	6 and 5	2.51	4.93
	2	T				

The predictability is also reasonable for the percentage of fine particles ($R^2 > 75\%$), a parameter indicative of process yield (Table 2). However, adequate accuracy was not achieved with such a small number of degrees of freedom. The model shows a main effect for the interaction pressure-nozzle, but temperature also affects process yield.

Variables studied do not explain sufficiently the variations in the standard deviation of the particle size distribution ($R^2 < 75\%$). The particle size distributions with PGSS® technique are broad and characterized by high standard deviations, probably higher than the variations promoted by the processing parameters (temperature, pressure and nozzle diameter) used in this research. Therefore, the ANN cannot define a good model for this standard deviation.

IF ... THEN rules, generated by the neurofuzzylogic software allows acquiring knowledge in an easy way (Figure A1). According to these rules, IF the temperature is low (up to 62 °C) THEN the mean particle size obtained is high (over 144.8 μm). The increase in temperature over 62 °C produces a decrease in particle size (Figure 3).

On the other hand, (IF) the pressure increase (... THEN) promotes a decrease in the particle size of the microparticles (Figure 4). This rule applies for both small and large nozzle diameters, being the variations in particle size wider when the large nozzle is used. Figure 5 represents the predicted results by the model for mean particle size for the large (Figure 5A) and small (Figure 5B) nozzle. This effect was related to the increased solubility of CO_2 in molten GMS. At higher pressures CO_2 solubility will increase and, upon depressurization, more nucleation bubbles will form due to CO_2 supersaturation, breaking the lipid into smaller particles (Figure 4) [42,46]. Using the large nozzle diameter, pressure variations produced a more pronounced effect on the mean particle diameter.

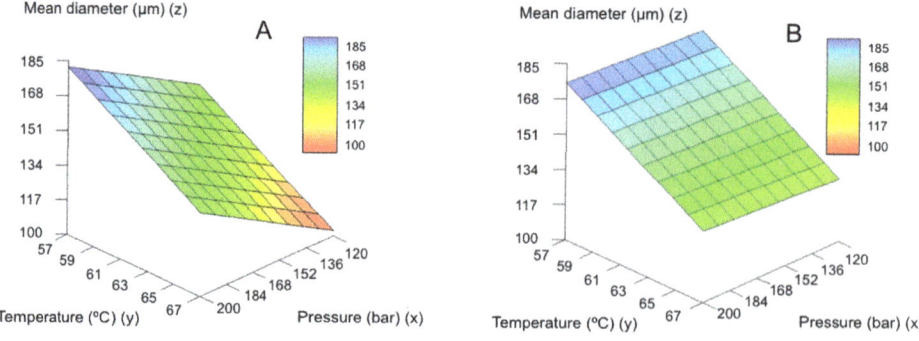

Figure 5. Predicted results by the model for mean particle size for the (**A**) large and (**B**) small nozzles.

Figure 6 shows the predicted values for the percentage of fine particles as a function of pressure and temperature. The increase in temperature leads to a reduction in the process yield, being especially important up to 62 °C. In the temperature range of the experimental design (57–67 °C), the Joule-Thomson coefficient is very similar for the 0–200 bar pressure range [47]. At higher temperatures, the positive Joule-Thomson effect contribution may not be enough to solidify the GMS when exiting the nozzle. Under these conditions, a significant fraction of GMS is in a semi-molten state when it reaches the precipitator and forms a crust in the walls of the vessel instead of forming SLMPs that deposit on the collector.

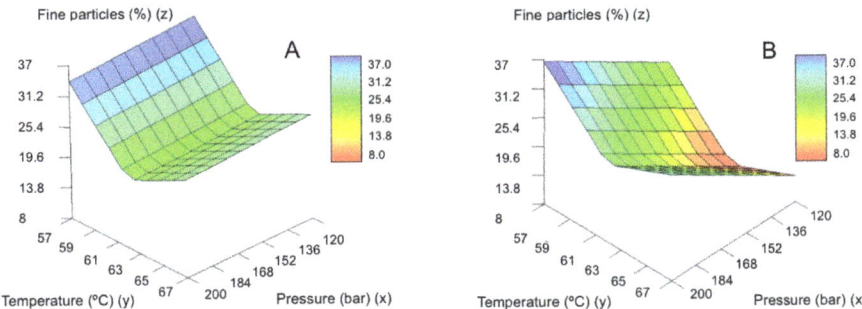

Figure 6. Influence of the parameters pressure and temperature on the yield of fine particle formation using: (**A**) the large nozzle diameter and (**B**) the smaller nozzle diameter.

The diameter of the nozzle also influenced the fine particle yield production. In general, the process performs better when using the small size nozzle. It has been reported that lower nozzle diameters led to smaller particle sizes for other lipid-based systems [48]. Differences in the effect of pressure were also detected depending on the size of the nozzle used. When a nozzle of smaller size is used, the increase in pressure causes a slight reduction in the percentage of fines obtained. This may be related to the production of even smaller particles that remain suspended in the CO_2 and are therefore vented out. However, when the nozzle has a larger diameter, the effect is the opposite, and the process performance is improved with increasing pressure. The pressure drop of the lipid-CO_2 melt through the nozzle is lower with larger nozzle diameters, leading to a decreased Joule-Thomson cooling effect. At higher pressures, this pressure drop effect is compensated by a higher CO_2 content in the lipid melt and particles are able to solidify and reach the collector leading to higher fine particle yield [49].

The experimental values were compared with the values predicted with the model, showing high accuracy of the models for fine particle fraction (Figure 7A) and mean diameter (Figure 7B).

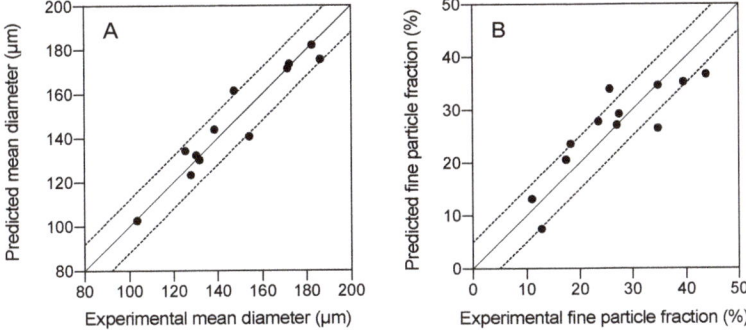

Figure 7. Parity plots of the predicted and experimental values of (**A**) mean particle size and (**B**) % of fine particles. Continuous diagonal line is a 45°-slope line; dotted lines correspond to an envelope of tolerance of 10%.

3. Materials and Methods

3.1. Materials

Kolliwax® GMS II (glycerylmonostearate 40–55 type II, powder, Tm = 54–64 °C) was supplied by BASF GmbH (Ludwigshafen am Rhein, Germany). CO_2 for the PGSS® technique (purity 99.8%) and for the melting point determination (purity 99.998%) were purchased from Praxair (Madrid, Spain) and Air Liquide (Santiago de Compostela, Spain), respectively.

3.2. Determination of the Melting Point of GMS in the Presence of Compressed CO_2 at Different Pressures

The melting point of the GMS in the presence of compressed CO_2 in a 0–200 bar pressure range was determined. A sample of GMS (approximately 3.5 mg) on a glass vial was placed inside a variable volume high-pressure cell, consisting of a horizontal stainless-steel cylinder with an internal diameter of 2 cm and a piston to adjust the volume from 7.9 to 29.5 cm^3. The cell was equipped with a sapphire window (1.6 cm diameter) that allowed the detection of phase transitions through an endoscope (Olympus 5 series, Olympus, Tokyo, Japan) connected to a CCD-camera (Moticam 2000, Motic Asia, Hong Kong, China). In one sidewall of the cylinder, a second sapphire window (6 mm in diameter) made it possible to illuminate the interior of the cell through an optical fiber. A Pt100 probe with an uncertainty of 0.02 °C was used to measure the temperature in the cell wall. The pressure was measured with a Heise model DXD series digital pressure transducer, with an operating range 0–500 bar and an uncertainty of 0.02% of the full scale (FS).

For the experimental trials, the cell at its maximum volume was filled with CO_2 at room temperature and supply pressure of 60–65 bar. Afterwards, the system was heated to the selected temperature (from 52 to 61 °C) and the pressure was gradually increased moving the piston (i.e., reducing the volume of the chamber) until the solid was completely molten to determine the melting point value. Thus, the melting pressure of the GMS at the selected temperature was determined. Subsequently, another temperature was selected and the procedure was repeated to obtain another value of the melting curve. Temperature measurements were carried out by triplicate. Results were expressed as the mean value ± standard deviation (SD). At a fixed temperature, this device shows repeatability for the pressure lower than 11.4%. The melting point temperature of the GMS at atmospheric pressure in the same equipment was also determined.

3.3. SLMPs Production by the PGSS Technique

For the particle formation protocol, 6 g of GMS powder were placed into a 250-mL high-pressure autoclave (saturator) (Eurotechnica GmbH, Bargteheide, Germany). After heating the saturator to the desired temperature (T), CO_2 entered the equipment at a constant flow of 7 g/min until the desired pressure (P) was reached. After 1 h of contact between the molten lipid and the compressed CO_2 under stirring at 400 rpm, the system was depressurized by opening the valve placed at the bottom of the saturator. When the molten lipid leaves the saturator through a nozzle, rapid depressurization causes lipid microparticles precipitation within a 2.7 L borosilicate autoclave (precipitator).

Batches of GMS particles were produced following a D-optimal experimental design for three variables: nozzle diameter (2 levels), operating temperature (3 levels) and pressure (3 levels) (Table 3) carried out by DataForm® v.3.1 software (Intelligensys Ltd., Stokesley, UK). GMS particles processed under different pressure and temperature conditions were denoted as GMS-x-y-z, where x is the nozzle diameter in mm, y the processing temperature in degrees Celsius and z the processing pressure in bar.

Table 3. Nozzle diameters and processing temperatures (T) and pressures (P) tested for the preparation of SLMPs of GMS using the PGSS® technique.

SLMPs	Nozzle (mm)	T (°C)	P (bar)
GMS-4-57-120	4	57	120
GMS-4-57-200	4	57	200
GMS-4-62-120	4	62	120
GMS-4-62-200	4	62	200
GMS-4-67-120	4	67	120
GMS-4-67-200	4	67	200
GMS-1-57-120	1	57	120
GMS-1-57-160	1	57	160
GMS-1-57-200	1	57	200
GMS-1-67-120	1	67	120
GMS-1-67-160	1	67	160
GMS-1-67-200	1	67	200

Microparticles were collected and weighed to determine the process yield according to Equation (1):

$$\% \text{ fine particles} = \frac{W_f}{W_0} \times 100 \qquad (1)$$

where W_0 is the initial weight of GMS added to the saturator and W_f is the final weight of fine particles collected. Also, the amount of GMS remaining on the walls of the precipitator and the interior of the tubing was weighed to verify all the GMS had left the saturator, and what amount had not precipitated into SLMPs.

3.4. Morphological Analysis, Physicochemical Characterization and Particle Size Distribution (PSD)

Four aliquots of each batch were characterized in terms of particle size distribution by optical microscopy using a camera (EP50, Olympus, Tokyo, Japan) provided with the software EP View (Olympus, Tokyo, Japan). The images were analyzed using the freeware ImageJ 1.49v. Calculated particle diameters correspond to the projected area equivalent diameter. The particle size distributions were fitted to a normal distribution, and mean particle size and standard deviations were obtained. The circularity of the particles was also evaluated by image analysis.

X-ray diffraction (XRD) and attenuated total reflectance/fourier transform infrared spectroscopy were used to test possible physicochemical modifications in GMS caused by PGSS® processing. XRD patterns were collected (PW-1710, Philips, Eindhoven, The Netherlands) in the 2–50° 2θ-range using a 0.02° step and CuKα_1 radiation. ATR/FT-IR spectra (Gladi-ATR, Pike, Madison, WI, USA) were obtained in the 400–4000 cm^{-1} spectrum range from 32 scans and at a resolution of 2 cm^{-1}.

Particles were also analyzed by scanning electron microscopy (SEM Zeiss EVO LS 15; Zeiss, Oberkochen, Germany) to evaluate their morphology and surface texture. Particles were previously sputtered-coated with a layer of 10 nm of iridium to improve the contrast (Q150 T S/E/ES, Quorum Technologies, Lewes, UK). Bulk density of the particles was determined by a volumetric method and the skeletal density was evaluated using helium pycnometry (MPY-2; Quantachrome, Delray Beach, FL, USA).

3.5. Modeling

The generated database (inputs from Table 3 and outputs from Table 1) was modeled using the commercial software FormRules® v4.03 (Intelligensys Ltd., Stokesley, UK) which is a hybrid system that combines Artificial Neural Networks (ANN) and fuzzy logic. Nozzle diameter, pressure and temperature were introduced as inputs, while percentage of fine particles, mean particle size and standard deviation were introduced as outputs. A separate model was developed for each output. These models are split into different submodels, when it is possible, to generate simple and understandable rules.

Among the fitness criteria included by FormRules® (cross validation, minimum description length, structural risk minimization, leave one out cross validation and Bayesian information criterion), minimum description length was selected because it gives the best R-squared as well as the simpler and more intelligible rules. Modeling was carried out using the parameters shown in Table 4.

Table 4. Training parameters setting with FormRules® v4.03.

Minimization parameters
Ridge Regression Factor: 10^{-6}
Model Selection Criteria
Minimum Description Length
Number of Set Densities: 2
Set Densities: 2.3
Adapt Nodes: TRUE
Max. Inputs Per SubModel: 2
Max. Nodes Per Input: 10

Three sets of "IF...THEN" rules were subsequently generated to express the model, one set for each output. IF...THEN rules are made up of two parts: the initial one, which includes the input or inputs explaining a specific output, followed by the second part describing the output characteristics, which are defined by a word and its corresponding membership degree (Table A1) [36].

The predictability of the models was assessed using the determination coefficient (R^2) defined by Equation (2):

$$R^2 = \left(1 - \frac{\sum_{i=1}^{n}(y_i - y_i')^2}{\sum_{i=1}^{n}(y_i - y_i'')^2}\right) \times 100 \quad (2)$$

where y_i is the actual point in the data set, y_i' is the value calculated by the model and y_i'' is the mean of the dependent variable. Values of R^2 must be lower than 99.9%, otherwise there is a risk of overtraining the neural network [50]. The larger the value of the train set R^2, the more the model captured the variation in the training data. Values for $R^2 > 70\%$ are indicative of reasonable model predictabilities.

The accuracy of the models was evaluated with the analysis of variance to compare predicted and experimental results, respectively. Computed f ratio values higher than critical f values for the degrees of freedom of the model, indicate no statistical significance between predicted and experimental results and hence, model accuracy.

4. Conclusions

PGSS® is an advantageous processing technique that allows for the manufacturing of molten substances into solid microparticles, with a special interest for the processing of thermolabile compounds. Melting point measurements of GMS were essential to preliminarily determine the feasible PGSS® operating pressure and temperature conditions. The melting point depletion of GMS lipid under compressed CO_2 of up to 9 °C is especially relevant from the energy savings and process economics points of view. SLMPs were thus obtained at operating temperatures (57 °C) well below the normal melting point of GMS (61 °C). Artificial intelligence tools combining artificial neural networks and fuzzy logic was as a successful analytical duo to model the production of SLMPs by the PGSS® process. The obtained models served to simplify the understanding of the SLMPs processing through linguistic rules. The model unveiled that the processing pressure and temperature, as well as the nozzle diameter, had a certain influence on the particle size distribution of the SLMPs and yield of particle production. These operating conditions influenced remarkably the mean diameter of the particles, with smaller particles obtained at high temperatures and pressures and small nozzle diameter.

Author Contributions: Conceptualization, C.L.-I. and C.A.G.-G.; methodology, C.L.-I. and E.R.L.; software, M.L.; investigation, C.L.-I.; data curation, M.L; writing—original draft preparation, C.L.-I.; writing—review and editing, E.R.L., J.F., M.L. and C.A.G.-G.; supervision, C.A.G.-G.; funding acquisition, J.F., M.L. and C.A.G.-G. All authors have read and agreed to the published version of the manuscript.

Funding: This work was supported by Xunta de Galicia [ED431F 2016/010, ED431C 2020/17 & GRC ED431C 2020/10], MCIUN [RTI2018-094131-A-I00], Agrupación Estratégica de Materiales [AeMAT- BIOMEDCO2, ED431E 2018/08], Agencia Estatal de Investigación [AEI] and FEDER funds. C.A.G.-G. acknowledges to MINECO for a Ramón y Cajal Fellowship [RYC2014-15239]. Work carried out in the frame of the COST Action CA18224 (GREENERING) and funded by the European Commission.

Conflicts of Interest: The authors declare no conflict of interest.

Appendix A

Table A1. IF … THEN rules generated by FormRules® software. Membership degrees are in parenthesis.

Parameter	Submodel	Rule
Mean diameter	1	IF T is low THEN mean diameter is high (1.0) IF T is high THEN mean diameter is low (0.79)
	2	IF P is low and nozzle is large THEN mean diameter is low (1.0) IF P is low and nozzle is small THEN mean diameter is high (0.69) IF P is high and nozzle is large THEN mean diameter is high (0.69) IF P is high and nozzle is small THEN mean diameter is high (0.53)
Standard deviation	1	IF P is low and nozzle is large THEN SD is low (0.63) IF P is low and nozzle is small THEN SD is high (0.85) IF P is high and nozzle is large THEN SD is high (0.85) IF P is high and nozzle is small THEN SD is high (0.78)
% fine particles	1	IF nozzle is large and P is low THEN % particles is low (1.0) IF nozzle is large and P is high THEN % particles is high (0.67) IF nozzle is small and P is low THEN % particles is high (0.58) IF nozzle is small and P is high THEN % particles is high (0.50)
	2	IF T is low THEN % particles is high (0.90) IF T is medium THEN % particles is low (0.90) IF T is high THEN % particles is low (0.56)

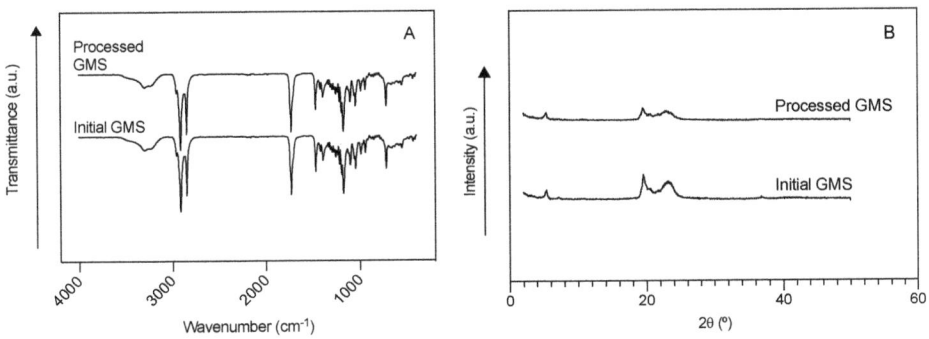

Figure A1. (**A**) ATR/FT-IR spectra and (**B**) XRD patterns of raw GMS particles and GMS particle processed by PGSS®.

References

1. Rashid, M.; Kaur, V.; Hallan, S.S.; Sharma, S.; Mishra, N.K. Microparticles as controlled drug delivery carrier for the treatment of ulcerative colitis: A brief review. *Saudi Pharm. J.* **2016**, *24*, 458–472. [CrossRef]
2. Saghazadeh, S.; Rinoldi, C.; Schot, M.; Kashaf, S.S.; Sharifi, F.; Jalilian, E.; Nuutila, K.; Giatsidis, G.; Mostafalu, P.; Derakhshandeh, H.; et al. Drug delivery systems and materials for wound healing applications. *Adv. Drug Deliv. Rev.* **2018**, *127*, 138–166. [CrossRef] [PubMed]
3. Lengyel, M.; Kállai-Szabó, N.; Antal, V.; Laki, A.J.; Antal, I. Microparticles, Microspheres, and Microcapsules for Advanced Drug Delivery. *Sci. Pharm.* **2019**, *87*, 20. [CrossRef]
4. Galogahi, F.M.; Zhu, Y.; An, H.; Nguyen, N.-T. Core-shell microparticles: Generation approaches and applications. *J. Sci. Adv. Mater. Devices* **2020**. [CrossRef]
5. Sagis, L.M.C. *Microencapsulation and Microspheres for Food Applications*; Elsevier: Amsterdam, The Netherlands, 2015.
6. Kohane, D.S. Microparticles and nanoparticles for drug delivery. *Biotechnol. Bioeng.* **2006**, *96*, 203–209. [CrossRef] [PubMed]
7. Perry, S.L.; McClements, D.J. Recent Advances in Encapsulation, Protection, and Oral Delivery of Bioactive Proteins and Peptides using Colloidal Systems. *Molecules* **2020**, *25*, 1161. [CrossRef]
8. Dalpiaz, A.; Cacciari, B.; Mezzena, M.; Strada, M.; Scalia, S. Solid Lipid Microparticles for the Stability Enhancement of a Dopamine Prodrug. *J. Pharm. Sci.* **2010**, *99*, 4730–4737. [CrossRef]
9. Willerth, S. *Engineering Neural Tissue from Stem Cells*; Academic Press: Cambridge, MA, USA, 2017; pp. 159–180.
10. El-Sherbiny, I.M.; El-Baz, N.M.; Yacoub, M.H. Inhaled nano- and microparticles for drug delivery. *Glob. Cardiol. Sci. Pr.* **2015**, *2015*, 2. [CrossRef]
11. Li, J.; Ghatak, S.; El Masry, M.S.; Das, A.; Liu, Y.; Roy, S.; Lee, R.J.; Sen, C.K. Topical Lyophilized Targeted Lipid Nanoparticles in the Restoration of Skin Barrier Function following Burn Wound. *Mol. Ther.* **2018**, *26*, 2178–2188. [CrossRef]
12. Davis, S.S. Coming of age of lipid-based drug delivery systems. *Adv. Drug Deliv. Rev.* **2004**, *56*, 1241–1242. [CrossRef]
13. Shrestha, H.; Bala, R.; Arora, S. Lipid-Based Drug Delivery Systems. *J. Pharm.* **2014**, *2014*, 1–10. [CrossRef]
14. Jaspart, S.; Piel, G.; Delattre, L.; Evrard, B. Solid lipid microparticles: Formulation, preparation, characterisation, drug release and applications. *Expert Opin. Drug Deliv.* **2005**, *2*, 75–87. [CrossRef] [PubMed]
15. López-Iglesias, C.; Quílez, C.; Barros, J.; Velasco, D.; Alvarez-Lorenzo, C.; Jorcano, J.L.; Monteiro, F.J.; García-González, C. Lidocaine-Loaded Solid Lipid Microparticles (SLMPs) Produced from Gas-Saturated Solutions for Wound Applications. *Pharmaceutics* **2020**, *12*, 870. [CrossRef]
16. Esfandiari, N. Production of micro and nano particles of pharmaceutical by supercritical carbon dioxide. *J. Supercrit. Fluids* **2015**, *100*, 129–141. [CrossRef]
17. Melgosa, R.; Benito-Román, Ó.; Sanz, M.T.; De Paz, E.; Beltrán, S. Omega-3 encapsulation by PGSS-drying and conventional drying methods. Particle characterization and oxidative stability. *Food Chem.* **2019**, *270*, 138–148. [CrossRef]
18. Weidner, E.; Steiner, R.; Knez, Ž. Powder generation from polyethyleneglycols with compressible fluids. In *High Pressure Chemical Engineering, Proceedings of the 3rd International Symposium on High Pressure Chemical Engineering*; Rohr, R.V., Trepp, C., Eds.; Elsevier BV: Zürich, Switzerland, 1996; Volume 12, pp. 223–228.
19. Weidner, E.; Knez, Z.; Novak, Z. A process and equipment for production and fractionation of fine particles from gas saturated solutions. World Patent WO **1994**, *95*, 21688.
20. Santos-Rosales, V.; Gallo, M.; Jaeger, P.; Alvarez-Lorenzo, C.; Gómez-Amoza, J.L.; García-González, C.A. New insights in the morphological characterization and modelling of poly(ε-caprolactone) bone scaffolds obtained by supercritical CO_2 foaming. *J. Supercrit. Fluids* **2020**, *166*, 105012. [CrossRef]
21. García-González, C.; Argemí, A.; De Sousa, A.S.; Duarte, C.; Saurina, J.; Domingo, C. Encapsulation efficiency of solid lipid hybrid particles prepared using the PGSS® technique and loaded with different polarity active agents. *J. Supercrit. Fluids* **2010**, *54*, 342–347. [CrossRef]
22. Fraile, M.; Martínez, Á.M.; Deodato, D.; Rodriguez-Rojo, S.; Nogueira, I.; Simplício, A.; Cocero, M.; Duarte, C. Production of new hybrid systems for drug delivery by PGSS (Particles from Gas Saturated Solutions) process. *J. Supercrit. Fluids* **2013**, *81*, 226–235. [CrossRef]

23. Ciftci, O.N.; Temelli, F. Formation of solid lipid microparticles from fully hydrogenated canola oil using supercritical carbon dioxide. *J. Food Eng.* **2016**, *178*, 137–144. [CrossRef]
24. Shekunov, B.Y.; Chattopadhyay, P.; Seitzinger, J.; Huff, R. Nanoparticles of Poorly Water-Soluble Drugs Prepared by Supercritical Fluid Extraction of Emulsions. *Pharm. Res.* **2006**, *23*, 196–204. [CrossRef] [PubMed]
25. Sodeifian, G.; Sajadian, S.A.; Ardestani, N.S.; Razmimanesh, F. Production of Loratadine drug nanoparticles using ultrasonic-assisted Rapid expansion of supercritical solution into aqueous solution (US-RESSAS). *J. Supercrit. Fluids* **2019**, *147*, 241–253. [CrossRef]
26. Akolade, J.O.; Nasir-Naeem, K.O.; Swanepoel, A.; Yusuf, A.A.; Balogun, M.; Labuschagne, P. CO_2-assisted production of polyethylene glycol/lauric acid microparticles for extended release of Citrus aurantifolia essential oil. *J. CO_2 Util.* **2020**, *38*, 375–384. [CrossRef]
27. Pascual, C.D.; Subra-Paternault, P. *Supercritical Fluid Nanotechnology*; Pan Stanford Publishing: Singapore, 2015.
28. Tokunaga, S.; Ono, K.; Ito, S.; Sharmin, T.; Kato, T.; Irie, K.; Mishima, K.; Satho, T.; Harada, T.; Aida, T.M.; et al. Microencapsulation of drug with enteric polymer Eudragit L100 for controlled release using the particles from gas saturated solutions (PGSS) process. *J. Supercrit. Fluids* **2021**, *167*, 105044. [CrossRef]
29. Haq, M.; Chun, B.-S. Microencapsulation of omega-3 polyunsaturated fatty acids and astaxanthin-rich salmon oil using particles from gas saturated solutions (PGSS) process. *LWT* **2018**, *92*, 523–530. [CrossRef]
30. Perinelli, D.R.; Bonacucina, G.; Cespi, M.; Naylor, A.; Whitaker, M.; Palmieri, G.; Giorgioni, G.; Casettari, L. Evaluation of P(L)LA-PEG-P(L)LA as processing aid for biodegradable particles from gas saturated solutions (PGSS) process. *Int. J. Pharm.* **2014**, *468*, 250–257. [CrossRef]
31. Pedro, A.S.; Villa, S.D.; Caliceti, P.; De Melo, S.A.V.; Cabral-Albuquerque, E.C.; Bertucco, A.; Salmaso, S. Curcumin-loaded solid lipid particles by PGSS technology. *J. Supercrit. Fluids* **2016**, *107*, 534–541. [CrossRef]
32. Chakravarty, P.; Famili, A.; Nagapudi, K.; Al-Sayah, M.A. Using Supercritical Fluid Technology as a Green Alternative During the Preparation of Drug Delivery Systems. *Pharmaceutics* **2019**, *11*, 629. [CrossRef] [PubMed]
33. Pestieau, A.; Krier, F.; Lebrun, P.; Brouwers, A.; Streel, B.; Evrard, B. Optimization of a PGSS (particles from gas saturated solutions) process for a fenofibrate lipid-based solid dispersion formulation. *Int. J. Pharm.* **2015**, *485*, 295–305. [CrossRef]
34. Strumendo, M.; Bertucco, A.; Elvassore, N. Modeling of particle formation processes using gas saturated solution atomization. *J. Supercrit. Fluids* **2007**, *41*, 115–125. [CrossRef]
35. de Azevedo, E.G.; Jun, L.; Matos, H. *Proceedings of 6th International Symposium on Supercritical Fluids*; Institut National Polytechnique de Lorraine: Versailles, France, 2003.
36. Landin, M.; Rowe, R.C. Artificial neural networks technology to model, understand, and optimize drug formulations. In *Formulation Tools for Pharmaceutical Development*; Aguilar, J.E., Ed.; Woodhead Publishing, Ltd.: Sawston, UK, 2013; pp. 7–37.
37. Rodríguez-Dorado, R.; Landin, M.; Altai, A.; Russo, P.; Aquino, R.P.; Del Gaudio, P. A novel method for the production of core-shell microparticles by inverse gelation optimized with artificial intelligent tools. *Int. J. Pharm.* **2018**, *538*, 97–104. [CrossRef] [PubMed]
38. Jara, M.O.; Catalan-Figueroa, J.; Landin, M.; Morales, J. Finding key nanoprecipitation variables for achieving uniform polymeric nanoparticles using neurofuzzy logic technology. *Drug Deliv. Transl. Res.* **2017**, *8*, 1797–1806. [CrossRef] [PubMed]
39. Rouco, H.; Alvarez-Lorenzo, C.; Rama-Molinos, S.; Remuñán-López, C.; Landin, M. Delimiting the knowledge space and the design space of nanostructured lipid carriers through Artificial Intelligence tools. *Int. J. Pharm.* **2018**, *553*, 522–530. [CrossRef]
40. Shah, M.; Agrawal, Y. Ciprofloxacin hydrochloride-loaded glyceryl monostearate nanoparticle: Factorial design of Lutrol F68 and Phospholipon 90G. *J. Microencapsul.* **2012**, *29*, 331–343. [CrossRef] [PubMed]
41. Mu, H.; Holm, R. Solid lipid nanocarriers in drug delivery: Characterization and design. *Expert Opin. Drug Deliv.* **2018**, *15*, 771–785. [CrossRef]
42. De Sousa, A.S.; Simplício, A.L.; De Sousa, H.C.; Duarte, C.M. Preparation of glyceryl monostearate-based particles by PGSS®—Application to caffeine. *J. Supercrit. Fluids* **2007**, *43*, 120–125. [CrossRef]
43. García-González, C.A.; Da Sousa, A.S.; Argemí, A.; Periago, A.L.; Saurina, J.; Duarte, C.; Domingo, C. Production of hybrid lipid-based particles loaded with inorganic nanoparticles and active compounds for prolonged topical release. *Int. J. Pharm.* **2009**, *382*, 296–304. [CrossRef]

44. Weidner, E. High pressure micronization for food applications. *J. Supercrit. Fluids* **2009**, *47*, 556–565. [CrossRef]
45. Van Ginneken, L.; Weyten, H. Particle Formation Using Supercritical Carbon Dioxide. In *Carbon Dioxide Recovery and Utilization*; Aresta, M., Ed.; Springer Science and Business Media LLC: Berlin, Germany, 2003; pp. 123–136.
46. Yun, J.-H.; Lee, H.-Y.; Asaduzzaman, A.; Chun, B.-S. Micronization and characterization of squid lecithin/polyethylene glycol composite using particles from gas saturated solutions (PGSS) process. *J. Ind. Eng. Chem.* **2013**, *19*, 686–691. [CrossRef]
47. Roebuck, J.R.; Murrell, T.A.; Miller, E.E. The Joule-Thomson Effect in Carbon Dioxide. *J. Am. Chem. Soc.* **1942**, *64*, 400–411. [CrossRef]
48. Sampaio de Sousa, A.R. Development of Functional Particles Using Supercritical Fluid Technology. Ph.D. Thesis, Universidade Nova de Lisboa, Oeiras, Portugal, 2007.
49. Montes, A.; Litwinowicz, A.A.; Gradl, U.; Gordillo, M.D.; Pereyra, C.; De La Ossa, E.J.M.; Fernández-Ponce, M.T. Exploring High Operating Conditions in the Ibuprofen Precipitation by Rapid Expansion of Supercritical Solutions Process. *Ind. Eng. Chem. Res.* **2013**, *53*, 474–480. [CrossRef]
50. Colbourn, E.; Rowe, R. Neural Computing and Pharmaceutical Formulation. In *Encyclopedia of Pharmaceutical Technology*; Swarbrick, J., Ed.; Marcel Dekker: New York, NY, USA, 2005; pp. 145–157.

Sample Availability: Samples of the compounds before and after processing are available from the authors.

Publisher's Note: MDPI stays neutral with regard to jurisdictional claims in published maps and institutional affiliations.

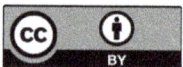

© 2020 by the authors. Licensee MDPI, Basel, Switzerland. This article is an open access article distributed under the terms and conditions of the Creative Commons Attribution (CC BY) license (http://creativecommons.org/licenses/by/4.0/).

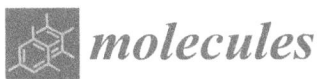

Review

Technologies and Formulation Design of Polysaccharide-Based Hydrogels for Drug Delivery

Giulia Auriemma [1], Paola Russo [1], Pasquale Del Gaudio [1], Carlos A. García-González [2], Mariana Landín [2] and Rita Patrizia Aquino [1,*]

[1] Department of Pharmacy, University of Salerno, Via Giovanni Paolo II 132, I—84084 Fisciano (SA), Italy; gauriemma@unisa.it (G.A.); paorusso@unisa.it (P.R.); pdelgaudio@unisa.it (P.D.G.)
[2] Department of Pharmacy and Pharmaceutical Technology, University of Santiago de Compostela, 15782 Santiago de Compostela, Spain; carlos.garcia@usc.es (C.A.G.-G.); m.landin@usc.es (M.L.)
* Correspondence: aquinorp@unisa.it; Tel.: +39-089-969395; Fax: +39-089-969602

Academic Editor: Derek McPhee
Received: 5 June 2020; Accepted: 2 July 2020; Published: 10 July 2020

Abstract: Polysaccharide-based hydrogel particles (PbHPs) are very promising carriers aiming to control and target the release of drugs with different physico-chemical properties. Such delivery systems can offer benefits through the proper encapsulation of many drugs (non-steroidal and steroidal anti-inflammatory drugs, antibiotics, etc) ensuring their proper release and targeting. This review discusses the different phases involved in the production of PbHPs in pharmaceutical technology, such as droplet formation (SOL phase), sol-gel transition of the droplets (GEL phase) and drying, as well as the different methods available for droplet production with a special focus on prilling technique. In addition, an overview of the various droplet gelation methods with particular emphasis on ionic cross-linking of several polysaccharides enabling the formation of particles with inner highly porous network or nanofibrillar structure is given. Moreover, a detailed survey of the different inner texture, in xerogels, cryogels or aerogels, each with specific arrangement and properties, which can be obtained with different drying methods, is presented. Various case studies are reported to highlight the most appropriate application of such systems in pharmaceutical field. We also describe the challenges to be faced for the breakthrough towards clinic studies and, finally, the market, focusing on the useful approach of safety-by-design (SbD).

Keywords: polysaccharides; hydrogels; prilling; droplets; ionotropic gelation; drying; xerogels; cryogels; aerogels

1. Introduction

In the last three decades, there has been a constant development of polysaccharide-based hydrogel particles (PbHPs) as smart tools to release drugs with the right kinetic and target. The encapsulation of an active pharmaceutical ingredient (API) inside these polymeric micro-particles

- gives the possibility to realize controlled release according to specific therapeutic needs
- ensures the protection against the action of environmental and physiological agents
- can modify pharmacokinetic and bio-distribution profiles
- can reduce clearance and side effects
- improve drug targeting.

Several techniques can be used for the preparation of PbHPs. Many methods are based on the preparation of spherical droplets made by mixtures of the API and the polymeric excipients. For the development of such PbHPs is crucial the polysaccharide droplet formation phase (Figure 1) that in turn defines the size and the size distribution of the resulting microparticles, the two primary factors affecting drug release [1–3].

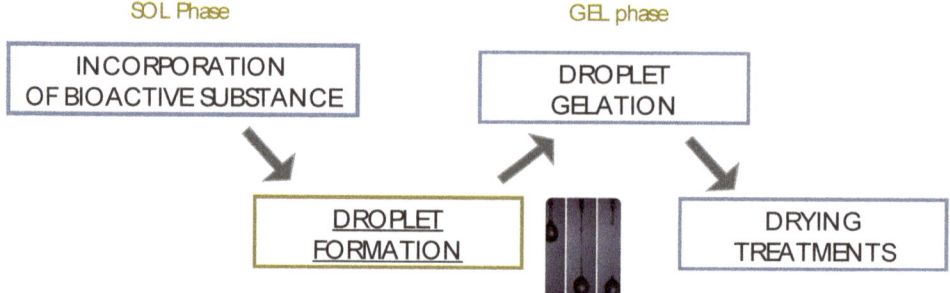

Figure 1. Illustration of the general way for producing hydrogels in form of particles: transition from polysaccharide solution (SOL phase) to a gel particle (GEL phase) followed by possible drying treatments.

In general, the processes used to prepare monodispersed particles starting from polysaccharide-droplets can be divided into:

(1) Formation of droplets in a gaseous phase with following fall in a gelling medium.
(2) Formation of droplets in a liquid phase that is immiscible with the polymeric solution; in this case, the mixing leads to an emulsion.

For both methodologies, the critical parameters able to determine size and shape of the liquid droplets, are the following: the viscosity of each phase, the surface tension of the polysaccharide solution compared to the surrounding medium (gas/air or liquid) and the dynamic interactions of the droplets with the matrix fluid (laminar or turbulent flow). In case (a), where the liquid is pushed through a nozzle at a constant flow rate, surface tension between droplet and air (liquid-air interface) is essential. In the second case (b), the liquid is broken down in an immiscible fluid system in form of droplets and the interfacial tension between dispersed and continuous phases is usually controlled by surfactants [4].

As shown in Figure 2, the main processes involving droplet formation in gaseous phase can be grouped according to the mechanism of liquid jet break-up in: simple extrusion (conventional dripping, Figure 2a), vibrating nozzle (Figure 2b), electrostatic (Figure 2c) and mechanical cutting method (Figure 2d).

Conventional dripping has been widely used to produce mainly alginate particles able to encapsulate cells, enzymes, probiotics, plant extracts, oils and flavours [5–14]. This method involves the manual extrusion of polymeric droplets from a fluid filled syringe or pipette into a gelation or coagulation bath (Figure 2a). When the polysaccharide solution flows out, a droplet is formed at the orifice. The polymeric droplet grows in size until it detaches from the orifice under the influence of gravity, falling toward the gelling medium. In this method, there is no precise control on the formation of the droplets that, during the falling, have the tendency to become spherical due to the surface tension of the liquid before being gelified. Although extrusion by syringe or pipette is the simplest way to produce polysaccharide gel particles, this method generally leads to large gel particles that are polydisperse and not always spherical in shape [4,15,16]. This happens because gravity is the main driving force to generate the droplet from the orifice. In addition, several scale-up difficulties limit this method to a lab scale setup [4,17,18]. Another limitation is represented by the possibility to process only low viscosity feed solutions due to pumping problems and needle blockage [19].

Considering the other technologies illustrated in Figure 2b–d, the breaking up of the polysaccharide liquid jet into droplets is determined by specific devices that give the possibility to strictly control droplet formation [4]. Among them, vibrating nozzle method, also known as prilling or laminar jet break-up, has been widely reported in literature for its great versatility, reproducibility and high scalability potential [20–23].

The present review surveys the main results gained in prilling technology addressing: (i) the basic aspects of the droplet formation technique, its possible implementations and the ionic crosslinking as main gelation method of the droplets formed by prilling, (ii) the main polysaccharides suitable for PbHPs production by prilling; (iii) the possible approaches exploitable for the ionic gelation, e.g. external, internal or inverse, (iv) the influence of the applied drying method on polymer matrix characteristics and hence on its properties affecting the release of the entrapped drug.

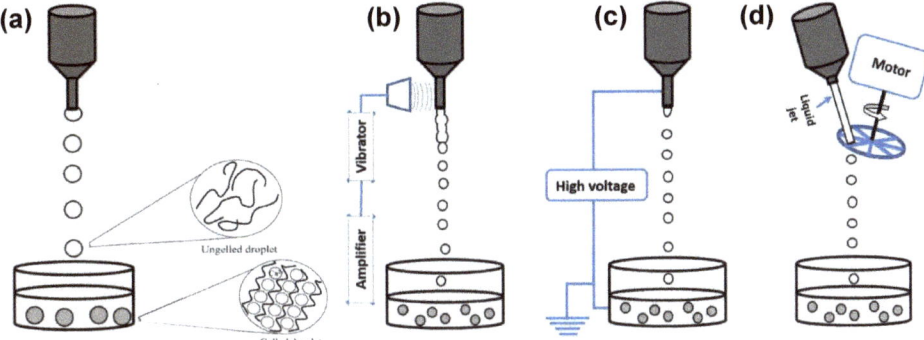

Figure 2. Illustration of dripping devices: (**a**) conventional dripping method influenced by gravity, surface tension and viscosity; breaking up of liquid jets into droplets stimulated by (**b**) vibrating nozzle method, (**c**) electrostatic forces and (**d**) a mechanical cutting device. Reprinted (with some modifications) from [4]. Copyright (2018) Ganesan, Budtova, Ratke, Gurikov, Baudron, Preibisch, Niemeyer, Smirnova, Milow.

2. Prilling Technique to Produce Polymeric Droplets

Prilling or Laminar Jet Break-Up

Prilling process is based on the mechanical dispersion of the feed solution through pressure-controlled injection in a specific gelation or coagulation medium after breaking apart into mono-sized drops by means of a vibrating nozzle device [23,24]. The technology has been shown especially suitable to immobilize microorganisms or entrap bioactive substances in polymeric beads; these are formed by fall of a mixed host-polymer liquid formulation into an appropriate polymer gelling solution [25–28]. Recently, many pharmaceutical applications of such beads have been developed in order to control the drug release in orally administered formulations [29,30] or the colon targeting [31,32].

In the vibrating nozzle method (Figure 3), the monodispersed droplets are formed from a laminar liquid jet by applying superimposed vibrations with an optimal frequency either on the nozzle or on the liquid that is approaching the nozzle. The vibrations can be generated using sound waves (ultrasound) [4,33]; the acoustic jet excitation process involved in prilling was patented to produce uniform microspheres of alginate [34], collagen [35] and PLGA [36]. Practically, polymeric feed solution is pressurized using a pump or gas through a nozzle in order to generate the liquid jet. The superimposed vibrations destabilize the liquid jet (Rayleigh instability) and the jet is disintegrated into monodispersed liquid droplets [3].

Several variables, such as density, dynamic viscosity and flow rate of the feed solution, nozzle geometry and diameter, frequency of vibration as well as falling distance, can affect shape, size and size distribution of the droplets and consequently of the resulting hydrogel particles [16,37–40].

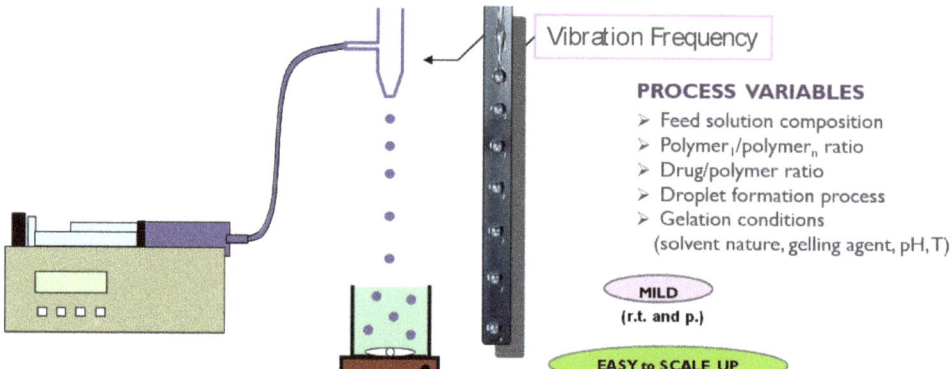

Figure 3. Schematic illustration of prilling technology with the indication of the main process variables.

Viscosity is certainly one of the most important variable of this technique; prilling is able to process only solutions with viscosity values lower than few hundreds of mPa·s [21] and it is essential to study the so-called nozzle viscosity (dynamic viscosity) using appropriate theoretical model [23].

As regards to the droplet size, it is estimated to be at least twice the nozzle inner diameter and can be varied by changing the flow rate of the liquid and nozzle diameter [40]. In addition, particle sphericity can be highly influenced by the distance between the vibrating nozzle and the gelling bath. In fact, when the droplets hit the surface of the gelation medium, their spherical shape can be deformed if the droplet viscosity and surface tension forces are unable to overcome the surface tension exerted by the gelling solution [17,41]. Different papers have demonstrated that the liquid droplets are generally able to overcome the impact forming spherical gel particles when the falling distance is greater than 10 cm [15,16]. Uniformity of the polymeric gel particles can also be improved by reducing the surface tension of the gelling bath by the addition of surfactants [15,42]. Moreover, smaller nozzle diameters and higher frequencies increase the possibility of coalescence [24]. For this reason, frequency is usually kept as low as possible in order to avoid the formation of satellite droplets leading to a broader size distribution [29].

Prilling technology can be also used in the co-axial configuration (Figure 4) to obtain droplets with multiple layers formed by different polysaccharides, in a single manufacturing step [43,44]. Core-shell beads can be easily fabricated by prilling in co-axial configuration designing formulations able to obtain a drug controlled release and to diminish the effect of the GI environment. The appropriate combination of two or more polysaccharides may be, for example, an effective way to produce a polymer-drug core (e.g., pectin) enveloped by gastroresistant shell (e.g., alginate) able to prevent the early release of the drug in the upper part of the gastro-intestinal tract (GIT) [45–48]. An enteric shell may release the drug in a specific district of the organism (intestinal/colonic tract); moreover, from the use of bioadhesive polymers may increase the gastric retention time and, therefore, improve the localized action in GI tract or even delay the release in a precise moment of the day as required, for example, for the treatment of severe chronic mucosal inflammations such as Inflammatory bowel disease IBD [31].

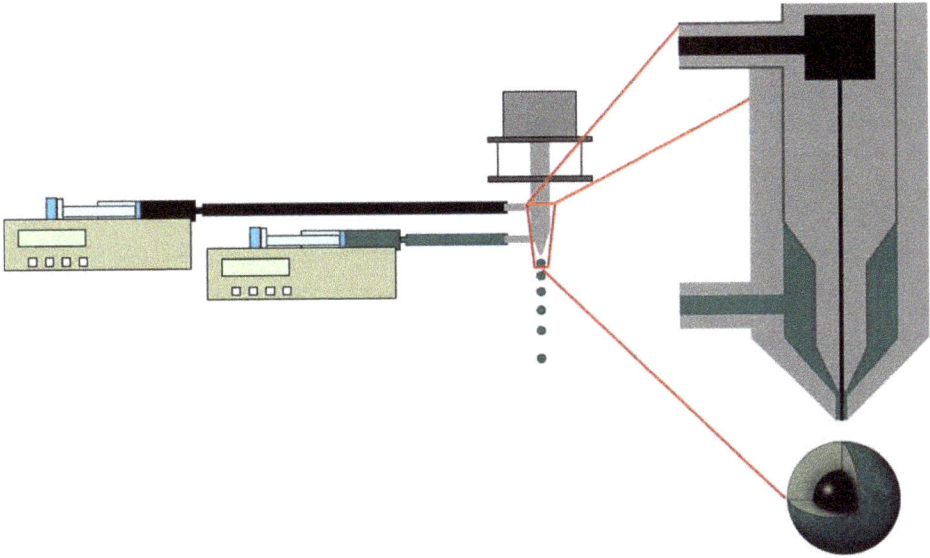

Figure 4. Schematic reproduction of prilling process in co-axial configuration. Reprinted from [43] with permission from Elsevier. Copyright (2014).

Particle manufacturing through the vibrating nozzle device is easily to scale up e.g., by using a multi-nozzle system (Figure 5) without changing other process parameters such as flow rate and the vibration frequency [21,26]. The most important element is about the arrangement of the nozzles which must ensure equal jet formation and equal pressure drops between the nozzles [26]. The pilot apparatus using this technique is now being sold by some companies such as Brace GmbH (Karlstein am Main, Bavaria, Germany), Nisco Inc. (Zurich, Switzerland), EncapBioSystems AG (Greifensee, Switzerland) [24,49].

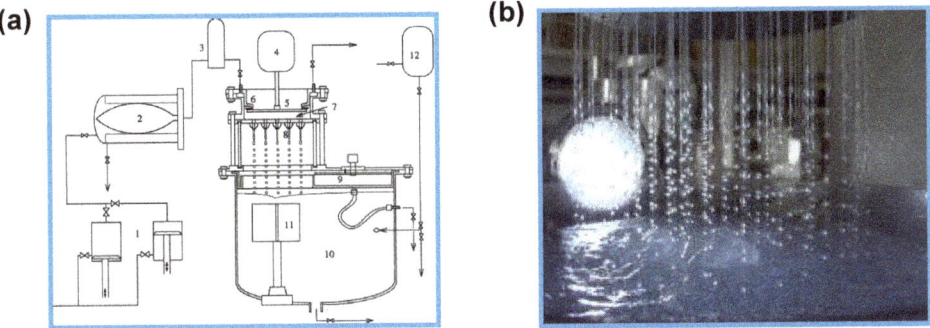

Figure 5. (**a**) Schematic illustration representing a multi-nozzle encapsulator (1, double piston pump; 2, sterile barrier; 3, damper; 4, vibrator; 5, membrane of pulsation chamber; 6, concentric split; 7, pulsation chamber; 8, nozzle plate; 9, bypass system; 10, reaction vessel; 11, stirrer; and 12, input hardening solution). Reprinted from [26] with permission from Elsevier. Copyright (1998). (**b**) Picture showing the equipment supplied by Brace GmbH (https://www.brace.de).

Once the droplets are formed, the SOL-GEL transition in hydrogels (gel network formation) must take place as soon as possible to prevent either the aggregation of polymer droplets or the undesired leakage of encapsulated drugs. The chemical nature of the droplets (dispersed phase) determines the subsequent consolidation step, in which the droplets are transformed into solid particles known as gel-beads, involving: (i) non-solvent induced phase separation (NIPS), (ii) temperature or pH modifications, (iii) chemical reactions or ionic cross-linking for water soluble polymers or solvent evaporation/extraction for oil soluble polymers [24]. During the hardening process, the droplets can shrink. The shrinkage is influenced by the type of polysaccharide, its concentration and nature of the hardening medium.

3. Methods for the Gelation of Polymeric Droplets to Produce Gel-Particles

Figure 6 shows the main mechanisms involved in the gelation of polysaccharide droplets to produce gel particles.

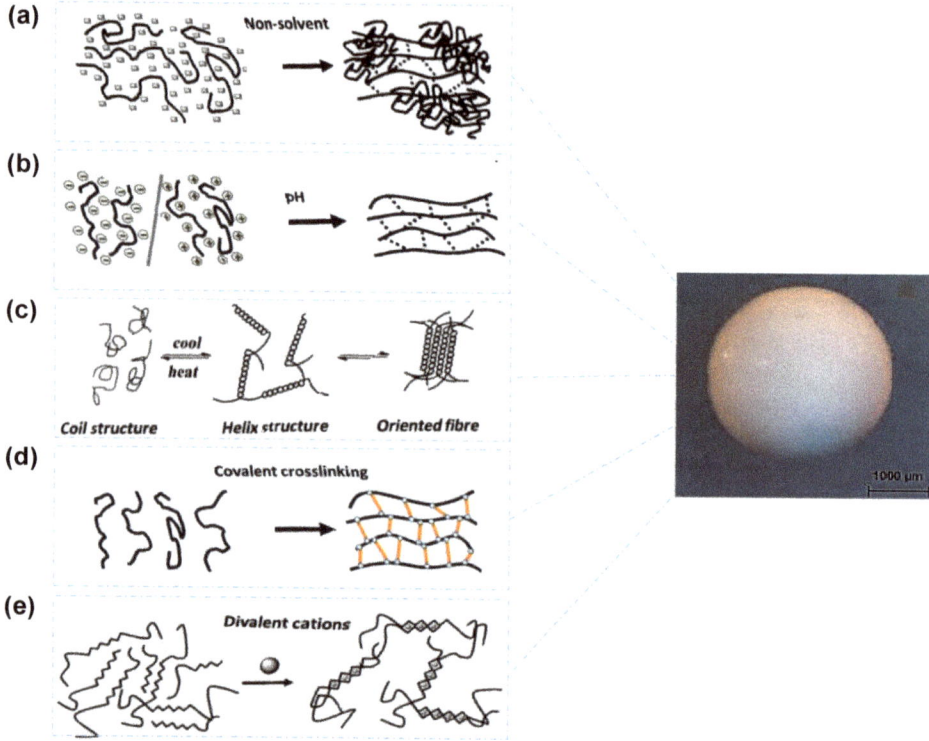

Figure 6. Illustration of the main mechanisms to induce SOL-GEL transition of polysaccharide droplets: (**a**) non-solvent approach to produce a non-solvent filled gel network, (**b**) pH-induced gelation, (**c**) temperature-induced (thermotropic) gelation in which the polysaccharides undergo structural transition from coil to helix and then to double helix, (**d**) covalent crosslinking approach in which the polysaccharide chains are covalently crosslinked to form gel network and (**e**) ions-induced (ionotropic) gelation in which the polysaccharide molecules are crosslinked by ions. Reprinted (with some modifications) from [4]. Copyright (2018) Ganesan, Budtova, Ratke, Gurikov, Baudron, Preibisch, Niemeyer, Smirnova, Milow.

3.1. Non-Solvent Induced Phase Separation

Non-solvent induced phase separation (NIPS) is also known as coagulation or immersion precipitation. In this case, the polymer is dissolved in a specific solvent and when this solution is extruded into the coagulation bath containing the non-solvent, there is a rapid decrease of polymer solubility leading to phase separation. Polymer chains self-associate and form a 3D self-standing network with the non-solvent in the pores (see Figure 6a). Generally, polysaccharide macromolecules shrink upon the addition of non-solvent, but not completely collapse if polymer concentration is above the overlap concentration. The NIPS process has been applied from several authors to a diverse set of polysaccharides, such as cellulose [50,51], alginate [52,53], pectin [54] and chitin [55]. In these publications, different liquids were exploited as non-solvents to induce phase separation. Pérez-Madrigal et al. studied the ability of aqueous sodium alginates to gelify upon mixing with dimethyl sulfoxide (DMSO) and other organic solvents such as dimethylformamide, methanol, ethanol etc. Gel formation was shown to depend on nature of the non-solvent, solution viscosity (which is correlate to polymer molecular weight and concentration) and gelation time. Similar results were obtained by Tkalec et al. [56,57]. Chitin and chitin-graft-poly(4-vinyl pyridine) were coagulated in ethanol [58,59]; in this case the gelation occurs for the increase of the hydrophobic interactions between the polysaccharide chains, an effect depending on the polymer type. The obtained gel particles are usually defined "alcogels", an attractive opportunity for aerogels processing by supercritical drying [57,60] as we will discuss in the next paragraphs.

The non-solvent properties of ethanol have been also utilized for hardening of alginate and pectin hydrogel microparticles prepared with other techniques such as emulsion gelation [61,62] and ionic cross-linking [61–64] with the aim to further stabilize the polymeric gel network by a combination of hydrogen bonds and hydrophobic interactions [53].

3.2. pH-Induced Gelation

The pH-induced gelation can be promoted changing pH value of some polysaccharide solvent; at the contact point of each droplet of polymeric solution with the acidic or alkaline bath, the gelation starts forming first a shell, and becomes later complete thanks to the diffusion of the ions through the shell (see Figure 6b). This method is often used alone or in combination with other gelation methods to prepare gel particles of chitosan, pectin and alginic acid [15]. For example, alginic acid gels are formed when pH of the solution is brought down below the disassociation constant (pKa) of the polymer [65]. As reported by Draget et al. [66] also the rate of decrease in pH can affect gel properties; in fact, a rapid decrease in pH results in precipitation of alginic molecules in the form of aggregates while a slow and steady drop in pH results in the formation of a continuous alginic acid bulk gel. Unlike ionic gels, acid gels of alginate are stabilized by intermolecular hydrogen bonds between carboxylic groups of different chains and M-blocks residues have been shown to play a part in gelation. This also applies to pectin, for which the gelation is stabilized by hydrophobic interactions of methylated groups [67,68]. By contrast, chitosan gel particles are prepared at higher pH values. Chitosan is firstly dissolved under mild acidic condition (usually realized using acetic acid) by protonating the amine functional group, and then gel particles are produced under alkaline medium (usually with NaOH solution); the pH value of the alkaline solution must be maintained above the pKa value (6.3) of -NH_2 functional groups in order to deprotonate the amine groups [4]. Cellulose is instead coagulated using strong acidic solutions of H_2SO_4 [69], HNO_3 [70] or HCl [71–73] that, acting as non-solvents, induce the formation of a gel-like structure [4].

3.3. Temperature-Induced Gelation

Temperature-induced gelation is also called thermotropic- or cryo-gelation. In this case, the polysaccharide molecules associate themselves often into oriented form, e.g., from coil to helix and then to double helix, in response to temperature, usually upon cooling. The association of these helices leads to double helix formation, then proceeding to a gel network (Figure 6c). Temperature-induced gelation as well as gel properties are highly depending upon polysaccharide typology. In fact, different mechanisms are discussed in the literature, e.g., for agar [74–76], κ-carrageenan [76,77], starch [78,79], cellulose [80–82] and chitosan [83].

3.4. Chemical Gelation

Chemical gelation can be mediated by ionotropic or covalent crosslinking. In the first case, the polysaccharides are crosslinked by ions forming a gel network (Figure 6e). In the second case, gels are formed via covalent cross-linking which leads to irreversible chemical networks (Figure 6d). The main problem is that the majority of covalent cross-linking agents are not biocompatible [4,84]. Among them, glutaraldehyde is certainly that with the longest history; it has been widely used to cross-link several biopolymers such as chitosan [85,86], sodium alginate [87–89], cellulose [90,91], guar gum [92,93], collagen [94], collagen-chitosan [95], alginate-guar gum [96], and carrageenan [97,98]. For instance, chitosan microspheres can be produced by mixing chitosan and glutaraldehyde solutions in oil containing surfactants [99,100]. In this case, a Schiff base reaction between amine and aldehyde occurs and as a result, chitosan chains are covalently cross-linked by the glutaraldehyde molecules. With the same mechanism, other aldehydes such as glyoxal and formaldehyde are able to crosslink chitosan chains [101–103]. Glutaraldehyde has been highly used also for alginate reticulation. Other covalent gelling agents used for this polymer are adipic dihydrazide, lysine, and poly(ethylene glycol)-diamines [104]. Clearly, the type of cross-linking molecule and the cross-linking density determines both the mechanical properties and the degree of swelling in alginate hydrogels. Usually, cellulose is chemically cross-linked in aqueous solution by using epichlorohydrin, dichlorohydroxytriazine, 1,3,5-triacryloylhexahydrotriazine, 2,4-diacrylamido-benzenesulphonic acid, N-methylol resins or dialdehydes [4].

As confirmed by the high number of papers present in the literature, among all gelation techniques, ionotropic cross-linking of polysaccharide solutions is the most investigated for the fabrication of biocompatible systems used in biomedical field, due to its affordability, versatility and high reproducibility [105,106].

3.5. Ionotropic Cross-Linking

Ionotropic gelation exploits the capability of polysaccharide-based polyelectrolytes to crosslink in the presence of counter ions under specific ranges of concentration and/or pH [107]. The ionic cross-linking of polysaccharide droplets in aqueous solution gives rise to hydrogel particles (or beads) characterized by a microstructure with interconnected nanofibrillar network [108–111]. Hydrogel physicochemical properties depend upon chemical composition of the selected polysaccharide, its concentration as well as the size (i.e., ionic radius) and the valence (i.e., coordination number) of counter ions and eventually, the presence of water of hydration surrounding cross-linking ions [2,112].

Biocompatible and biodegradable alginate, pectin, chitosan are polyelectrolytes having active functional groups, such as carboxylate, sulphate and amine that can be involved in the ionotropic gelation mechanism [113]. Obviously, the type of counter ion and the gelling conditions must be chosen in relation to the specific polysaccharide used for droplet formation. Alginate and pectin, being polyanionic polysaccharides, tend to cross-link in presence of polyvalent cations. In this case, the gelation is induced by the electrostatic interactions establishing between cations and the polymer anion blocks [114]. On the contrary, chitosan with its amine functional group can undergo ionotropic gelation in presence of anionic counter ions such as tripolyphosphate (TPP), sulphate and citrate. The gel network formation is due to the electrostatic interactions established between anionic counter ions and the chitosan cationic blocks [115–117].

3.5.1. Alginate Ionic Cross-Linking

Alginate is certainly the most well-known and studied example of polysaccharide that can be cross-linked via a ionotropic mechanism [118]. It is a linear polysaccharide copolymer consisting of α-L-guluronic acid (**G**) and β-D-mannuronic acid (**M**) repeating units forming regions of **M**- and **G**-blocks and alternating structure (**MG**-blocks) [65,119,120] (Figure 7).

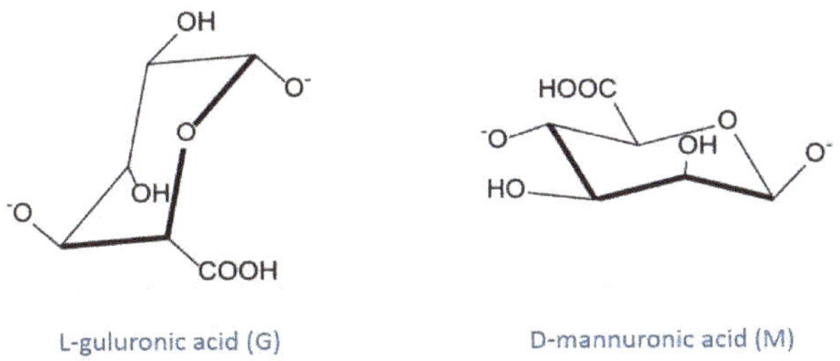

L-guluronic acid (G)   D-mannuronic acid (M)

Figure 7. Chemical structure of alginate monomers: L-guluronic acid and D-mannuronic acid.

Alginate can be obtained from different brown seaweed species or from certain bacterial strains (e.g., *Pseudomonas aeruginosa*) [121]. The alginate source defines the **G**-to-**M** ratio and the molecular weight of the polysaccharide leading to significant differences in the physicochemical and mechanical properties of the resulting gels [119]. Commercially, alginates are available as alginic acid or in the form of sodium, potassium, or ammonium salts. Generally, most of divalent cations (Ca^{2+}, Sr^{2+}, Cd^{2+}, Co^{2+}, Cu^{2+}, Mn^{2+}, Ni^{2+}, Pb^{2+} and Zn^{2+}) and some trivalent cations (Fe^{3+}, Cr^{3+}, Al^{3+}, Ga^{3+}, Sc^{3+} and La^{3+}) can interact with **G**-blocks regions of alginate in a highly cooperative manner, generating a 3D network according to the so-called "egg-box" model [122]. Alginate affinity towards such polyvalent cations is directly dependent on the amount of G-blocks present in the alginate structure [123,124]. As demonstrated in [125] by numerous competitive inhibition studies, the main involved gelation mechanism is the dimerization of **G** residues. In detail, the addition of polyvalent cations (often Ca^{2+} ions) to the alginate solution determines the binding of two **G**-blocks on opposite sides; the result is a diamond shaped hole consisting of a hydrophilic cavity that binds the cations by multicoordination using the oxygen atoms from the carboxyl functional groups. This arrangement causes the formation of a junction zone shaped like an "egg-box" (Figure 8).

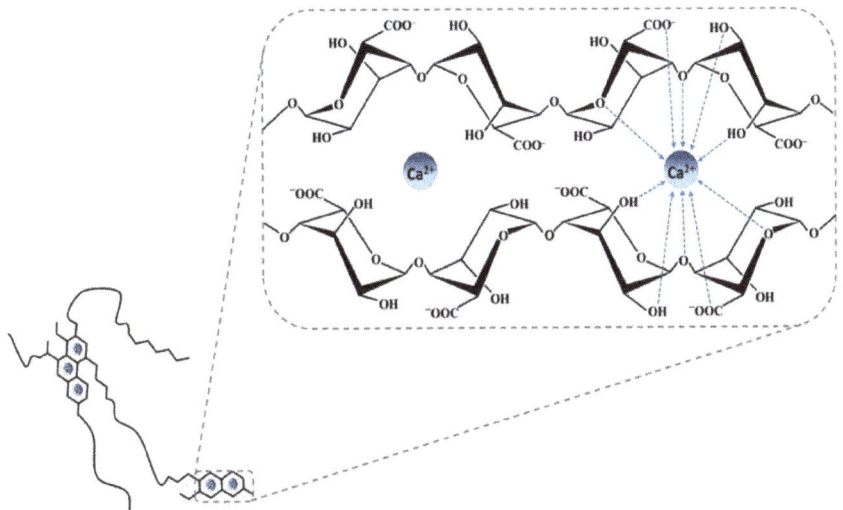

Figure 8. Egg-box model representing the interactions between alginate **G**-blocks and calcium ions. Reprinted from [113]. Copyright (2019) Martău, Mihai, Vodnar.

Each cation binds with four **G** residues in the egg-box formation to form a 3D hydrogel network of these interconnected regions [15,126]. It has been reported that in the case of Ca^{2+}, the formation of a stable junction requires eight to twenty adjacent **G** unites [65].

Generally, the greater the atomic radius of the cation, the stronger is the cross-linked polymeric matrix. In fact, as reported by [123,127–129], divalent ions of larger ionic radii such as Ba^{2+} and Sr^{2+} are able to produce stronger alginate gel particles than the Ca^{2+}-based ones (Figure 8). By contrast, having a smaller atomic radius, Mg^{2+} is not able to cross-link alginate [112,130]. Overall, alginate affinity to cations increases in the following order: Mn^{2+} < Zn^{2+}, Ni^{2+}, Co^{2+} < Fe^{3+} < Ca^{2+} < Sr^{2+} < Ba^{2+} < Cd^{2+} < Cu^{2+} < Pb^{2+} [123]. For practical applications, the use of highly toxic cations such as Pb^{2+}, Cu^{2+}, and Cd^{2+} is limited. The use of Sr^{2+} and Ba^{2+}, which are mildly toxic, has been reported in cell immobilization applications although only at low concentrations [131]. Ca^{2+} is certainly the divalent cation most used to form ionic alginate gels for its good binding affinity to alginate and lack of toxicity under normal conditions of use [15]. Although it is generally recognized that most divalent and trivalent cations are able to form alginate gels according to the pioneering "egg-box" model (valid mainly for **GG** sequences), it is important to consider that the chemical composition of such polymers and hence the **M/G** ratio can significantly vary [132]. This means that binding affinity with cations as well as polymeric conformation can vary too. Some binding studies have shown that Sr^{2+} is able to bind to G-blocks only, Ca^{2+} to both **G-** as well as **MG**-blocks, and Ba^{2+} to both **G-** and **M**-blocks [65,123]. In general, binding affinity with cations is lower for both **MM** and alternating **MG** blocks, requiring a rather high polyvalent ion concentration to be more efficiently complexed. Compared to **GG** blocks, both **MM** and **MG** ones present a more open geometry that make them more available for interchain aggregations along polymer (self-assembly of alginate chains) causing significant irregularities in the arrangement of uronic units in alginate chains; this happens for the gels cross-linked by relatively low ion radius cations [125]. Since in the pharmaceutical field the ionotropic gelation is commonly used to entrap an API between the polymer chains, this arrangement can affect the drug release in a controlled manner.

3.5.2. Pectin Ionic Cross-Linking

Pectin is a linear polysaccharide mainly consisting of galacturonic acid units which are connected via α-(1–4) bonds and with a certain degree of methyl esterification of carboxyl groups (Figure 9) (DE, degree of esterification) depending on the polysaccharide quality and source [133]. It is commonly extracted from apple pomace and citrus peels under slightly acidic conditions. There are currently three commercially types of pectins: (1) low methoxyl (LM) pectin, where less than 50% of galacturonic acid groups are esterified with methyl groups; (2) high methoxyl (HM) pectin, where more than 50% of existing galacturonic acid groups are esterified with methyl groups; and (3) amidated pectin (A), where acid groups are partly amidated. Gelling properties highly depend on the ratio of esterified and amidated acid groups [134].

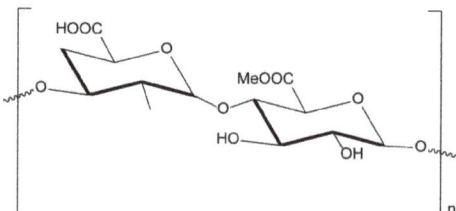

Figure 9. Pectin structure.

As reported by Braccini and Perez [114], despite the structural analogy between polyguluronate and polygalacturonate chains, the egg box model valid for alginates (guluronate system) cannot be directly transposed to the pectate gels. In this case, the most favorable antiparallel associations of galacturonate chains may, at best, be considered as "shifted egg boxes". The observed "shift" seems to lead to an efficient association with several van der Waals contacts; it reduces the original large cavity and provides two symmetrical sub-cavities of appropriate size for binding a cation and it creates an efficient periodic intermolecular hydrogen bonding network. Generally, the methyl esterification of carboxyl groups weakens the crosslinker-pectate interaction and might hamper subsequent dimer-dimer. Therefore, ionotropic gelation is more pronounced for lower-methylated pectins and at pH around 3–3.5; increasing the pH leads to deprotonation of acidic groups which prevents aggregation of chains and eventually gelation. Pectin has been also mixed with alginate to form in presence of cross-linking ions an interpenetrated network made up by heterogeneous interactions [135–137].

3.5.3. Chitosan Ionic Cross-Linking

Among several polysaccharides amenable to ionotropic cross-linking, chitosan is another noteworthy example even if by far less investigated than negatively charged polysaccharides such as alginate and pectin [138]. Chitosan is typically obtained from the alkaline deacetylation of the highly abundant, naturally occurring polymer chitin, but other sources can directly provide it as such (e.g., yeasts) [113]. Chitosan is composed of β-1,4-linked glucosamine and N-acetylglucosamine residues [139]. Both the degree of acetylation (DA) and the degree of polymerisation (DP) of chitosan are crucial factors determining the structural and functional properties of this family of polymers and their resulting engineered materials [140]. Commercially available chitosans vary in their DA, usually between 5 and 20%, and in their DP or molecular weight, typically ranging between 10 and 500 kDa. Unlike chitin, chitosan is soluble in water under mild acidic conditions thanks to the protonation of its amino groups (pKa = 6.2–7) able to promote the solvation of polymer chains. In these conditions, chitosan behaves as a polycation and, consequently, can form a gel by ionic interaction in presence of multivalent anions. Tripolyphosphate (TPP) is by far the most employed cross-linker to ionically reticulate chitosan due to its high net negative charges (ranging from one to five depending on pH) per monomeric unit and nontoxicity [116,141,142]. TPP has been widely exploited in pharmaceutical field to obtain chitosan microparticles [143–145], nanoparticles [143,146] and nano/micro-gels [147,148] intended for controlled drug delivery [149].

3.6. Different Approaches to Hydrogel Formation by Ionotropic Cross-Linking

Hydrogels can be generated using ionotropic gelation technique by three main methods that differ in the way crosslinking ions are introduced to the polymer, realizing the so-called external, internal or inverse gelation [18,150].

In the external gelation or diffusion controlled method, polysaccharide solution is added dropwise into the gelling bath. The hydrogel matrix is formed through the diffusion of the cross-linking agents from the external continuous phase into the inner structure of polymeric droplets [151]. As expected, at the outermost layer of the hydrogel, gelling kinetics is rapid and gel formation is instantaneous. Then, counter-ions start to diffuse towards the center of the particle creating an inhomogeneous gelation profile in which the interaction between ions and polymer functional groups is maximum at the surface and zero at the core [152,153].

The internal gelation also called in situ gelation is an approach widely used to produce calcium alginate particles [154]. In this case, an insoluble calcium salt (e.g., $CaCO_3$ and $CaSO_4$) is mixed with the polysaccharide solution, and the obtained mixture is then extruded into an acidic gelling bath [155–157]. The acidic environment increases the solubility of calcium salt, allowing its release that leads to the formation of the polysaccharide gel network. This mechanism guarantees a controlled and homogeneous alginate exposure to cations and hence a uniform gel network formation [120]. Despite the good homogeneity, the internal cross-linked matrices results less dense, with larger pore sizes and thus more permeable than those obtained for external gelation, with lower encapsulation efficiencies and faster release rates [157,158]. This happens because matrix permeability is affected by competition between Ca^{2+} and H^+ ions due to the acid added. It seems that while the acid in the gelling bath liberates Ca^{2+} from the insoluble salt, it also competes with Ca^{2+} for interaction with the alginate/polymer. This drawback can be overcome by manipulating the pH of the medium and the amount of calcium salt employed [150].

Another approach is the inverse gelation, based on the dripping of the medium containing the cross-linking agents into the polysaccharide solution. This method is usually applied to emulsions for producing alginate microcapsules with an oily content and soft shell [5,159,160]. In comparison to other cross-linking methods, it exploits low amounts of biopolymer leading to the formation of a soft particle shell. Clearly, as highlighted by Martins at al. [161] in a recent published paper, the properties of the obtained microcapsules (e.g., mechanical resistance and release of bioactive substances) can vary based on the type of emulsion used (W/O or O/W) for the inverse gelation

4. Influence of Drying Process on Gel Particle Characteristics

As discussed above, polysaccharide-based hydrogel particles can be used in the hydrated form for different applications [119,162–166]. However, to avoid their chemical or microbiological degradation a drying step is often required [167,168]. Hydrogel particles can be dried using several techniques such as conventional, dielectric, freeze or supercritical drying, each one with a significant impact on the physicochemical and textural properties of the final dried beads [169]. Phenomena such as modifications of the highly interconnected hydrogel network, solute migration, polymorphism, damages by overheating and many other effects can occur [170]. Therefore, the choice of the drying method represents one of the critical step on the pathway to the production of PbHPs. As illustrated in Figure 10, each drying process leads to polymeric material with different inner structure; conventional or dielectric methods allow to obtain "xerogels" whereas freeze and supercritical drying generally allow to achieve "cryogels" and "aerogels", respectively [171–175].

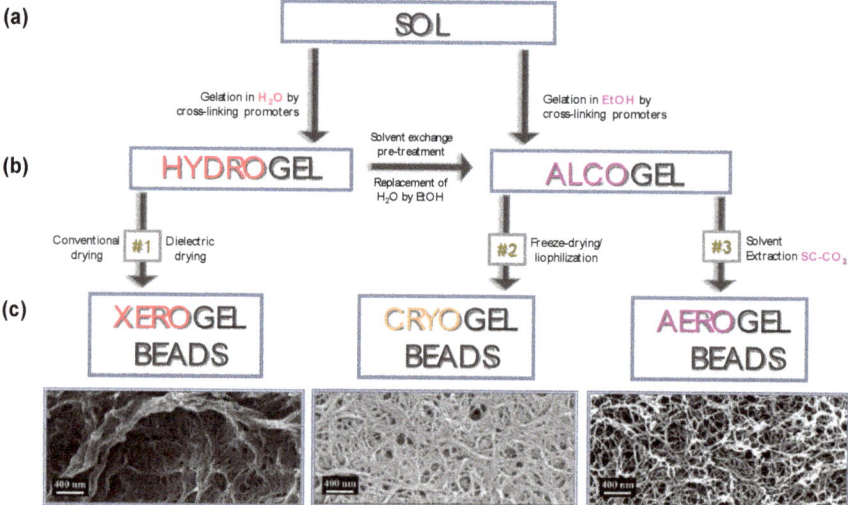

Figure 10. Pathway for the production of xerogels, cryogels and aerogels from polysaccharide based hydrogels via several steps including: (**a**) gelation (SOL→GEL), (**b**) solvent exchange pre-treatment, if required (e.g., the replacement of the water contained in the pores of the hydrogel with a suitable organic solvent), (**c**) drying final step with a specific technology. The images of xerogel, cryogel and aerogel beads were here reprinted (with some modifications) from [176] with permission from Elsevier. Copyright (2016).

Each drying method presents specific advantages and disadvantages (Table 1), and the choice must be done based on the desired performances for the final product, system cost-effectiveness and realizable scale-up.

In the following paragraphs, production and properties of xerogel, cryogel and aerogel particles are discussed.

Table 1. Main characteristics of the drying methods for polysaccharide hydrogels.

Drying Method	Particle Inner Structure	Advantages	Disadvantages
Conventional Dielectric Drying	XEROGEL	■ Simple, rapid and cheap ■ High shrinkage	■ Presence of capillary forces that destroy part of the inner structure
Supercritical-Assisted Drying	AEROGEL	■ No shrinkage of the porous inner texture	■ High cost ■ Need of aqueous/organic solvent exchange
Freeze-Drying	CRYOGEL	■ Low shrinkage ■ Higher pore Diameter	■ High cost ■ Need of aqueous/organic solvent exchange

4.1. Conventional and Dielectric Drying to Produce Xerogels

Conventional drying (e.g., using ambient air and an oven) as well as dielectric treatments generally cause the collapse of the nanoporous structure of the parent hydrogel due to the high capillary pressure gradient established during the solvent removal. The collapsing of the polymer structure produces a massive volume shrinkage leading to the formation of a highly aggregated and densely packed material without pores; the formed compact structure is known as "xerogel". However, as discussed in a large number of papers [175,177–179], porous texture of the dried material can be tuned by a proper selection of solvent, temperature, carrier gas used during evaporation and, specifically for microwave heating, the irradiating regimen. These parameters alone or in combination can allow to obtain either microporous, micro-mesoporous or micro-macroporous textures of the dried beads. For instance, as reported by [176] the porous structure of cellulose-based wet gels may resist to collapse to a certain limit when alcohol, having low surface tension and low vapor pressure, is used as organic solvent. In addition, an interesting study of [180] showed that degree of substitution (DS) of cellulose can play an important role for the production, via ambient drying, of low density, open porous and hydrophobic cellulose material defined "Xerocellulose". During this research, tritylcellulose with different DS was synthesized in homogeneous conditions and then subjected to dissolution-coagulation-drying producing "Xerocellulose". Results showed that, depending on DS, the chemical modification leads to the development of unusual microstructure due to the different manner of self-assembly of cellulose molecules and lack of hydrogen bonding.

Xerogel porosity may be specifically tuned, as demonstrated by studies of our research group aimed to verify the feasibility of the tandem technique Prilling/Microwave assisted drying for the production of alginate-based beads loaded with non-steroidal anti-inflammatory drugs (NSAIDs) [181,182]. Microwaves at different regimens of irradiation affected matrix porosity, solid state of the loaded drug (i.e., ketoprofen or piroxicam) and drug-polymer interaction, leading to beads with significant differences in drug release profiles. Interestingly, high MW irradiation level led to dried beads with highly porous and swellable inner matrix able to rapidly release the encapsulated drug in the simulated gastrointestinal fluids. By contrast, low MW irradiation levels produced beads with few pores in the inner matrix acting as NSAID delayed delivery systems.

4.2. Freeze-Drying to Produce Cryogels

During the freeze drying, the liquid entrapped into the hydrogel body is frozen and sublimed under regulated vacuum [118,183] reducing the volume shrinkage of the beads to 40%–50%. Unless special precautions are often taken to prevent the growth of ice crystals, freezing may destroy the pore structure and damage the nanostructured gel matrix as freezing always implies the growth of crystals [184]. The increase of the solvent volume upon crystallization induces the formation of a dendritic network of the crystalline solvent phase. The dendrites are, depending on the cooling rate, typically in the range of few up to a few tens of micrometers' size; they push the walls of the network at the crystal boundaries destroying the morphology/inner structure [185–189]. The resulting material is open porous product with a pore size in the range of several micrometers termed "cryogels".

In certain cases, modifying the freeze-drying conditions it is possible to modulate the ultrastructure of the porous matrix, moving from nanofibrillar to sheet-like skeletons with hierarchical micro- and nanoscale morphology. For instance, by increasing the cooling rate of the hydrogel precursors with e.g., liquid propane, or by using the spraying freeze drying approach, it is possible to avoid the macroporous 2D-sheet morphology of cellulose cryogels, producing aerogel-like dried systems with intermediate textural properties (BET-specific surface areas of 70–100 m^2/g) [190]. Interestingly, the freeze drying of alcogels from resorcinol-formaldehyde using t-butanol as solvent resulted in a significant improvement of the mesoporosity of the resulting dried gels if compared to the freeze drying of hydrogel counterparts [187].

4.3. Supercritical Assisted Drying to Produce Aerogels

Supercritical drying is the best method to preserve the porous texture and structural properties of the wet gel network in a dry form without cracks as well as without substantial volume reduction or packed network structure due to the intrinsic absence of surface tension in the pores of the gel. Supercritical drying produces nanostructured materials with low-density (typically <0.2 g cm^{-3}), high-porosity (>96% v/v) in the mesoporous range, with full pore interconnectivity and large surface area (>250 m^2/g), commonly called "aerogels". Aerogels have been designed in a several morphologies (e.g., cylinders, beads, microparticles) and configurations (e.g., only core, core-shell, coated particles) with an attractive processing versatility [191–194].

During supercritical drying, the organic solvent in the hydrogel pores (deriving from the pre-treatment named solvent exchange procedure, see Figure 10), is removed under supercritical conditions. As well known, a fluid reaches its supercritical state when it is compressed and heated above its critical point. Supercritical fluids have liquid-like densities and gas-like viscosities [195]. Supercritical carbon dioxide is the most commonly used fluid for supercritical drying due to its mild critical point conditions (304 K, 7.4 MPa), nontoxicity (it is considered to be Generally Recognized as Safe or GRAS), environmental friendliness, widely availability and cheapness/cost-effectiveness [191,196,197]. Generally, prior to the supercritical drying, the solvent exchange (that is the replacement of the water contained in the pores of the hydrogel with a suitable organic solvent) is needed due to the low affinity of water to supercritical carbon dioxide (SC-CO$_2$) [196,198]. The presence of even small amounts of water in the pores of the wet gel can cause a dramatic change in the initially highly porous polysaccharide network upon supercritical drying. The usual approach in SC-CO$_2$ drying procedure is the displacement of the water using a solvent with high solubility in CO$_2$, commonly alcohol or acetone [191] and then the immersion of the gel in SC-CO$_2$. The extraction time depends mainly on the thickness of the gel samples. Therefore, it can be still reduced from the several hours needed for thick monoliths to only few minutes for polysaccharide particles of millimeter size.

5. Case-Studies: Polysaccharide-Based Hydrogel Particles Produced by Prilling/Ionotropic Gelation and Their Application as Drug Delivery Systems (DDS)

Polysaccharide-based hydrogel particles can be used as drug carriers, which application in pharmaceutics depends on the characteristics of the polysaccharides and the drugs, the particle configuration, as well as on the inner structure, namely xerogels, cryogels and aerogels. Table 2 summarizes the different kinds of PbHPs produced via prilling/ionotropic gelation, particle configuration (only core or core-shell), their main physico-chemical and technological properties, and the potential pharmaceutical applications.

As shown in Table 2, hydrogels can be obtained as simple monolayered (only core) or multi-layered (core-shell) systems, in the hydrated or in the dried form. Based on the specific drying treatment, hydrogel beads can be transformed into xerogel, cryogel or aerogel form. The choice of a specific polysaccharide and particle system must be driven by the final desired application and performance requirements. Prior to any process design, it is necessary to study physico-chemical characteristics of the polymeric materials, like viscosities, densities, gelation and, physico-chemical and biopharmaceutical properties of the carried drug.

Table 2. Overview of PbHPs (polysaccharide-based hydrogel particles) produced by prilling/inotropic crosslinking/drying methods.

Polysaccharide	Prilling Configuration	Ionic Cross-Linking Conditions	Drying Method	Type of Particle/ Inner Structure	Pharmaceutical Application	References
Alginate	Basic Apparatus	Inverse gelation Ca^{2+}	None	Soft alginate capsules	Topical administration	[199]
Alginate	Coaxial system	Inverse gelation Ca^{2+}	None	Hydrated core-shell beads loaded with hydrophobic substances	Microencapsulation of hydrophobic compounds into a hydrophilic matrix	[200]
Alginate	Basic Apparatus	External gelation Ca^{2+}, Zn^{2+}, Ca^{2+} plus Zn^{2+}	Conventional	Only core Xerogels	Delayed DDS for oral administration	[23,29,201–203]
Alginate	Basic Apparatus	External gelation Ca^{2+}	Dielectric	Only core Xerogels	Controlled DDS for oral administration	[181,182]
Pectin	Basic Apparatus	External gelation Zn^{2+}	Conventional	Only core Xerogels	Delayed DDS for oral administration	[204]
Pectin	Basic Apparatus plus enteric coating ES100	External gelation Zn^{2+}	Conventional	Core/shell beads Xerogels	Colon targeted DDS for oral administration	[32,205]
Pectin and Alginate	Coaxial system	External gelation Zn^{2+}	Conventional	Core/shell beads Xerogels	Colon targeted DDS for oral administration	[31,43]
Alginate, Pectin and HPMC	Basic Apparatus	External gelation: Zn^{2+}	Conventional	Floating Hollow Beads	Floating and sustained release DDS for oral administration	[206]
Alginate	Basic Apparatus	(a) External gelation Zn^{2+} (b) Internal gelation Ca^{2+}	Conventional	Floating Hollow Beads	Floating and sustained release DDS for oral administration	[207]
Alginate	Basic Apparatus	External gelation Ca^{2+}	Supercritical-CO_2	Only core Aerogels	Immediate release DDS for oral administration	[208,209]
Alginate and Pectin	Coaxial system	External gelation Ca^{2+}	Supercritical-CO_2	Core/shell Aerogels	Topical application (Wound Healing)	[44]
Alginate	Basic Apparatus	External gelation Ca^{2+}	▪ Conventional ▪ Freeze-drying ▪ Supercritical-CO_2	▪ Xerogels ▪ Cryogels ▪ Aerogels	Controlled DDS for oral administration or topical application	[169]

5.1. Design of PbHPs in Form of Xerogels

As reported in Table 2, successful outcomes have been achieved through a formulation design based on prilling in tandem with conventional drying that provide efficient drug delivery of both steroidal (e.g., prednisolone and betamethasone) and non-steroidal (e.g., ketoprofen, ketoprofen lysine salt and piroxicam) anti-inflammatory drugs, targeting chronic inflammation and early morning pathologies.

The accurate selection of biopolymer, the opportune set-up of process parameters and gelling conditions allowed to produce interesting delivery systems in the xerogel form with controlled drug release both for low soluble and highly soluble NSAIDs. Zn^{2+} as external cross-linking agent for alginate/ketoprofen (K) solutions gave PbHPs with good technological properties such as drug loading, particle size, morphology, hardness of cross-linked matrix [202]. In vitro and in vivo release behavior resulted to be strongly influenced by the amount of NSAID loaded inside the polymer; the loading of high amount of drug into feed solutions promotes, during the gelling phase, the formation of a compact gel polymeric network via intermolecular interactions, as hydrophobic or hydrogen bonding, which stabilize the well-known alginate "egg-box" structure. This phenomenon leads to tough polymer beads (Figure 11a), reducing the leaching of the drug from the drops into the gelling medium. Accordingly, the formulation obtained with the highest drug content (F20, K/alginate ratio 1:5) showed the highest entrapment of the drug within the matrix (encapsulation efficiency, 53%) and a delayed release of the drug in simulated intestinal fluid (see Figure 11b). This in vitro release pattern was clearly reflected in the in vivo prolonged anti-inflammatory effect evaluated using a modified carrageenan-induced acute edema assay in rat paw. F20, administered 3 h before edema induction, showed a significant anti-inflammatory activity, reducing maximum paw volume in response to carrageenan injection, whereas no response was observed for pure ketoprofen (see Figure 11c).

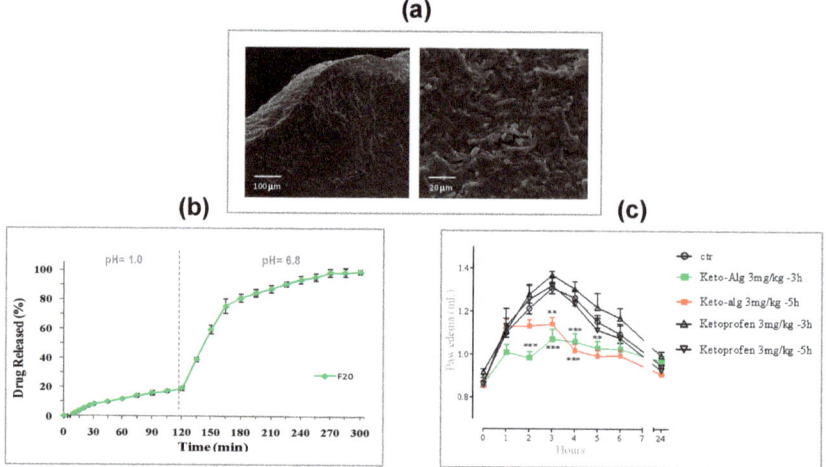

Figure 11. Main in vitro and in vivo results obtained for Zn-alginate-based xerogel beads loaded with ketoprofen: (**a**) SEM microphotographs showing the compact inner matrix; (**b**) relese profile performed by USP Apparatus 4 and, (**c**) edema volume reduction in rats (** p-value $\leq$ 0.01, *** p-value $\leq$ 0.001 compared with control). These images were here reprinted (with some modifications) from [202] with permission from Elsevier. Copyright (2015).

Zn^{2+} as external cross-linking agent for pectin solutions was able to produce PbHPs containing ketoprofen lysine salt (KL), a highly soluble NSAID [204]. In this case, the best results were obtained using amidated low methoxyl pectin (esterification degree 24% and amidation degree 23%) producing beads with good morphological properties and size, high drug content and encapsulation efficiency (93.5%), and interesting KL sustained release profiles.

5.2. Investigation on the Effect of Different Cations on Gelation Process

Many researchers evaluated the influence of different divalent cations on PbHP properties. For instance, Chan et al. [210] studied the ability of calcium chloride and zinc sulphate to cross-link alginate microspheres prepared by emulsification.

In this study, the aqueous phase, consisting of 2.5% *w/w* sodium alginate and 1% *w/w* sulphaguanidine was dispersed in isooctane with the aid of surfactants and a mechanical stirrer. The fine globules of sodium alginate produced were gelified by addition of calcium chloride and zinc sulphate, alone or in combination. The microspheres formed were collected by filtration, washed and oven dried at 40 °C. The results of characterization studies showed that the simultaneous use of these two salts led to different particle morphology and slower drug release compared to particles cross-linked by the calcium salt alone. These effects were attributed to a greater extent of interaction between zinc cations and the alginate molecules able to produce a less permeable alginate matrix. Cerciello et al. also investigated the specific effect of these two divalent cations, i.e., Ca^{2+} and Zn^{2+}, used alone or blended in different ratios ($Ca^{2+}:Zn^{2+}$, ratio 1:1, 1:4 or 4:1), on the properties of alginate beads obtained via prilling/external gelation [201]. The synergistic effect of the two cations, when used in the gelling bath in the ratio $Ca^{2+}:Zn^{2+}$ 1:4; positively affected particle morphology, size, inner structure, ability to encapsulate the model drug (SAID, prednisolone, P) and to control its release from the polymer matrix. Figure 12 shows SEM and SEM-EDS microphotographs of cryofractured blank beads obtained using the different ratios Ca^{2+}/Zn^{2+} in the gelling solution. As showed, formulations gelified using $Ca^{2+}:Zn^{2+}$ in the ratios 1:1 and 4:1 exhibited an internal structure enriched in Ca^{2+}, due to the higher diffusivity of this cation, compared to Zn^{2+}. Only with a ratio Ca^{2+}/Zn^{2+} 1:4 was possible to observe an equilibrium between the two cations quantities into the polymeric matrix. This specific ratio, in fact, exploited the Ca^{2+} ability to establish quicker electrostatic interactions with **G** groups of alginate and the Zn^{2+} ability to establish covalent-like bonds with both **M** and **G** blocks of alginate. Drug release profiles clearly reflected the advantages deriving from the simultaneous use of both cations. Their proper mixing allowed to produce a polymeric matrix tougher and more resistant compared to those obtained with a single cation (zinc or calcium) and with an interesting P prolonged release.

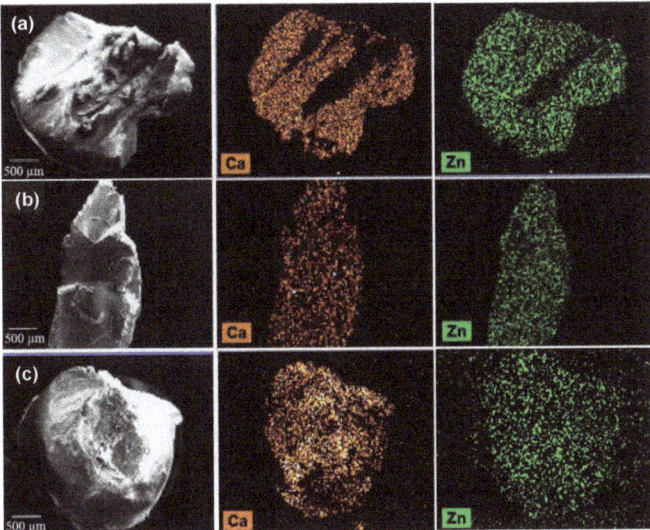

Figure 12. SEM and SEM-EDS microphotographs of cryofractured blank xerogel beads produced with different Ca^{2+}/Zn^{2+} ratios: (**a**) 1:1, (**b**) 1:4 and (**c**) 4:1. Reprinted from [201] with permission from Elsevier. Copyright (2017).

5.3. Prilling to Obtain Floating PbHPs

A significant number of studies was conducted to develop floating PbHPs, mainly alginate based particles, using gas-forming agents such as $CaCO_3$ or $NaHCO_3$. In the most of them, calcium has been used as external cross-linker for the gelation phase [157,211,212]. More recently, an important milestone was achieved with the simultaneous use of two different divalent cations to produce floating and prolonged release alginate PbHPs for the oral administration of prednisolone, P [207]. Critical parameters were established: prilling/ionotropic gelation was used as microencapsulation technique, zinc acetate in the gelling solution as the alginate external crosslinker, and calcium carbonate in the feed acting as the internal crosslinking agent able to generate gas when in contact with the acidic zinc acetate solution. The double gelation process (internal- and external) promoted by Ca^{2+} and Zn^{2+} ions gave alginate beads with extremely high encapsulation efficiency values (up to 94%) and a very porous inner matrix conferring buoyancy in vitro in simulated gastric fluid up to 5 h. Particularly, the best formulation F4 (P/Alginate ratio 1:5; Alg/$CaCO_3$ ratio 1:0.50) was able to control the drug release in acidic medium for the entire time corresponding to the floating period. Although porous, the tougher matrix obtained thanks to the double gelation process is able to reduce swelling and erosion processes in simulated gastric fluid (SGF). F4 was also able to prolong the in vivo anti-inflammatory effect up to 15 h compared with raw prednisolone. Therefore, this alginate-based system has been proposed as a new technological platform able to extend the anti-inflammatory efficacy of SAID such as prednisolone (characterized by high efficacy and high tolerability, but short half-life) for many hours and successfully treat patient suffering from chronic inflammatory diseases, also reducing the frequency of the oral administration.

An interesting production innovation was obtained designing floating PbHPs with controlled release properties without using any gas-generating agent. Our research group designed a hollow multipolymer matrix made up of alginate, ALM-pectin and HPMC. Results showed that particle shape and sphericity can be correlated to nozzle viscosity of the feed solutions; the higher the nozzle viscosity, the slower the break-up of the polymeric laminar-jet and, thus, droplet formation. The high entanglement existing between the chains of three different polymers makes the polymeric jet highly cohesive (viscoelastic stresses dominate) delaying drops detachment from the nozzle. At the lowest feed concentration (4.75 *w/w*), corresponding to a nozzle viscosity of 24.4 mPa·s, polymer chains are relaxed and surface tension dominates, allowing the formation of droplets that, falling in the gelation bath, give rise to spherical particles. Optimized formulation F4 (Drug/Polymers ratio 1:15; $Pol_1/Pol_2/Pol_3$ ratio 1.25:3:0.5) showed beads spherical in shape with a sphericity coefficient mean value of 0.94 and a mean diameter around 2200 μm. This formulation acts as a floating-system able to release the encapsulated model drug (piroxicam, PRX) in a controlled and delayed manner.

Floating properties of F4 are due both to the swelling of the hydrocolloid particles and to hollow inner structure (Figure 13). The hydration of the hydrocolloid particle surface in SGF results in an increased bulk volume and, at the same time, the presence of internal pores make beads able to entrap air. As a result beads had bulk density <1, and, therefore, remained buoyant on the acidic medium. In addition, the inner cross-linked multi-polysaccharide matrix acts as reservoir for slow and sustained PRX. Drug release was controlled by a diffusion mechanism process through the swollen polymers gel layer, as shown by in vitro release assay. Figure 14 shows the presence of pores and air bubbles entrapped within the gel barrier after 60 min of floating in acidic medium.

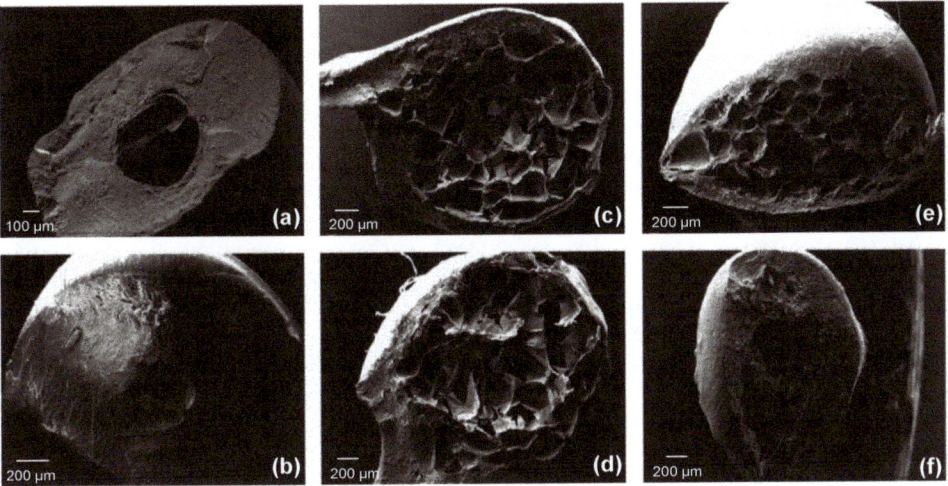

Figure 13. SEM microphotographs showing the hollow inner matrix of polysaccharide-based floating beads produced with different $Pol_1/Pol_2/Pol_3$ ratios: (**a,b**) 1.75:4:1, (**c,d**) 1.75:3:0.5 and (**e,f**) 1.25:3:0.5. Reprinted from [206] with permission from Elsevier. Copyright (2018).

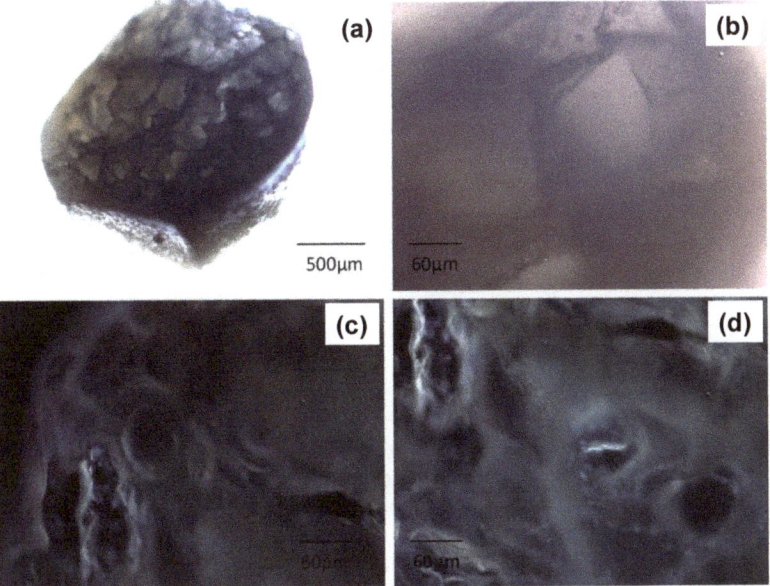

Figure 14. Microphotographs obtained using bright-field (**a,b**) and fluorescent microscopy (**c,d**) showing the presence of pores and air bubbles entrapped within the gel matrix of hydrated beads, able to confer their floating ability in SGF. Reprinted from [206] with permission from Elsevier. Copyright (2018).

As expected by morphology and results from in vitro assays, a promising application of floating PbHPs is the treatment of chronic inflammatory-diseases in elderly patients needing a rapid onset of drug action followed by a maintenance dose. In this regard, the in vivo anti-inflammatory activity of this type of new floating PbHPs, evaluated using the modified protocol of carrageenan-induced acute edema in rat paw previously developed [202], showed an incredible extension, up to 48 h, of the anti-inflammatory effect compared to standard PRX, as effect of both floating and sustaining release abilities.

5.4. Core-Shell PbHPs

Generally, the production of core-shell PbHPs through a generic dripping device can be easily conducted exploiting coacervation. The major driving force for the coacervation method is electrostatic attraction between cationic and anionic water-soluble polysaccharides. The resultant "coacervate" generally forms the particle shell. The power of the interaction between the polysaccharides and the nature of the complex is affected by many factors such as pH, concentration, ionic strength, biopolymer type, and the ratio of biopolymers [213]. With this method several core-shell PbHPs have been produced [214–216]. For instance, alginate and chitosan can be used together because of their opposite charges to form alginate particles coated with chitosan. The electrostatic interaction of carboxylic groups of alginate with the amine groups of chitosan results in the formation of a membrane surrounding the surface of the core particles and reduces their porosity [47,217,218]. Ren et al. [219] exploited this method to prepare alginate-chitosan microcapsules for protein delivery via oral route. This study confirmed that such systems are pH sensitive; in acidic solution, due to the ionic bond between the chitosan and alginate as well as the physical barrier provided by the interphasic membrane itself, microcapsules maintained integrity well, and effectively prevented the direct exposure of protein to the gastric fluid. In fact, less than 10% of protein (i.e., IgG) was released in SGF and 80% of its activity was preserved; during the first hour of permanence into simulated intestinal fluid, a burst release of IgG was observed.

In general, to increase the performances of such particle systems and make more efficient the delivery of macromolecules as well as drugs throughout the GIT, the manufacturing phase should provide a major control on shell formation process. To this regard, an important achievement was the design and the development of multiparticulate beads in core-shell configuration using (a) prilling apparatus in its basic configuration followed by an enteric coating process [32,205] and (b) prilling apparatus in coaxial configuration [31,43]. This latter is certainly the most innovative approach; it employs multiple concentric nozzles to produce a smooth coaxial jet comprising polymer annular shell and core material, which are broken up by acoustic excitation into uniform core-shell droplets and gelled into a cross-linking solution. PbHPs in core-shell configuration consisting of zinc-ALM pectinate as core and zinc-alginate as shell were produced. Both NSAID (piroxicam, PRX) and SAID (betamethasone, B) were respectively loaded as model drug within the pectin core. The aim was to combine the pH dependent solubility (gastro-resistance) of zinc alginate and the colon targeted selectivity of zinc-ALM pectinate [220,221] in a unique system to obtain an enteric carrier targeting colon. The most critical process parameter to obtain uniform double-layered particles was identified in the ratio between the nozzle viscosity of the inner and outer polymer solutions. In fact, beads with homogeneous layered, good spherical shape and smooth particle surface were obtained when this ratio was above 6. Moreover, optimization of other process parameters such as selection of the cross-linker, pH of the gelling solution as well as cross-linking time was necessary to obtain well-formed and homogeneously coated microcapsules (see Figure 15, panel a) with strong drug/polymer core showing a tailored control of drug release in the gastrointestinal tract (see Figure 15, panel b).

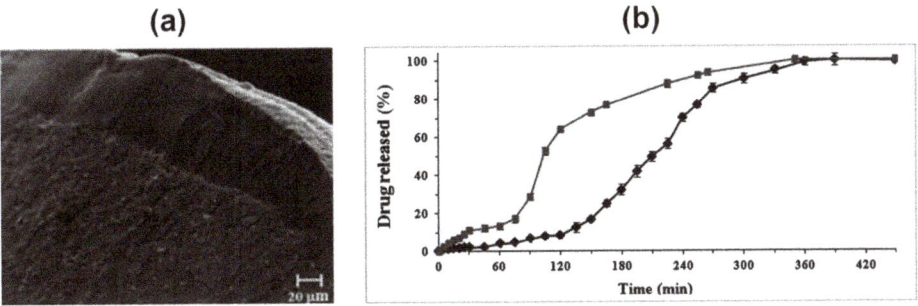

Figure 15. Main in vitro results obtained for core-shell (Pectin/Alginate) beads loaded with piroxicam: (**a**) SEM microphotographs showing the complete and homogeneous alginate shell surrounding the pectin core; (**b**) Release profiles of mono-layered "only core" (Pectin) beads (-■-) and bi-layered "core-shell" (Pectin/Alginate) beads (-♦-), performed in simulated intestinal fluid by using USP Apparatus 2. Reprinted from [43] with permission from Elsevier. Copyright (2014).

5.5. Design of PbHPs in Form of Aerogels

The application of biopolymer aerogels as drug delivery systems has gained increased interest during the last decade since these structures have large surface area and accessible pores allowing for, e.g., high drug loadings. Examples of oral, mucosal, and most recently pulmonary drug delivery routes have been highly discussed in the literature. Furthermore, thanks to high pore volume and swelling ability both pristine and drug-loaded polysaccharide aerogel particles have been suggested as superabsorbent and for wound healing applications [44,222]. Being largely mesoporous solids, aerogels can accommodate drugs in the amorphous state suppressing re-crystallization [223]. This feature along with the high specific surface area and rapid pore collapse upon contact with liquid media gives rise to unusually fast drug release.

Reverchon et al. [208,209] produced alginate-based aerogels as carriers for the fast delivery of slightly soluble NSAIDs in the upper gastrointestinal tract by prilling of drug/alginate feed solutions followed by cross-linking in ethanol or aqueous $CaCl_2$ solutions, water replacement and, supercritical-CO_2-assisted drying. The selected techniques allowed to successfully produce spherical aerogels (sphericity coefficient 0.97–0.99) in narrow size distribution with reduced particle shrinkage and smooth surface (surface roughness 1.10–1.13); the internal porous texture of the parent hydrogels was preserved and appeared as a network of nanopores with diameters around 200 nm (see Figure 16a).

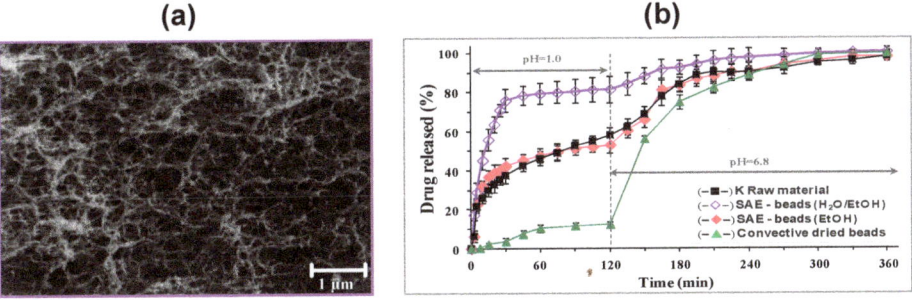

Figure 16. Main in vitro results obtained for alginate-based aerogel beads loaded with ketoprofen: (**a**) SEM microphotographs showing the inner nanoporous structure; (**b**) Release profiles of beads dried by both supercritical-CO_2 and conventional drying, performed in simulated gastro-intestinal fluids by using USP Apparatus 2. Reprinted from [208] with permission from Elsevier. Copyright (2012).

Recently, we verified the influence of the alginate molecular weight, the solvent used in the gelation solution on porosity, textural properties and stability of the alginate aerogel beads produced via prilling/ionotropic gelation/SC-CO_2 drying route [169]. Gelation in ethanolic media promoted the formation of aerogels with higher textural properties compared to the aerogels derived from particle crosslinked in aqueous media. As expected, the textural properties of aerogels were far higher than those obtained from cryogels and xerogels obtained by freeze-drying and oven drying, respectively. This study also highlighted that the use of medium molecular weight alginate led to aerogels with reduced shrinkage and enhanced porosity. By contrast, the use of high molecular weight alginate promoted the formation of aerogels with higher surface area. Finally, stability studies showed non-significant variations in aerogels weight and specific surface area after 3 months of storage, especially, in the case of aerogels produced with medium molecular weight alginate. Overall, this study allowed to highlight the suitability of such materials for wound dressing applications. In fact, thanks to their high surface area, aerogels can rapidly absorb the exudate once applied on a wound and at the same time, they can promote a controlled release of the active substance eventually embedded within the polymer network.

Several other researchers developed aerogel-based formulations for the management of chronic wounds. For instance, with this aim López-Iglesias and coworkers [224] produced vancomycin-loaded chitosan aerogel beads, starting from the simple dripping of a chitosan solution into a basic NaOH 0.1 M solution. In this sol-gel method, the gelation took place immediately after contact with the medium. After that, the productive process continues with the solvent exchange carried out using absolute EtOH, and it ends with the SC drying. The dried particles showed a fibrous structure characterized by a high porosity (>96%) and large surface area (>200 m^2/g); they preserved their initial spherical structure, with an overall volume shrinkage of 57.0 ± 4.5% attributable to the flexibility of the polymeric chains of chitosan that are brought closer after the extraction of the solvent.

A significant number of investigations also focused on the possibility to produce layered aerogels. Veronovsky et al. [225] prepared multilayer amidated LM pectin aerogel particles via ionotropic gelation by dripping 2% Wt pectin solutions through a needle into calcium chloride solution. The obtained hydrogels were then dripped into a 1% Wt pectin solution for obtaining membranes around the core particles, and again were crosslinked in $CaCl_2$ solution. Three-membrane hydrogel particles were produced by repeating the process. After solvent exchange, particles were dried with supercritical CO_2. To verify the ability of such materials to act as carriers for drug delivery, two model drugs that is theophylline and nicotinic acid were loaded within the core. The selected operative conditions allowed obtaining multilayer pectin aerogel particles with diameter of 8.0 and 9.8 mm, depending on the source of pectin (apple and citrus, respectively). Specific surface area varied from 469 to 593 m^2/g based on pectin source and its concentration. The release of both loaded drugs turned out to be controlled by swelling and dissolution of pectin matrix. Aerogels from citrus pectin showed more controlled release behavior than those from apple. Moreover, core-shell aerogels have been designed to delivery antibiotics. De Cicco et al. [44] combined amidated LM pectin with alginate to produce core-shell aerogels loaded with doxycycline hyclate, by means of prilling technique in coaxial configuration. Ionotropic gelation was conducted via diffusion method (external gelation) in an ethanolic $CaCl_2$ solution. The obtained aerogels showed spherical shape, smooth surface and an apparent density of around 0.3 g/cm^3.

5.6. Design of Experiments (DoE) and Artificial Intelligence (AI) for the Productionof PbHP by Inverse Gelation Technique

Recently, our research group exploited the possibility to apply the Design of Experiment for the development of wet alginate soft-capsules with a hydrophilic core through inverse gelation [199]. Soft-capsules, designed for topical administration, were produced through a vibrating nozzle device, dripping a thickened calcium chloride solution into an alginate bath. The experimental design applied revealed the effect of several critical process parameters such as the solution's composition, frequency and flow-rate onto critical quality attributes of the produced soft-capsules as e.g., drug content, encapsulation efficiency, size, shape and mechanical strength. The overall knowledge gained through the DoE exercise showed that the inverse gelation process was capable of producing PbHPs as soft-capsules with the desired attributes, resistant enough to allow handling during storage, but also very easy to break when applied onto the skin.

Process optimization may be gained by integration of several methods into the process of the formulation design of PbHPs. Artificial intelligence (AI) is one of the possibilities to predict the optimal process conditions, reproducibility and great precision and accuracy in data analysis. In the last years, we proposed inverse gelation for the production of PbHPs as wet core-shell microcapsules using AI tools for the process optimization [200]. A w/o emulsion containing aqueous calcium chloride solution in sunflower oil pumped through the inner nozzle of a prilling encapsulator apparatus gave the core while an aqueous alginate solution, coming out from the annular nozzle, produced the particle shell (see Figure 17). The numerous operative conditions such as w/o constituents, polymer concentrations, flow rates and frequency of vibration were optimized by two commercial software, FormRules® and INForm®, which implement neurofuzzy logic and artificial neural networks together with genetic algorithms, respectively. The optimized parameters by AI tools allowed to manufacturing of spherical core-shell beads (sphericity coefficient about 0.98) with diameter about 1.1 mm and a narrow size distribution containing the oily droplet wrapped by a thin and regular alginate layer (about 95 µm). This technique certainly represents an innovative approach to produce PbHPs in form of core-shell particles with different hardness loaded with oil or drugs dispersed into lipids.

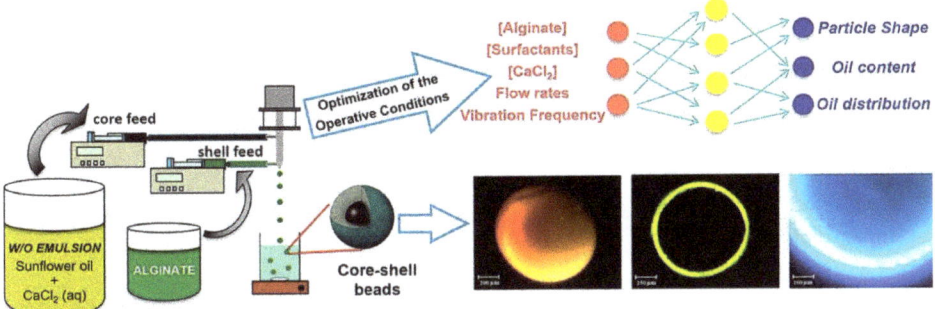

Figure 17. Schematic illustration of the method employed for the production of core-shell microparticles by inverse gelation optimized with artificial intelligent tools. Reprinted from [200] with permission from Elsevier. Copyright (2018).

6. PbHPs: Safety by Design and Clinical Translations

Despite the largely evolving knowledge and techniques for the development of PbHPs as controlled DDS able to improve biopharmaceutical properties of various bioactive molecules (e.g., small molecules, protein, oligonucleotides), their clinical study remains very limited [2]. As it always happens, opportunities are accompanied by challenges, and for new process technologies in pharmaceutical field, the main issue is the insecurity concerning their safe implementation. The main difficulty to translate such systems into clinical studies is due to a general lack of:

(1) understanding how properties of such materials influence the adsorption of bioactive molecules and their effect on cellular reactions,
(2) standardized methods assessing material characteristics as well as biological reactions,

both aspects falling in the field of safety. In particular, it is important to consider that natural-based polysaccharides are not a single discrete chemical system, as they vary in number and distribution of repeating building blocks along the backbone [2]. Since polymer molecular weight and composition can significantly vary, their main physicochemical properties such as solubility, chain flexibility, intra- and intermolecular forces, carrier size/shape, loading capacity, surface charge, and degradation profile can vary, and consequently also the in vivo performances. These aspects must be taken into account by regulatory authorities during control phases for a successful translation of PbHPs from bench to bedside.

In this contest, the safety-by-design (SbD) approach acquires a significant relevance. In general, SbD concepts foresee the risk identification and reduction as well as uncertainties regarding human health and environmental safety during the early stages of product development, by altering its design and by ensuring safety along its lifecycle. The SbD concept is therefore different from conventional risk assessment approaches, which only consider safety when the product is already fully developed. As well known, while the concept of quality-by-design (QbD) is widely used by pharmaceutical industry and its implementation is foreseen by the pharmaceutical development guidelines [226,227], that of SbD is new, and it is not yet included in ICH, EMA, or FDA guidelines. This means that even if safety is taken into account during the pharmaceutical development, there is still no systematic SbD approach in place, yet. As the QbD requires for its application the definition of the critical quality attributes (CQA) that will lead to the achievement of a product with proven effectiveness, in the same way the SbD has to establish CQA leading to a product with low safety concerns. Few papers focus on this intriguing and complex topic involving multidisciplinary knowledge (i.e., life science, clinical medicine, material science, chemistry, and engineering) as well as active collaboration among regulatory authorities, pharmaceutical companies, academics, and governments.

Recently, Schmutz et al. [228] elaborated a useful methodological SbD approach (referred as GoNanoBioMat SbD approach) focusing on polymeric biomaterials widely used to prepare nanoparticles and microparticles for drug delivery. Such approach allows identifying and addressing the relevant safety aspects to face with when developing biopolymeric-based DDS during design, characterization, assessment of human health and environmental risk, manufacturing and handling. As shown in Figure 18, the pillars of such approach are the following:

(1) Material Design, Characterization, Human Health and Environmental Risks
(2) Manufacturing and control
(3) Storage and Transport.

For the Human Health Risks step, the route of administration/exposure, the dosage, the duration and frequency should be determined as safety of polymeric biomaterials depends on the route of administration/exposure and the resulting respective pharmacokinetic profile. If one final candidate has been selected, the developer of such materials should go to the Manufacturing and Control step to ensure product safety and quality. The goal of this step is to scale-up the production by applying Good Manufacturing Practices (GMPs), preventing contamination and ensuring uniformity between the batches. In this step, CQAs of nanobiomaterials must be identified as well as Critical Process Parameters. These are defined as the "process parameters that influence CQAs and therefore should be monitored or controlled to ensure the process produces the desired quality" (ICH Q8 (R2), 2009). The goal of the final step is guarantee safe storage and transport.

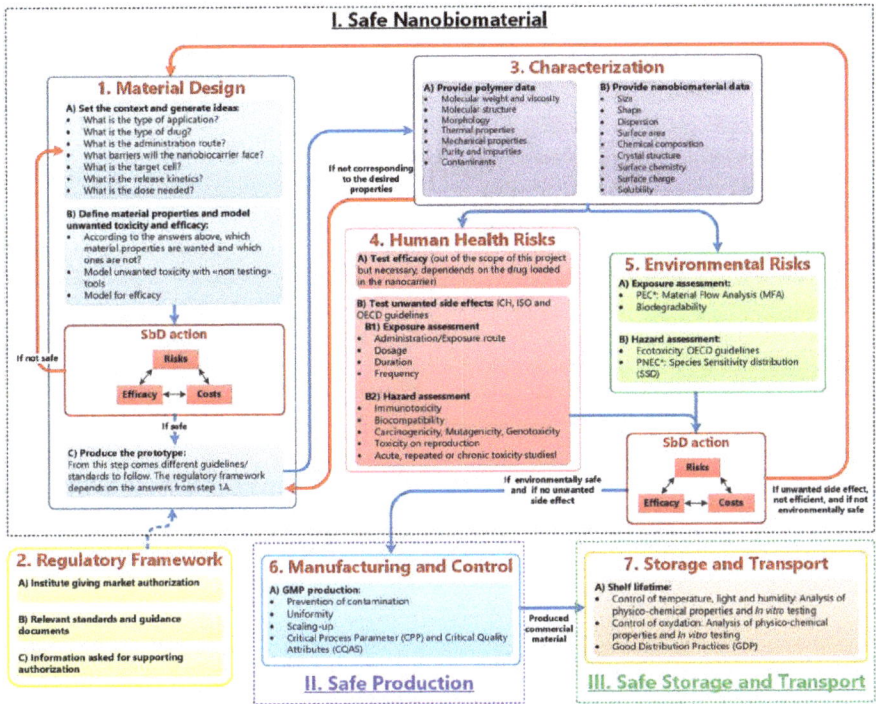

Figure 18. Safety-by-Design approach. Blue arrows correspond to the flow of polymeric nanobiomaterials as drug delivery systems from design to storage and transport, red arrows are feedback loops uses whenever the nanobiomaterial product is unsafe, inefficient or has unwanted side effects, and bullet points represent the methods/tools or endpoints at each step. Reprinted from [228]. Copyright (2020) Schmutz, Borges, Jesus, Borchard, Perale, Zinn, Sips, Soeteman-Hernandez, Wick and Som.

A recent paper by Poel and Robay [229] highlights the usefulness to "design for the responsibility for safety", rather than directly for safety, and propose some heuristics to use in deciding how to share and distribute responsibility for safety through design; in summary, designers should think where the responsibility for safety is best situated and design technologies, accordingly. The solution to safety issues is not to be sought in transferring all responsibility to the users of a technology (or to other stakeholders) but rather in a model of responsibility shared among the various actors involved, such as operators and users. The authors state that it is better to accept indeterminacy and to use it as potential source for safety rather to design it out in an attempt to achieve absolute safety, which is unattainable; in many real-world situations, human actions should be considered not a source of risks but of safety. Reason argues that the human possibility to improvise may be crucial to react to (unexpected) risks and is, therefore a source of safety [230]. Based on these considerations, indeterminacy is not only a liability but also an asset as it opens the possibility to use the expertise and insights of the actors in the value chain to identify risks unknown during the design phase.

To date, there are still many open questions on safety and conformity assessment. From this point of view, an early and deep dialogue between experts from academic community, industry and regulatory authorities is of utmost importance to "anticipate" quality and safety requirements of PbHPs. In general, regulatory requirements as well as regulatory/scientific guidance on new technologies and nanomaterials applied in medicinal products as well as medical devices are emerging. A new regulatory framework for medical devices was recently published in Europe [231]. The new regulation contains several provisions for nanomaterials, including a definition, specific attention for safety of nanomaterials and classification rules leading to different routes for conformity assessment. For the implementation of such aspects, more guidance is needed.

7. Conclusions

In this review, a comprehensive description of the theoretical and practical aspects behind the production of different polysaccharide-based hydrogel particles (PbHPs) by prilling technology in tandem with several curing technique is given. PbHPs, depending on the designed characteristics, can be produced as drug delivery systems exerting a number of functions as to control drug release and targeting. Beads with modular inner structure and tailored texture (xerogel, aerogel, cryogel) and with different configurations (mono-layered "only core" or multi-layered "core-shell") may be obtained by a proper selection of the droplet formation technique and the subsequent gelation step. However, the choice of the drying method for the hydrogel is a critical step allowing to obtain carriers with specific morphology and inner structure and hence with controlled release properties, mainly of anti-inflammatory and antibiotic drugs.

Several studies in literature highlight that prilling is a versatile technique to develop polysaccharide-based particles loaded with different drugs (i.e., NSAIDs and SAIDs), both with poor and high solubility, intended for oral or topical applications and intended as fast or prolonged/sustained drug release formulations. The added value of this technique is related to its versatility and scalability. In fact, such technique is already approved for large scale by some companies. In general, the pathway for PbHP production through prilling comprises a deep knowledge of various formulation and process parameters, starting from biopolymer concentration, type of solvent, feed solution viscosity, gelling methods and properties of cation or cations for ionotropic gelation. Moreover, drying conditions play an important role in determining the characteristics of the final material.

Despite the promising pharmaceutical applications, these are some challenges correlated to the numerous critical parameters influencing size, shape, morphology and structure (i.e., homogeneity, density, strength, flexibility, pore size, permeability) of the final material and hence the release profile of the entrapped drug and its in vivo activity. The possibility to apply the Design of Experiment for the development of PbHPs and the use of artificial intelligent (AI) tools for the process optimization may reduce the time and make more efficient the process design. Another important aspect to consider is the possibility of including safety in the design of PbHPs as useful tool to enhance the medical translation of such innovative DDS.

Author Contributions: All authors contributed equally to this paper. All authors have read and agreed to the published version of the manuscript.

Funding: This research was funded by: -Regione Campania Italy—POR Campania FESR 2014-2020 Technology Platform for Therapeutic Strategies Against Resistant Cancer Project "Campania Oncoterapie", Combattere la Resistenza Tumorale: Piattaforma Integrata Multidisciplinare per un Approccio Tecnologico Innovativo alle Oncoterapie. -Xunta de Galicia [ED431F 2016/010], MCIUN [RTI2018-094131-A-I00], Agrupación Estratégica de Materiales [AeMAT-BIOMEDCO2, ED431E 2018/08], Agencia Estatal de Investigación [AEI] and FEDER funds.

Acknowledgments: C.A. García-González acknowledges to MINECO for a Ramón y Cajal Fellowship [RYC2014-15239].

Conflicts of Interest: The authors declare no conflict of interest.

References

1. Kim, K.K.; Pack, D.W. Microspheres for drug delivery. In *Biomems and Biomedical Nanotechnology*; Springer: Boston, MA, USA, 2006; pp. 19–50.
2. Miao, T.; Wang, J.; Zeng, Y.; Liu, G.; Chen, X. Polysaccharide-Based Controlled Release Systems for Therapeutics Delivery and Tissue Engineering: From Bench to Bedside. *Adv. Sci. (Weinh)* **2018**, *5*, 1700513. [CrossRef] [PubMed]
3. Dormer, N.H.; Berkland, C.J.; Singh, M. Monodispersed microencapsulation technology. In *Microencapsulation in the Food Industry*; Elsevier Science: Amsterdam, The Netherlands, 2014; pp. 111–123.

4. Ganesan, K.; Budtova, T.; Ratke, L.; Gurikov, P.; Baudron, V.; Preibisch, I.; Niemeyer, P.; Smirnova, I.; Milow, B. Review on the production of polysaccharide aerogel particles. *Mater. (Basel)* **2018**, *11*, 2144. [CrossRef] [PubMed]
5. Chan, E.-S. Preparation of Ca-alginate beads containing high oil content: Influence of process variables on encapsulation efficiency and bead properties. *Carbohydr. Polym.* **2011**, *84*, 1267–1275. [CrossRef]
6. Smidsrød, O.; Skja, G. Alginate as immobilization matrix for cells. *Trends Biotechnol.* **1990**, *8*, 71–78. [CrossRef]
7. Fundueanu, G.; Nastruzzi, C.; Carpov, A.; Desbrieres, J.; Rinaudo, M. Physico-chemical characterization of Ca-alginate microparticles produced with different methods. *Biomaterials* **1999**, *20*, 1427–1435. [CrossRef]
8. Zohar-Perez, C.; Chet, I.; Nussinovitch, A. Irregular textural features of dried alginate-filler beads. *Food Hydrocoll.* **2004**, *18*, 249–258. [CrossRef]
9. Chan, E.-S.; Lim, T.-K.; Voo, W.-P.; Pogaku, R.; Tey, B.T.; Zhang, Z. Effect of formulation of alginate beads on their mechanical behavior and stiffness. *Particuology* **2011**, *9*, 228–234. [CrossRef]
10. Burey, P.; Bhandari, B.R.; Howes, T.; Gidley, M.J. Hydrocolloid Gel Particles: Formation, Characterization, and Application. *Crit. Rev. Food Sci. Nutr* **2008**, *48*, 361–377. [CrossRef]
11. Krasaekoopt, W.; Bhandari, B.; Deeth, H. The influence of coating materials on some properties of alginate beads and survivability of microencapsulated probiotic bacteria. *Int. Dairy J.* **2004**, *14*, 737–743. [CrossRef]
12. Krasaekoopt, W.; Bhandari, B.; Deeth, H.C. Survival of probiotics encapsulated in chitosan-coated alginate beads in yoghurt from UHT- and conventionally treated milk during storage. *Lwt-Food Sci. Technol.* **2006**, *39*, 177–183. [CrossRef]
13. Nedovic, V.; Willaert, R. Alginate as a carrier for cell immobilisation. In *Fundamentals of Cell Immobilisation Biotechnology*; Springer Science & Business Media: Dordrecht, The Netherlands, 2013; Volume 8.
14. Chan, E.-S.; Yim, Z.-H.; Phan, S.-H.; Mansa, R.F.; Ravindra, P. Encapsulation of herbal aqueous extract through absorption with ca-alginate hydrogel beads. *Food Bioprod. Process.* **2010**, *88*, 195–201. [CrossRef]
15. Ching, S.H.; Bansal, N.; Bhandari, B. Alginate gel particles–A review of production techniques and physical properties. *Crit. Rev. Food Sci. Nutr* **2017**, *57*, 1133–1152. [CrossRef] [PubMed]
16. Blandino, A.; Macías, M.; Cantero, D. Formation of calcium alginate gel capsules: Influence of sodium alginate and CaCl2 concentration on gelation kinetics. *J. Biosci. Bioeng* **1999**, *88*, 686–689. [CrossRef]
17. Chan, E.-S.; Lee, B.-B.; Ravindra, P.; Poncelet, D. Prediction models for shape and size of ca-alginate macrobeads produced through extrusion–dripping method. *J. Colloid Interface Sci.* **2009**, *338*, 63–72. [CrossRef]
18. Leong, J.-Y.; Lam, W.-H.; Ho, K.-W.; Voo, W.-P.; Lee, M.F.-X.; Lim, H.-P.; Lim, S.-L.; Tey, B.-T.; Poncelet, D.; Chan, E.-S. Advances in fabricating spherical alginate hydrogels with controlled particle designs by ionotropic gelation as encapsulation systems. *Particuology* **2016**, *24*, 44–60. [CrossRef]
19. Prüsse, U.; Bilancetti, L.; Bučko, M.; Bugarski, B.; Bukowski, J.; Gemeiner, P.; Lewińska, D.; Manojlovic, V.; Massart, B.; Nastruzzi, C.; et al. Comparison of different technologies for alginate beads production. *Chem. Pap.* **2008**, *62*, 364. [CrossRef]
20. Zvonar, A.; Kristl, J.; Kerč, J.; Grabnar, P.A. High celecoxib-loaded nanoparticles prepared by a vibrating nozzle device. *J. Microencapsul.* **2009**, *26*, 748–759. [CrossRef]
21. Whelehan, M.; Marison, I.W. Microencapsulation using vibrating technology. *J. Microencapsul.* **2011**, *28*, 669–688. [CrossRef]
22. Del Gaudio, P.; De Cicco, F.; Sansone, F.; Aquino, R.P.; Adami, R.; Ricci, M.; Giovagnoli, S. Alginate beads as a carrier for omeprazole/SBA-15 inclusion compound: A step towards the development of personalized paediatric dosage forms. *Carbohydr. Polym.* **2015**, *133*, 464–472. [CrossRef]
23. Del Gaudio, P.; Colombo, P.; Colombo, G.; Russo, P.; Sonvico, F. Mechanisms of formation and disintegration of alginate beads obtained by prilling. *Int. J. Pharm.* **2005**, *302*, 1–9. [CrossRef]
24. Tran, V.-T.; Benoît, J.-P.; Venier-Julienne, M.-C. Why and how to prepare biodegradable, monodispersed, polymeric microparticles in the field of pharmacy? *Int. J. Pharm.* **2011**, *407*, 1–11. [CrossRef] [PubMed]
25. Seifert, D.B.; Phillips, J.A. Production of small, monodispersed alginate beads for cell immobilization. *Biotechnol. Prog.* **1997**, *13*, 562–568. [CrossRef]
26. Brandenberger, H.; Widmer, F. A new multinozzle encapsulation/immobilisation system to produce uniform beads of alginate. *J. Biotechnol.* **1998**, *63*, 73–80. [CrossRef]

27. Heinzen, C.; Marison, I.; Berger, A.; von Stockar, U. Use of vibration technology for jet break-up for encapsulation of cells, microbes and liquids in monodisperse microcapsules. *Landbauforsch. VölkenrodeSh241* **2002**, 19–25.
28. Eckert, C.; Agnol, W.D.; Dallé, D.; Serpa, V.G.; Maciel, M.J.; Lehn, D.N.; de Souza, C.F.V. Development of alginate-pectin microparticles with dairy whey using vibration technology: Effects of matrix composition on the protection of Lactobacillus spp. from adverse conditions. *Food Res. Int.* **2018**, *113*, 65–73. [CrossRef]
29. Del Gaudio, P.; Russo, P.; Rosaria Lauro, M.; Colombo, P.; Aquino, R.P. Encapsulation of ketoprofen and ketoprofen lysinate by prilling for controlled drug release. *Aaps Pharmscitech* **2009**, *10*, 1178–1185. [CrossRef]
30. Lascol, M.; Bourgeois, S.; Barratier, C.; Marote, P.; Lantéri, P.; Bordes, C. Development of pectin microparticles by using ionotropic gelation with chlorhexidine as cross-linking agent. *Int. J. Pharm.* **2018**, *542*, 205–212. [CrossRef]
31. Auriemma, G.; Cerciello, A.; Aquino, R.P.; Gaudio, P.D.; Fusco, B.M.; Russo, P. Pectin and zinc alginate: The right inner/outer polymer combination for core-shell drug delivery systems. *Pharmaceutics* **2020**, *12*, 87. [CrossRef]
32. Auriemma, G.; Mencherini, T.; Russo, P.; Stigliani, M.; Aquino, R.P.; Del Gaudio, P. Prilling for the development of multi-particulate colon drug delivery systems: Pectin vs. pectin–alginate beads. *Carbohydr. Polym.* **2013**, *92*, 367–373. [CrossRef]
33. Ghosal, S.K.; Talukdar, P.; Pal, T.K. Standardization of a newly designed vibrating capillary apparatus for the preparation of microcapsules. *Chem. Eng. Technol.* **1993**, *16*, 395–398. [CrossRef]
34. Alisch, G.; Brauneis, E.; Pirstadt, B.; Iffland, N.; Brandau, E. Process and Plant for the Production of Spherical Alginate Pellets. U.S. Patent 5472648A, 5 December 1995.
35. Dumas, H.; Tardy, M.; Rochat, M.; Tayot, J. Prilling process applied to collagen solutions. *Drug Dev. Ind. Pharm.* **1992**, *18*, 1395–1409. [CrossRef]
36. Kim, K.; Pack, D.W.; Berkland, C. Microparticles. U.S. Patent 6669961B2, 30 December 2003.
37. Ouwerx, C.; Velings, N.; Mestdagh, M.M.; Axelos, M.A.V. Physico-chemical properties and rheology of alginate gel beads formed with various divalent cations. *Polym. Gels Netw.* **1998**, *6*, 393–408. [CrossRef]
38. Mazzitelli, S.; Tosi, A.; Balestra, C.; Nastruzzi, C.; Luca, G.; Mancuso, F.; Calafiore, R.; Calvitti, M. Production and characterization of alginate microcapsules produced by a vibrational encapsulation device. *J. Biomater. Appl.* **2008**, *23*, 123–145. [CrossRef] [PubMed]
39. Berkland, C.; Kim, K.K.; Pack, D.W. Fabrication of PLG microspheres with precisely controlled and monodisperse size distributions. *J. Control. Release* **2001**, *73*, 59–74. [CrossRef]
40. Poncelet, D. Microencapsulation: Fundamentals, methods and applications. In *Surface Chemistry in Biomedical and Environmental Science*; Springer Dordrecht: Berlin, Germany, 2006; pp. 23–34.
41. Davarcı, F.; Turan, D.; Ozcelik, B.; Poncelet, D. The influence of solution viscosities and surface tension on calcium-alginate microbead formation using dripping technique. *Food Hydrocoll.* **2017**, *62*, 119–127. [CrossRef]
42. Thu, B.; Smidsrod, O.; Skjåk-Bræk, G. Alginate gels-Some structure-function correlations relevant. *Immobil. Cells Basics Appl.* **1996**, *11*, 19–30.
43. Del Gaudio, P.; Auriemma, G.; Russo, P.; Mencherini, T.; Campiglia, P.; Stigliani, M.; Aquino, R.P. Novel co-axial prilling technique for the development of core–shell particles as delayed drug delivery systems. *Eur. J. Pharm. Biopharm.* **2014**, *87*, 541–547. [CrossRef]
44. De Cicco, F.; Russo, P.; Reverchon, E.; García-González, C.A.; Aquino, R.P.; Del Gaudio, P. Prilling and supercritical drying: A successful duo to produce core-shell polysaccharide aerogel beads for wound healing. *Carbohydr. Polym.* **2016**, *147*, 482–489. [CrossRef]
45. Hiorth, M.; Versland, T.; Heikkilä, J.; Tho, I.; Sande, S.A. Immersion coating of pellets with calcium pectinate and chitosan. *Int. J. Pharm.* **2006**, *308*, 25–32. [CrossRef]
46. Wong, T.W.; Nurjaya, S. Drug release property of chitosan–pectinate beads and its changes under the influence of microwave. *Eur. J. Pharm. Biopharm.* **2008**, *69*, 176–188. [CrossRef]
47. Zhang, Y.; Wei, W.; Lv, P.; Wang, L.; Ma, G. Preparation and evaluation of alginate–chitosan microspheres for oral delivery of insulin. *Eur. J. Pharm. Biopharm.* **2011**, *77*, 11–19. [CrossRef] [PubMed]
48. Luo, Y.; Wang, Q. Recent development of chitosan-based polyelectrolyte complexes with natural polysaccharides for drug delivery. *Int. J. Biol. Macromol.* **2014**, *64*, 353–367. [CrossRef]

49. Brandau, T. Preparation of monodisperse controlled release microcapsules. *Int. J. Pharm.* **2002**, *242*, 179–184. [CrossRef]
50. Lin, C.-x.; Zhan, H.-y.; Liu, M.-h.; Fu, S.-y.; Lucia, L.A. Novel preparation and characterization of cellulose microparticles functionalized in ionic liquids. *Langmuir* **2009**, *25*, 10116–10120. [CrossRef]
51. Braun, M.; Guentherberg, N.; Lutz, M.; Magin, A.; Siemer, M.; Swaminathan, V.N.; Linner, B.; Ruslim, F.; Ramierz, G.A.F. Process for Producing Cellulose Beads from Solutions of Cellulose in Ionic Liquid. U.S. Patent 2708690A, 30 December 2010.
52. Pérez-Madrigal, M.M.; Torras, J.; Casanovas, J.; Häring, M.; Alemán, C.; Díaz, D.D. Paradigm shift for preparing versatile m2+-free gels from unmodified sodium alginate. *Biomacromolecules* **2017**, *18*, 2967–2979. [CrossRef] [PubMed]
53. Gurikov, P.; Smirnova, I. Non-conventional methods for gelation of alginate. *Gels* **2018**, *4*, 14. [CrossRef]
54. Groult, S.; Budtova, T. Tuning structure and properties of pectin aerogels. *Eur. Polym. J.* **2018**, *108*, 250–261. [CrossRef]
55. Ratanajiajaroen, P.; Ohshima, M. Preparation of highly porous β-chitin structure through nonsolvent–solvent exchange-induced phase separation and supercritical CO_2 drying. *J. Supercrit. Fluids* **2012**, *68*, 31–38. [CrossRef]
56. Tkalec, G.; Kranvogl, R.; Uzunalić, A.P.; Knez, Ž.; Novak, Z. Optimisation of critical parameters during alginate aerogels' production. *J. Non-Cryst. Solids* **2016**, *443*, 112–117. [CrossRef]
57. Tkalec, G.; Knez, Ž.; Novak, Z. Formation of polysaccharide aerogels in ethanol. *Rsc Adv.* **2015**, *5*, 77362–77371. [CrossRef]
58. Silva, S.S.; Duarte, A.R.C.; Mano, J.F.; Reis, R.L. Design and functionalization of chitin-based microsphere scaffolds. *Green Chem.* **2013**, *15*, 3252–3258. [CrossRef]
59. Oylum, H.; Yilmaz, E.; Yilmaz, O. Preparation of Chitin-g-poly (4-vinylpyridine) Beads. *J. Macromol. Sci. Part. A* **2013**, *50*, 221–229. [CrossRef]
60. Tkalec, G.; Knez, Ž.; Novak, Z. Fast production of high-methoxyl pectin aerogels for enhancing the bioavailability of low-soluble drugs. *J. Supercrit. Fluids* **2015**, *106*, 16–22. [CrossRef]
61. Wan, L.; Heng, P.; Chan, L. Drug encapsulation in alginate microspheres by emulsification. *J. Microencapsul.* **1992**, *9*, 309–316. [CrossRef] [PubMed]
62. Paharia, A.; Yadav, A.K.; Rai, G.; Jain, S.K.; Pancholi, S.S.; Agrawal, G.P. Eudragit-coated pectin microspheres of 5-fluorouracil for colon targeting. *Aaps Pharmscitech* **2007**, *8*, E87–E93. [CrossRef]
63. Vicini, S.; Mauri, M.; Wichert, J.; Castellano, M. Alginate gelling process: Use of bivalent ions rich microspheres. *Polym. Eng. Sci.* **2017**, *57*, 531–536. [CrossRef]
64. Li, J.; He, J.; Huang, Y.; Li, D.; Chen, X. Improving surface and mechanical properties of alginate films by using ethanol as a co-solvent during external gelation. *Carbohydr. Polym.* **2015**, *123*, 208–216. [CrossRef]
65. Donati, I.; Paoletti, S. Material properties of alginates. In *Alginates: Biology and Applications*; Springer: Berlin, Germany; Heidelberg, Germany, 2009; pp. 1–53.
66. Draget, K.I.; Skjåk-Bræk, G.; Stokke, B.T. Similarities and differences between alginic acid gels and ionically crosslinked alginate gels. *Food Hydrocoll.* **2006**, *20*, 170–175. [CrossRef]
67. Tsai, C.S. *Biomacromolecules: Introduction to Structure, Function and Informatics*; John Wiley & Sons: Hoboken, NJ, USA, 2007.
68. Finch, P. *Carbohydrates: Structures, Syntheses and Dynamics*; Springer Science & Business Media: Dordrecht, The Netherlands, 2013.
69. Gavillon, R. Preparation and Characterization of Ultra Porous Cellulosic Materials. Ph.D. Thesis, École Nationale Supérieure des Mines de Paris, Paris, France, 23 March 2007.
70. Trygg, J.; Fardim, P.; Gericke, M.; Mäkilä, E.; Salonen, J. Physicochemical design of the morphology and ultrastructure of cellulose beads. *Carbohydr. Polym.* **2013**, *93*, 291–299. [CrossRef] [PubMed]
71. Mohamed, S.M.K.; Ganesan, K.; Milow, B.; Ratke, L. The effect of zinc oxide (ZnO) addition on the physical and morphological properties of cellulose aerogel beads. *Rsc Adv.* **2015**, *5*, 90193–90201. [CrossRef]
72. Luo, X.; Zhang, L. Creation of regenerated cellulose microspheres with diameter ranging from micron to millimeter for chromatography applications. *J. Chromatogr. A* **2010**, *1217*, 5922–5929. [CrossRef]
73. Blachechen, L.S.; Fardim, P.; Petri, D.F. Multifunctional cellulose beads and their interaction with gram positive bacteria. *Biomacromolecules* **2014**, *15*, 3440–3448. [CrossRef] [PubMed]

74. Mao, B.; Divoux, T.; Snabre, P. Normal force controlled rheology applied to agar gelation. *J. Rheol.* **2016**, *60*, 473–489. [CrossRef]
75. Holland, S.; Tuck, C.; Foster, T. Fluid Gels: A New Feedstock for High Viscosity Jetting. *Food Biophys.* **2018**, *13*, 175–185. [CrossRef]
76. Alba, K.; Kontogiorgos, V. Seaweed polysaccharides (agar, alginate carrageenan). In *Encyclopedia of Food Chemistry*; Elsevier: Amsterdam, The Netherlands, 2018; pp. 240–250.
77. Takemasa, M.; Chiba, A.; Date, M. Gelation mechanism of κ-and ι-carrageenan investigated by correlation between the strain−optical coefficient and the dynamic shear modulus. *Macromolecules* **2001**, *34*, 7427–7434. [CrossRef]
78. Ratnayake, W.S.; Jackson, D.S. Starch gelatinization. *Adv. Food Nutr. Res.* **2009**, *55*, 221–268. [PubMed]
79. Alvarez, M.D.; Fuentes, R.; Canet, W. Effects of pressure, temperature, treatment time, and storage on rheological, textural, and structural properties of heat-induced chickpea gels. *Foods* **2015**, *4*, 80–114. [CrossRef] [PubMed]
80. Calabrese, V.; Muñoz-García, J.C.; Schmitt, J.; da Silva, M.A.; Scott, J.L.; Angulo, J.; Khimyak, Y.Z.; Edler, K.J. Understanding heat driven gelation of anionic cellulose nanofibrils: Combining saturation transfer difference (STD) NMR, small angle X-ray scattering (SAXS) and rheology. *J. Colloid Interface Sci.* **2019**, *535*, 205–213. [CrossRef] [PubMed]
81. Appaw, C.; Gilbert, R.D.; Khan, S.A.; Kadla, J.F. Phase separation and heat-induced gelation characteristics of cellulose acetate in a mixed solvent system. *Cellulose* **2010**, *17*, 533–538. [CrossRef]
82. Fatimi, A.; Tassin, J.-F.; Turczyn, R.; Axelos, M.A.V.; Weiss, P. Gelation studies of a cellulose-based biohydrogel: The influence of pH, temperature and sterilization. *Acta Biomater.* **2009**, *5*, 3423–3432. [CrossRef]
83. Qin, W.; Li, J.; Tu, J.; Yang, H.; Chen, Q.; Liu, H. Fabrication of porous chitosan membranes composed of nanofibers by low temperature thermally induced phase separation, and their adsorption behavior for Cu2. *Carbohydr. Polym.* **2017**, *178*, 338–346. [CrossRef] [PubMed]
84. Mi, F.L.; Tan, Y.C.; Liang, H.C.; Huang, R.N.; Sung, H.W. In vitro evaluation of a chitosan membrane cross-linked with genipin. *J. Biomater. Sci. Polym. Ed.* **2001**, *12*, 835–850. [CrossRef] [PubMed]
85. Mirzaei, B.E.; Ramazani, S.A.A.; Shafiee, M.; Danaei, M. Studies on glutaraldehyde crosslinked chitosan hydrogel properties for drug delivery systems. *Int. J. Polym. Mater. Polym. Biomater.* **2013**, *62*, 605–611. [CrossRef]
86. Dini, E.; Alexandridou, S.; Kiparissides, C. Synthesis and characterization of cross-linked chitosan microspheres for drug delivery applications. *J. Microencapsul* **2003**, *20*, 375–385. [CrossRef] [PubMed]
87. Kulkarni, A.R.; Soppimath, K.S.; Aralaguppi, M.I.; Aminabhavi, T.M.; Rudzinski, W.E. Preparation of cross-linked sodium alginate microparticles using glutaraldehyde in methanol. *Drug Dev. Ind. Pharm.* **2000**, *26*, 1121–1124. [CrossRef]
88. Almeida, P.F.; Almeida, A. Cross-linked alginate-gelatine beads: A new matrix for controlled release of pindolol. *J. Control. Release* **2004**, *97*, 431–439. [CrossRef]
89. Kumar, S.; Haq, I.; Prakash, J.; Raj, A. Improved enzyme properties upon glutaraldehyde cross-linking of alginate entrapped xylanase from Bacillus licheniformis. *Int. J. Biol. Macromol.* **2017**, *98*, 24–33. [CrossRef]
90. Jeon, J.G.; Kim, H.C.; Palem, R.R.; Kim, J.; Kang, T.J. Cross-linking of cellulose nanofiber films with glutaraldehyde for improved mechanical properties. *Mater. Lett.* **2019**, *250*, 99–102. [CrossRef]
91. Buhus, G.; Popa, M.; Desbrieres, J. Hydrogels based on carboxymethylcellulose and gelatin for inclusion and release of chloramphenicol. *J. Bioact. Compat. Polym.* **2009**, *24*, 525–545. [CrossRef]
92. Hongbo, T.; Yanping, L.; Min, S.; Xiguang, W. Preparation and property of crosslinking guar gum. *Polym. J.* **2012**, *44*, 211–216. [CrossRef]
93. Sandolo, C.; Matricardi, P.; Alhaique, F.; Coviello, T. Effect of temperature and cross-linking density on rheology of chemical cross-linked guar gum at the gel point. *Food Hydrocoll.* **2009**, *23*, 210–220. [CrossRef]
94. Usha, R.; Ramasami, T. Structure and conformation of intramolecularly cross-linked collagen. *Colloids Surf. B Biointerfaces* **2005**, *41*, 21–24. [CrossRef] [PubMed]
95. Wu, X.; Black, L.; Santacana-Laffitte, G.; Patrick Jr, C.W. Preparation and assessment of glutaraldehyde-crosslinked collagen-chitosan hydrogels for adipose tissue engineering. *J. Biomed. Mater. Res. Part. A* **2007**, *81*, 59–65. [CrossRef] [PubMed]
96. George, M.; Abraham, T. pH sensitive alginate-guar gum hydrogel for the controlled delivery of protein drugs. *Int. J. Pharm.* **2007**, *335*, 123–129. [CrossRef] [PubMed]

97. Distantina, S.; Rochmadi, S.; Fahrurrozi, M.; Wiratni, M. Preparation of hydrogel based on glutaraldehyde-crosslinked carrageenan. In Proceedings of the 3rd International Conference on Chemistry and Chemical Engineering IPCBEE, Singapore, 26–28 February 2012.
98. Distantina, S.; Rochmadi, R.; Fahrurrozi, M.; Wiratni, W. Preparation and characterization of glutaraldehyde-crosslinked kappa carrageenan hydrogel. *Eng. J.* **2013**, *17*, 57–66. [CrossRef]
99. Baki, E.; Denkbas, M.; Odabasi, E.; Kiliçay, N.O. Human serum albumin (HSA) adsorption with chitosan microspheres. *J. Appl. Polym. Sci.* **2002**, *86*, 3035–3039.
100. Nayak, U.Y.; Gopal, S.; Mutalik, S.; Ranjith, A.K.; Reddy, M.S.; Gupta, P.; Udupa, N. Glutaraldehyde cross-linked chitosan microspheres for controlled delivery of zidovudine. *J. Microencapsul.* **2009**, *26*, 214–222. [CrossRef] [PubMed]
101. Rinki, K.; Dutta, P.K.; Hunt, A.J.; Macquarrie, D.J.; Clark, J.H. Chitosan aerogels exhibiting high surface area for biomedical application: Preparation, characterization, and antibacterial study. *Int. J. Polym. Mater.* **2011**, *60*, 988–999. [CrossRef]
102. Thakkar, H.P.; Murthy, R.R. Effect of cross-linking agent on the characteristics of celecoxib loaded chitosan microspheres. *Asian, J. Pharm. (Ajp): Free Full Text. Artic. Asian J. Pharm.* **2014**, *2*. [CrossRef]
103. Gangurde, H.H.; Chavan, N.V.; Mundada, A.S.; Derle, D.V.; Tamizharasi, S. Biodegradable Chitosan-Based Ambroxol Hydrochloride Microspheres: Effect of Cross-Linking Agents. *J. Young Pharm.* **2011**, *3*, 9–14. [CrossRef]
104. Lee, K.Y.; Rowley, J.A.; Eiselt, P.; Moy, E.M.; Bouhadir, K.H.; Mooney, D.J. Controlling mechanical and swelling properties of alginate hydrogels independently by cross-linker type and cross-linking density. *Macromolecules* **2000**, *33*, 4291–4294. [CrossRef]
105. Pedroso-Santana, S.; Fleitas-Salazar, N. Ionotropic gelation method in the synthesis of nanoparticles/microparticles for biomedical purposes. *Polym. Int.* **2020**, *69*, 443–447. [CrossRef]
106. Racoviță, S.; Vasiliu, S.; Popa, M.; Luca, C. Polysaccharides based on micro-and nanoparticles obtained by ionic gelation and their applications as drug delivery systems. *Rev. Roum. De Chim.* **2009**, *54*, 709–718.
107. Giri, T.K.; Verma, S.; Alexander, A.; Ajazuddin, B.H.; Tripathy, M.; Tripathi, D. Crosslinked biodegradable alginate hydrogel floating beads for stomach site specific controlled delivery of metronidazole. *Farmacia* **2013**, *61*, 533–550.
108. Patil, P.; Chavanke, D.; Wagh, M. A review on ionotropic gelation method: Novel approach for controlled gastroretentive gelispheres. *Int J. Pharm Pharm Sci* **2012**, *4*, 27–32.
109. Laurienzo, P. Marine polysaccharides in pharmaceutical applications: An overview. *Mar. Drugs* **2010**, *8*, 2435–2465. [CrossRef]
110. Patil, J.; Kamalapur, M.; Marapur, S.; Kadam, D. Ionotropic gelation and polyelectrolyte complexation: The novel techniques to design hydrogel particulate sustained, modulated drug delivery system: A review. *Dig. J. Nanomater. Biostruct.* **2010**, *5*, 241–248.
111. Garner, J.; Park, K. Chemically modified natural polysaccharides to form gels. *Polysacch. Cham Springer Int. Publ.* **2015**, 1555–1582.
112. DeRamos, C.M.; Irwin, A.E.; Nauss, J.L.; Stout, B.E. 13C NMR and molecular modeling studies of alginic acid binding with alkaline earth and lanthanide metal ions. *Inorg. Chim. Acta* **1997**, *256*, 69–75. [CrossRef]
113. Mărțău, G.A.; Mihai, M.; Vodnar, D.C. The use of chitosan, alginate, and pectin in the biomedical and food sector—biocompatibility, bioadhesiveness, and biodegradability. *Polymers* **2019**, *11*, 1837. [CrossRef]
114. Braccini, I.; Pérez, S. Molecular basis of C(2+)-induced gelation in alginates and pectins: The egg-box model revisited. *Biomacromolecules* **2001**, *2*, 1089–1096. [CrossRef] [PubMed]
115. Shu, X.; Zhu, K. Chitosan/gelatin microspheres prepared by modified emulsification and ionotropic gelation. *J. Microencapsul.* **2001**, *18*, 237–245. [PubMed]
116. Shu, X.; Zhu, K. A novel approach to prepare tripolyphosphate/chitosan complex beads for controlled release drug delivery. *Int. J. Pharm.* **2000**, *201*, 51–58. [CrossRef]
117. Panos, I.; Acosta, N.; Heras, A. New drug delivery systems based on chitosan. *Curr. Drug Discov. Technol.* **2008**, *5*, 333–341. [CrossRef] [PubMed]
118. Smrdel, P.; Bogataj, M.; Mrhar, A. The influence of selected parameters on the size and shape of alginate beads prepared by ionotropic gelation. *Sci. Pharm.* **2008**, *76*, 77–90. [CrossRef]
119. Lee, K.Y.; Mooney, D.J. Alginate: Properties and biomedical applications. *Prog. Polym. Sci.* **2012**, *37*, 106–126. [CrossRef]

120. Draget, K.I. Alginates. In *Handbook of Hydrocolloids*; Elsevier: Amsterdam, The Netherlands, 2009; pp. 807–828.
121. Sabra, W.; Zeng, A.-P.; Deckwer, W.-D. Bacterial alginate: Physiology, product quality and process aspects. *Appl. Microbiol. Biotechnol.* **2001**, *56*, 315–325. [CrossRef]
122. d'Ayala, G.G.; Malinconico, M.; Laurienzo, P. Marine derived polysaccharides for biomedical applications: Chemical modification approaches. *Molecules* **2008**, *13*, 2069–2106. [CrossRef]
123. Mørch, Ý.A.; Donati, I.; Strand, B.L.; Skjåk-Bræk, G. Effect of Ca^{2+}, Ba^{2+}, and Sr^{2+} on Alginate Microbeads. *Biomacromolecules* **2006**, *7*, 1471–1480. [CrossRef]
124. Montanucci, P.; Terenzi, S.; Santi, C.; Pennoni, I.; Bini, V.; Pescara, T.; Basta, G.; Calafiore, R. Insights in behavior of variably formulated alginate-based microcapsules for cell transplantation. *Biomed. Res. Int.* **2015**, *2015*, 965804. [CrossRef]
125. Brus, J.; Urbanova, M.; Czernek, J.; Pavelkova, M.; Kubova, K.; Vyslouzil, J.; Abbrent, S.; Konefal, R.; Horský, J.; Vetchy, D. Structure and dynamics of alginate gels cross-linked by polyvalent ions probed via solid state NMR spectroscopy. *Biomacromolecules* **2017**, *18*, 2478–2488. [CrossRef]
126. BeMiller, J.N.; Whistler, R.L. *Industrial Gums: Polysaccharides and Their Derivatives*; Academic Press: Cambridge, MA, USA, 2012.
127. Clark, A.H.; Ross-Murphy, S.B. Structural and mechanical properties of biopolymer gels. *Biopolym. Adv. Polym. Sci.* **1987**, *83*, 57–192.
128. Chambin, O.; Dupuis, G.; Champion, D.; Voilley, A.; Pourcelot, Y. Colon-specific drug delivery: Influence of solution reticulation properties upon pectin beads performance. *Int. J. Pharm.* **2006**, *321*, 86–93. [CrossRef] [PubMed]
129. El-Gibaly, I. Oral delayed-release system based on Zn-pectinate gel (ZPG) microparticles as an alternative carrier to calcium pectinate beads for colonic drug delivery. *Int. J. Pharm.* **2002**, *232*, 199–211. [CrossRef]
130. Braccini, I.; Grasso, R.P.; Pérez, S. Conformational and configurational features of acidic polysaccharides and their interactions with calcium ions: A molecular modeling investigation. *Carbohydr. Res.* **1999**, *317*, 119–130. [CrossRef]
131. Willaert, R.; Nedovic, V. *Fundamentals of Cell Immobilisation Biotechnology*; Kluwer: Alfen am Rhein, The Netherlands, 2004.
132. Ahmed, S. *Alginates: Applications in the Biomedical and Food Industries*; John Wiley & Sons: Hoboken, NJ, USA, 2019.
133. Brejnholt, S.M. Pectin. Food StabilisersThick. *Gelling Agents* **2009**, 237–265.
134. Chan, S.Y.; Choo, W.S.; Young, D.J.; Loh, X.J. Pectin as a rheology modifier: Origin, structure, commercial production and rheology. *Carbohydr. Polym.* **2017**, *161*, 118–139. [CrossRef]
135. Rinaudo, M. Gelation of polysaccharides. *J. Intell. Mater. Syst. Struct.* **1993**, *4*, 210–215. [CrossRef]
136. Toft, K.; Grasdalen, H.; Smidsrød, O. *Synergistic Gelation of Alginates and Pectins*; ACS Publications: Washington, DC, USA, 1986.
137. Hasnain, M.S.; Nayak, A.K. *Natural Polysaccharides in Drug Delivery and Biomedical Applications*; Academic Press: Cambridge, MA, USA, 2019.
138. Sacco, P.; Paoletti, S.; Cok, M.; Asaro, F.; Abrami, M.; Grassi, M.; Donati, I. Insight into the ionotropic gelation of chitosan using tripolyphosphate and pyrophosphate as cross-linkers. *Int. J. Biol. Macromol.* **2016**, *92*, 476–483. [CrossRef]
139. Tharanathan, R.N.; Kittur, F.S. Chitin—The undisputed biomolecule of great potential. *Crit. Rev. Food Sci. Nutr.* **2003**, *43*, 61–87. [CrossRef]
140. Santander-Ortega, M.; Peula-García, J.; Goycoolea, F.; Ortega-Vinuesa, J. Chitosan nanocapsules: Effect of chitosan molecular weight and acetylation degree on electrokinetic behaviour and colloidal stability. *Colloids Surf. B Biointerfaces* **2011**, *82*, 571–580. [CrossRef] [PubMed]
141. Bodmeier, R.; Oh, K.-H.; Pramar, Y. Preparation and evaluation of drug-containing chitosan beads. *Drug Dev. Ind. Pharm.* **1989**, *15*, 1475–1494. [CrossRef]
142. Kim, S.-K. *Chitin and Chitosan Derivatives: Advances in Drug Discovery and Developments*; CRC Press: Boca Raton, FL, USA, 2013.
143. Sreekumar, S.; Goycoolea, F.M.; Moerschbacher, B.M.; Rivera-Rodriguez, G.R. Parameters influencing the size of chitosan-TPP nano- and microparticles. *Sci. Rep.* **2018**, *8*, 4695. [CrossRef] [PubMed]
144. Ko, J.; Park, H.J.; Hwang, S.J.; Park, J.; Lee, J. Preparation and characterization of chitosan microparticles intended for controlled drug delivery. *Int. J. Pharm.* **2002**, *249*, 165–174. [CrossRef]

145. Barakat, N.S.; Almurshedi, A.S. Preparation and characterization of chitosan microparticles for oral sustained delivery of gliclazide: In vitro/in vivo evaluation. *Drug Dev. Res.* **2011**, *72*, 235–246. [CrossRef]
146. Hassani, S.; Laouini, A.; Fessi, H.; Charcosset, C. Preparation of chitosan-TPP nanoparticles using microengineered membranes-Effect of parameters and encapsulation of tacrine. *Colloids Surf. A Physicochem. Eng. Asp.* **2015**, *482*, 34–43. [CrossRef]
147. Sacco, P.; Furlani, F.; De Marzo, G.; Marsich, E.; Paoletti, S.; Donati, I. Concepts for developing physical gels of chitosan and of chitosan derivatives. *Gels* **2018**, *4*, 67. [CrossRef]
148. Huang, Y.; Lapitsky, Y. Monovalent salt enhances colloidal stability during the formation of chitosan/tripolyphosphate microgels. *Langmuir* **2011**, *27*, 10392–10399. [CrossRef]
149. Periayah, M.H.; Halim, A.S.; Saad, A.Z.M. Chitosan: A promising marine polysaccharide for biomedical research. *Pharm. Rev.* **2016**, *10*, 39–42. [CrossRef]
150. Chan, L.W.; Lee, H.Y.; Heng, P.W. Mechanisms of external and internal gelation and their impact on the functions of alginate as a coat and delivery system. *Carbohydr. Polym.* **2006**, *63*, 176–187. [CrossRef]
151. Pavelková, M.; Kubová, K.; Vysloužil, J.; Kejdušová, M.; Vetchý, D.; Celer, V.; Molinková, D.; Lobová, D.; Pechová, A.; Vysloužil, J.; et al. Biological effects of drug-free alginate beads cross-linked by copper ions prepared using external ionotropic gelation. *Aaps Pharmscitech* **2017**, *18*, 1343–1354.
152. Zhang, H.; Tumarkin, E.; Peerani, R.; Nie, Z.; Sullan, R.M.; Walker, G.C.; Kumacheva, E. Microfluidic production of biopolymer microcapsules with controlled morphology. *J. Am. Chem. Soc.* **2006**, *128*, 12205–12210. [CrossRef] [PubMed]
153. Mikkelsen, A.; Elgsaeter, A. Density distribution of calcium-induced alginate gels. A numerical study. *Biopolym.: Orig. Res. Biomol.* **1995**, *36*, 17–41. [CrossRef]
154. Pawar, S.N.; Edgar, K.J. Alginate derivatization: A review of chemistry, properties and applications. *Biomaterials* **2012**, *33*, 3279–3305. [CrossRef]
155. Qun, L.; Ming, X.W.; Ting, Y.W.; Dong, L.X.; Yuan, Y.R.; Yun, L.J.; Jun, M.X. Studies on the membrane strength of alginate/chitosan microcapsule prepared by emulsification/internal gelation method. *Chem. Res. Chin. Univ.* **2002**, *7*.
156. Ahmed, M.M.; El-Rasoul, S.A.; Auda, S.H.; Ibrahim, M.A. Emulsification/internal gelation as a method for preparation of diclofenac sodium–sodium alginate microparticles. *Saudi Pharm. J.* **2013**, *21*, 61–69. [CrossRef]
157. Choi, B.; Park, H.J.; Hwang, S.; Park, J. Preparation of alginate beads for floating drug delivery system: Effects of CO_2 gas-forming agents. *Int. J. Pharm.* **2002**, *239*, 81–91. [CrossRef]
158. Vandenberg, G.W.; De La Noüe, J. Evaluation of protein release from chitosan-alginate microcapsules produced using external or internal gelation. *J. Microencapsul.* **2001**, *18*, 433–441. [CrossRef]
159. Martins, E.; Renard, D.; Davy, J.; Marquis, M.; Poncelet, D. Oil core microcapsules by inverse gelation technique. *J. Microencapsul* **2015**, *32*, 86–95. [CrossRef]
160. Abang, S.; Chan, E.-S.; Poncelet, D. Effects of process variables on the encapsulation of oil in ca-alginate capsules using an inverse gelation technique. *J. Microencapsul.* **2012**, *29*, 417–428. [CrossRef]
161. Martins, E.; Poncelet, D.; Rodrigues, R.C.; Renard, D. Oil encapsulation in core-shell alginate capsules by inverse gelation II: Comparison between dripping techniques using W/O or O/W emulsions. *J. Microencapsul.* **2017**, *34*, 522–534. [CrossRef] [PubMed]
162. Kabir, S.M.F.; Sikdar, P.P.; Haque, B.; Bhuiyan, M.A.R.; Ali, A.; Islam, M.N. Cellulose-based hydrogel materials: Chemistry, properties and their prospective applications. *Prog. Biomater.* **2018**, *7*, 153–174. [CrossRef] [PubMed]
163. Chirani, N.; Gritsch, L.; Motta, F.L.; Fare, S. History and applications of hydrogels. *J. Biomed. Sci.* **2015**, *4*.
164. Nicodemus, G.D.; Bryant, S.J. Cell encapsulation in biodegradable hydrogels for tissue engineering applications. *Tissue Eng Part. B Rev.* **2008**, *14*, 149–165. [CrossRef]
165. Jen, A.C.; Wake, M.C.; Mikos, A.G. Hydrogels for cell immobilization. *Biotechnol. Bioeng.* **1996**, *50*, 357–364. [CrossRef]
166. Bidarra, S.J.; Barrias, C.C.; Granja, P.L. Injectable alginate hydrogels for cell delivery in tissue engineering. *Acta Biomater.* **2014**, *10*, 1646–1662. [CrossRef]
167. Racheva, M.; Julich-Gruner, K.K.; Nöchel, U.; Neffe, A.T.; Wischke, C.; Lendlein, A. Influence of drying procedures on network formation and properties of hydrogels from functionalized gelatin. *Macromolecular Symposia* **2018**, *334*, 24–32. [CrossRef]

168. Hua, S.; Ma, H.; Li, X.; Yang, H.; Wang, A. pH-sensitive sodium alginate/poly(vinyl alcohol) hydrogel beads prepared by combined Ca^{2+} crosslinking and freeze-thawing cycles for controlled release of diclofenac sodium. *Int. J. Biol. Macromol.* **2010**, *46*, 517–523. [CrossRef]
169. Rodríguez-Dorado, R.; López-Iglesias, C.; García-González, C.A.; Auriemma, G.; Aquino, R.P.; Del Gaudio, P. Design of aerogels, cryogels and xerogels of alginate: Effect of molecular weight, gelation conditions and drying method on particles' micromeritics. *Molecules* **2019**, *24*, 1049. [CrossRef]
170. Auriemma, G.; Cerciello, A.; Aquino, R.P. NSAIDS: Design and development of innovative oral delivery systems. *Nonsteroidal Anti-Inflamm. Drugs* **2017**, *9*, 51000.
171. Al-Muhtaseb, S.A.; Ritter, J.A. Preparation and properties of resorcinol-formaldehyde organic and carbon gels. *Adv. Mater.* **2003**, *15*, 101–114. [CrossRef]
172. Job, N.; Pirard, R.; Marien, J.; Pirard, J.-P. Porous carbon xerogels with texture tailored by pH control during sol–gel process. *Carbon* **2004**, *42*, 619–628. [CrossRef]
173. Czakkel, O.; Marthi, K.; Geissler, E.; László, K. Influence of drying on the morphology of resorcinol–formaldehyde-based carbon gels. *Microporous Mesoporous Mater.* **2005**, *86*, 124–133. [CrossRef]
174. Zubizarreta, L.; Arenillas, A.; Menéndez, J.; Pis, J.J.; Pirard, J.-P.; Job, N. Microwave drying as an effective method to obtain porous carbon xerogels. *J. Non-Cryst. Solids* **2008**, *354*, 4024–4026. [CrossRef]
175. Zubizarreta, L.; Arenillas, A.; Domínguez, A.; Menéndez, J.; Pis, J. Development of microporous carbon xerogels by controlling synthesis conditions. *J. Non-Cryst. Solids* **2008**, *354*, 817–825. [CrossRef]
176. Ganesan, K.; Dennstedt, A.; Barowski, A.; Ratke, L. Design of aerogels, cryogels and xerogels of cellulose with hierarchical porous structures. *Mater. Des.* **2016**, *92*, 345–355. [CrossRef]
177. Léonard, A.; Job, N.; Blacher, S.; Pirard, J.-P.; Crine, M.; Jomaa, W. Suitability of convective air drying for the production of porous resorcinol-formaldehyde and carbon xerogels. *Carbon* **2005**, *43*, 1808–1811. [CrossRef]
178. Job, N.; Panariello, F.; Marien, J.; Crine, M.; Pirard, J.-P.; Léonard, A. Synthesis optimization of organic xerogels produced from convective air-drying of resorcinol-formaldehyde gels. *J. Non-Cryst. Solids* **2006**, *352*, 24–34. [CrossRef]
179. Menéndez, J.; Juárez-Pérez, E.; Ruisánchez, E.; Calvo, E.; Arenillas, A. A microwave-based method for the synthesis of carbon xerogel spheres. *Carbon* **2012**, *50*, 3555–3560. [CrossRef]
180. Pour, G.; Beauger, C.; Rigacci, A.; Budtova, T. Xerocellulose: Lightweight, porous and hydrophobic cellulose prepared via ambient drying. *J. Mater. Sci.* **2015**, *50*, 4526–4535. [CrossRef]
181. Auriemma, G.; Del Gaudio, P.; Barba, A.A.; d'Amore, M.; Aquino, R.P. A combined technique based on prilling and microwave assisted treatments for the production of ketoprofen controlled release dosage forms. *Int. J. Pharm.* **2011**, *415*, 196–205. [CrossRef]
182. Aquino, R.P.; Auriemma, G.; d'Amore, M.; D'Ursi, A.M.; Mencherini, T.; Del Gaudio, P. Piroxicam loaded alginate beads obtained by prilling/microwave tandem technique: Morphology and drug release. *Carbohydr. Polym.* **2012**, *89*, 740–748. [CrossRef] [PubMed]
183. Nussinovitch, A. *Polymer Macro- and Micro-Gel Beads: Fundamentals and Applications*; Springer Science & Business Media: Berlin, Germany, 2010.
184. Stefanescu, D.M. *Science and Engineering of Casting Solidification*; Springer: Midtown Manhattan, NY, USA, 2015.
185. Betz, M.; García-González, C.; Subrahmanyam, R.; Smirnova, I.; Kulozik, U. Preparation of novel whey protein-based aerogels as drug carriers for life science applications. *J. Supercrit. Fluids* **2012**, *72*, 111–119. [CrossRef]
186. Jiménez-Saelices, C.; Seantier, B.; Cathala, B.; Grohens, Y. Spray freeze-dried nanofibrillated cellulose aerogels with thermal superinsulating properties. *Carbohydr. Polym.* **2017**, *157*, 105–113. [CrossRef] [PubMed]
187. Tamon, H.; Ishizaka, H.; Yamamoto, T.; Suzuki, T. Influence of freeze-drying conditions on the mesoporosity of organic gels as carbon precursors. *Carbon* **2000**, *38*, 1099–1105. [CrossRef]
188. Babić, B.; Kaluđerović, B.; Vračar, L.; Krstajić, N. Characterization of carbon cryogel synthesized by sol-gel polycondensation and freeze-drying. *Carbon* **2004**, *42*, 2617–2624. [CrossRef]
189. Tonanon, N.; Siyasukh, A.; Tanthapanichakoon, W.; Nishihara, H.; Mukai, S.; Tamon, H. Improvement of mesoporosity of carbon cryogels by ultrasonic irradiation. *Carbon* **2005**, *43*, 525–531. [CrossRef]
190. Pääkkö, M.; Vapaavuori, J.; Silvennoinen, R.; Kosonen, H.; Ankerfors, M.; Lindström, T.; Berglund, L.A.; Ikkala, O. Long and entangled native cellulose I nanofibers allow flexible aerogels and hierarchically porous templates for functionalities. *Soft Matter* **2008**, *4*, 2492–2499. [CrossRef]

191. García-González, C.; Alnaief, M.; Smirnova, I. Polysaccharide-based aerogels—Promising biodegradable carriers for drug delivery systems. *Carbohydr. Polym.* **2011**, *86*, 1425–1438. [CrossRef]
192. Maleki, H.; Durães, L.; García-González, C.A.; del Gaudio, P.; Portugal, A.; Mahmoudi, M. Synthesis and biomedical applications of aerogels: Possibilities and challenges. *Adv. Colloid Interface Sci.* **2016**, *236*, 1–27. [CrossRef]
193. Smirnova, I.; Gurikov, P. Aerogels in chemical engineering: Strategies toward tailor-made aerogels. *Annu. Rev. Chem. Biomol. Eng.* **2017**, *8*, 307–334. [CrossRef] [PubMed]
194. Nita, L.E.; Ghilan, A.; Rusu, A.G.; Neamtu, I.; Chiriac, A.P. New trends in bio-based aerogels. *Pharmaceutics* **2020**, *12*, 449. [CrossRef]
195. Sanli, D.; Bozbag, S.; Erkey, C. Synthesis of nanostructured materials using supercritical CO_2: Part, I. Physical transformations. *J. Mater. Sci.* **2012**, *47*, 2995–3025. [CrossRef]
196. Diamond, L.W.; Akinfiev, N.N. Solubility of CO_2 in water from 1.5 to 100 C and from 0.1 to 100 MPa: Evaluation of literature data and thermodynamic modelling. *Fluid Phase Equilibria* **2003**, *208*, 265–290. [CrossRef]
197. Pasquali, I.; Bettini, R. Are pharmaceutics really going supercritical? *Int. J. Pharm.* **2008**, *364*, 176–187. [CrossRef] [PubMed]
198. Liu, N.; Zhang, S.; Fu, R.; Dresselhaus, M.S.; Dresselhaus, G. Carbon aerogel spheres prepared via alcohol supercritical drying. *Carbon* **2006**, *44*, 2430–2436. [CrossRef]
199. Russo, P.; Zacco, R.; Rekkas, D.M.; Politis, S.; Garofalo, E.; Del Gaudio, P.; Aquino, R.P. Application of experimental design for the development of soft-capsules through a prilling, inverse gelation process. *J. Drug Deliv. Sci. Technol.* **2019**, *49*, 577–585. [CrossRef]
200. Rodríguez-Dorado, R.; Landín, M.; Altai, A.; Russo, P.; Aquino, R.P.; Del Gaudio, P. A novel method for the production of core-shell microparticles by inverse gelation optimized with artificial intelligent tools. *Int. J. Pharm.* **2018**, *538*, 97–104. [CrossRef]
201. Cerciello, A.; Del Gaudio, P.; Granata, V.; Sala, M.; Aquino, R.P.; Russo, P. Synergistic effect of divalent cations in improving technological properties of cross-linked alginate beads. *Int. J. Biol. Macromol.* **2017**, *101*, 100–106. [CrossRef]
202. Cerciello, A.; Auriemma, G.; Morello, S.; Pinto, A.; Del Gaudio, P.; Russo, P.; Aquino, R.P. Design and in vivo anti-inflammatory effect of ketoprofen delayed delivery systems. *J. Pharm. Sci.* **2015**, *104*, 3451–3458. [CrossRef]
203. Cerciello, A.; Auriemma, G.; Morello, S.; Aquino, R.P.; Del Gaudio, P.; Russo, P. Prednisolone delivery platforms: Capsules and beads combination for a right timing therapy. *PLoS ONE* **2016**, *11*, e0160266. [CrossRef]
204. Cerciello, A.; Auriemma, G.; Del Gaudio, P.; Cantarini, M.; Aquino, R.P. Natural polysaccharides platforms for oral controlled release of ketoprofen lysine salt. *Drug Dev. Ind. Pharm.* **2016**, *42*, 2063–2069. [CrossRef] [PubMed]
205. Cerciello, A.; Auriemma, G.; Del Gaudio, P.; Sansone, F.; Aquino, R.P.; Russo, P. A novel core-shell chronotherapeutic system for the oral administration of ketoprofen. *J. Drug Deliv. Sci. Technol.* **2016**, *32*, 126–131. [CrossRef]
206. Auriemma, G.; Cerciello, A.; Sansone, F.; Pinto, A.; Morello, S.; Aquino, R.P. Polysaccharides based gastroretentive system to sustain piroxicam release: Development and in vivo prolonged anti-inflammatory effect. *Int. J. Biol. Macromol.* **2018**, *120*, 2303–2312. [CrossRef]
207. Russo, P.; Morello, S.; Pinto, A.; Del Gaudio, P.; Auriemma, G.; Aquino, R.P. Zinc and calcium cations combination in the production of floating alginate beads as prednisolone delivery systems. *Molecules* **2020**, *25*, 1140. [CrossRef] [PubMed]
208. Del Gaudio, P.; Auriemma, G.; Mencherini, T.; Della Porta, G.; Reverchon, E.; Aquino, R.P. Design of alginate-based aerogel for nonsteroidal anti-inflammatory drugs controlled delivery systems using prilling and supercritical-assisted drying. *J. Pharm. Sci.* **2013**, *102*, 185–194. [CrossRef] [PubMed]
209. Della Porta, G.; Del Gaudio, P.; De Cicco, F.; Aquino, R.P.; Reverchon, E. Supercritical drying of alginate beads for the development of aerogel biomaterials: Optimization of process parameters and exchange solvents. *Ind. Eng. Chem. Res.* **2013**, *52*, 12003–12009. [CrossRef]
210. Chan, L.W.; Jin, Y.; Heng, P.W.S. Cross-linking mechanisms of calcium and zinc in production of alginate microspheres. *Int. J. Pharm.* **2002**, *242*, 255–258. [CrossRef]

211. Rasel, M.A.T.; Hasan, M. Formulation and evaluation of floating alginate beads of diclofenac sodium. *Dhaka Univ. J. Pharm. Sci.* **2012**, *11*, 29–35. [CrossRef]
212. Celli, G.B.; Ghanem, A.; Brooks, M.S. Development and evaluation of floating alginate microspheres for oral delivery of anthocyanins—A preliminary investigation. *Food Sci. Nutr.* **2016**, *5*, 713–721. [CrossRef]
213. Timilsena, Y.P.; Akanbi, T.O.; Khalid, N.; Adhikari, B.; Barrow, C.J. Complex coacervation: Principles, mechanisms and applications in microencapsulation. *Int. J. Biol. Macromol.* **2019**, *121*, 1276–1286. [CrossRef]
214. Yadav, S.K.; Khan, G.; Bonde, G.V.; Bansal, M.; Mishra, B. Design, optimization and characterizations of chitosan fortified calcium alginate microspheres for the controlled delivery of dual drugs. *Artif. CellsNanomed. Biotechnol.* **2018**, *46*, 1180–1193. [CrossRef] [PubMed]
215. Butstraen, C.; Salaün, F. Preparation of microcapsules by complex coacervation of gum Arabic and chitosan. *Carbohydr. Polym.* **2014**, *99*, 608–616. [CrossRef] [PubMed]
216. Tiyaboonchai, W.; Ritthidej, G.C. Development of indomethacin sustained release microcapsules using chitosan-carboxymethyl-cellulose complex coacervation. *Development* **2003**, *25*, 246.
217. Lisuzzo, L.; Cavallaro, G.; Parisi, F.; Milioto, S.; Fakhrullin, R.; Lazzara, G. Core/shell gel beads with embedded halloysite nanotubes for controlled drug release. *Coatings* **2019**, *9*, 70. [CrossRef]
218. Lucinda-Silva, R.M.; Salgado, H.R.N.; Evangelista, R.C. Alginate-chitosan systems: In vitro controlled release of triamcinolone and in vivo gastrointestinal transit. *Carbohydr. Polym.* **2010**, *81*, 260–268. [CrossRef]
219. Ren, Z.; Zhang, X.; Guo, Y.; Han, K.; Huo, N. Preparation and in vitro delivery performance of chitosan–alginate microcapsule for IgG. *Food Agric. Immunol.* **2017**, *28*, 1–13. [CrossRef]
220. Assifaoui, A.; Loupiac, C.; Chambin, O.; Cayot, P. Structure of calcium and zinc pectinate films investigated by FTIR spectroscopy. *Carbohydr. Res.* **2010**, *345*, 929–933. [CrossRef]
221. Das, S.; Ng, K.-Y.; Ho, P.C. Formulation and optimization of zinc-pectinate beads for the controlled delivery of resveratrol. *Aaps Pharmscitech* **2010**, *11*, 729–742. [CrossRef]
222. Mallepally, R.R.; Bernard, I.; Marin, M.A.; Ward, K.R.; McHugh, M.A. Superabsorbent alginate aerogels. *J. Supercrit. Fluids* **2013**, *79*, 202–208. [CrossRef]
223. Gurikov, P.; Smirnova, I. Amorphization of drugs by adsorptive precipitation from supercritical solutions: A review. *J. Supercrit. Fluids* **2018**, *132*, 105–125. [CrossRef]
224. López-Iglesias, C.; Barros, J.; Ardao, I.; Monteiro, F.J.; Alvarez-Lorenzo, C.; Gómez-Amoza, J.L.; García-González, C.A. Vancomycin-loaded chitosan aerogel particles for chronic wound applications. *Carbohydr. Polym.* **2019**, *204*, 223–231. [CrossRef] [PubMed]
225. Veronovski, A.; Tkalec, G.; Knez, Ž.; Novak, Z. Characterisation of biodegradable pectin aerogels and their potential use as drug carriers. *Carbohydr. Polym.* **2014**, *113*, 272–278. [CrossRef] [PubMed]
226. Halamoda-Kenzaoui, B.; Baconnier, S.; Bastogne, T.; Bazile, D.; Boisseau, P.; Borchard, G.; Borgos, S.E.; Calzolai, L.; Cederbrant, K.; Di Felice, G.; et al. Bridging communities in the field of nanomedicine. *Regul. Toxicol. Pharmacol.* **2019**, *106*, 187–196. [CrossRef]
227. Dalwadi, C.; Patel, G. Implementation of "Quality by Design (QbD)" Approach for the Development of 5-Fluorouracil Loaded Thermosensitive Hydrogel. *Curr. Drug Deliv.* **2016**, *13*, 512–527. [CrossRef]
228. Schmutz, M.; Borges, O.; Jesus, S.; Borchard, G.; Perale, G.; Zinn, M.; Sips, Ä.A.; Soeteman-Hernandez, L.G.; Wick, P.; Som, C. A Methodological Safe-by-Design Approach for the Development of Nanomedicines. *Front. Bioeng. Biotechnol.* **2020**, *8*, 258. [CrossRef]
229. van de Poel, I.; Robaey, Z. Safe-by-Design: From Safety to Responsibility. *NanoEthics* **2017**, *11*, 297–306. [CrossRef]
230. Reason, J. Safety paradoxes and safety culture. *Inj. Control. Saf. Promot.* **2000**, *7*, 3–14. [CrossRef]
231. Maresova, P.; Hajek, L.; Krejcar, O.; Storek, M.; Kuca, K. New Regulations on Medical Devices in Europe: Are They an Opportunity for Growth? *Adm. Sci.* **2020**, *10*, 16. [CrossRef]

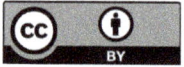

© 2020 by the authors. Licensee MDPI, Basel, Switzerland. This article is an open access article distributed under the terms and conditions of the Creative Commons Attribution (CC BY) license (http://creativecommons.org/licenses/by/4.0/).

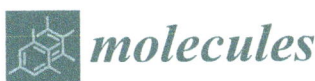

Article

Biobased Cryogels from Enzymatically Oxidized Starch: Functionalized Materials as Carriers of Active Molecules

Antonella Caterina Boccia [1,*], Guido Scavia [1], Ilaria Schizzi [2] and Lucia Conzatti [2]

[1] Institute for Chemical Sciences and Technologies-SCITEC "G. Natta", CNR, Via Corti, 12, 20133 Milano, Italy; guido.scavia@scitec.cnr.it
[2] Institute for Chemical Sciences and Technologies-SCITEC "G. Natta", CNR, Via De Marini, 6, 16149 Genova, Italy; ilaria.schizzi@scitec.cnr.it (I.S.); lucia.conzatti@cnr.it (L.C.)
* Correspondence: antonella.boccia@scitec.cnr.it; Tel.: +39-02-236-99-212

Academic Editors: Carlos A. García-González, Pasquale Del Gaudio and Ricardo Starbird
Received: 20 April 2020; Accepted: 28 May 2020; Published: 31 May 2020

Abstract: Starch recovered from an agrifood waste, pea pods, was enzymatically modified and used to prepare cryogels applied as drug carriers. The enzymatic modification of starch was performed using the laccase/(2,2,6,6-tetramethylpiperidin-1-yl)oxyl TEMPO system, at a variable molar ratio. The characterization of the ensuing starches by solution NMR spectroscopy showed partial conversion of the primary hydroxyl groups versus aldehyde and carboxyl groups and successive creation of hemiacetal and ester bonds. Enzymatically modified starch after simple freezing and lyophilization process provided stable and compact cryogels with a morphology characterized by irregular pores, as determined by atomic force (AFM) and scanning electron microscopy (SEM). The application of cryogels as carriers of active molecules was successfully evaluated by following two different approaches of loading with drugs: a) as loaded sponge, by adsorption of drug from the liquid phase; and b) as dry-loaded cryogel, from a dehydration step added to loaded cryogel from route (a). The efficiency of the two routes was studied and compared by determining the drug release profile by proton NMR studies over time. Preliminary results demonstrated that cryogels from modified starch are good candidates to act as drug delivery systems due to their stability and prolonged residence times of loaded molecules, opening promising applications in biomedical and food packaging scenarios.

Keywords: cryogel; starch; NMR spectroscopy; morphology; drug release

1. Introduction

Polysaccharides are natural and environmentally friendly polymers that have been used as starting materials for the production of a "new generation" of biobased materials because they are biocompatible, biodegradable, and nontoxic [1]. Native and modified polysaccharides, such as cellulose [2–5], hemicellulose [6,7], pectin [8,9], polygalactomannans [10–12], starch [13,14], and alginate [15] have been reported as promising matrices for producing bioaerogels via dissolution in water, retrodegradation, solvent exchange, drying via supercritical CO_2, and air–liquid phase replacement [1]; and for producing cryogels via conventional lyophilization [10,11]. Cryogels are supermacroporous gel networks derived from the cryogelation of monomers or polymeric precursor gel matrices at the subzero temperature. Being lightweight and very resistant to the breakage materials and characterized by interconnected and open porous structures, large surface area, high mechanical strength, and ultralow dielectric constant, they appear suitable for a wide range of applications in several fields [16,17]. Additionally, considering they may be obtained through a simplest approach and in aqueous medium, cryogels are suitable and fit for diverse biological and biomedical applications, such as for drug release, immobilization of molecules and cells, and matrices for cell separation [18,19].

The purpose of this paper is to describe the synthesis of modified starch via enzymatic oxidation and the production of cryogels suitable as carriers of active molecules. The oxidation reaction was carried out by using fungal laccase, from *Trametes versicolor* and the mediator TEMPO (2,2,6,6-tetramethyl-1-piperidinyl-1-oxy radical) at a variable molar ratio [20–22]. Starch from pea pods (*Pisum sativum*) was used as feedstock derived from an agrifood waste. Starch is a polysaccharide with high molecular weight whose principal components are amylose and amylopectin. Amylose is a linear polymer of D-glucose units linked through α-(1 → 4) glycosidic bonds. Amylopectin has a branched structure through both α-(1 → 6) and α-(1 → 4) glycosidic bonds [23]. The combined use of laccase enzyme and the mediator TEMPO is a well-known method for the suitable oxidation of the primary hydroxyl groups to aldehydes [24,25]. The consequential formation of hemiacetalic bonds between the newly formed carbonyl and carboxyl groups and the free hydroxyl groups supports the creation of a crosslinked network responsible for the modified material behavior and allows the modulation of the material properties [25]. After the oxidation reaction, the modified starches were thoroughly characterized by mono- and two-dimensional solution NMR spectroscopy to determine the degree of oxidation and the nature of newly formed functional groups. Applying a conventional lyophilization process to modified starch, cryogels were obtained, and the morphology was investigated using atomic force microscopy (AFM) and SEM. The sorption/desorption capability of the cryogels was evaluated using caffeine in water, chosen as a "model drug" for the presence of functional groups in the molecular structure able to interact with those on starch polymer chains, thus favoring a slower desorption phenomenon. Moreover, this being a molecule that is a natural antioxidant by scavenging hydroxyl radicals, it is appropriate for biomedical applications to support the use of the proposed carrier [26]. Two different approaches of cryogel loading were evaluated, as reported: (a) adsorption of caffeine from the liquid phase (sponge cryogel); and (b) adsorption of caffeine from the liquid phase followed by a dehydration process (dry-loaded cryogel). Profile studies of release were then conducted by collecting a series of proton NMR spectra over time, thus showing encouraging preliminary results for the use as carriers. Synthesized cryogels, due to their properties, could have a wide range of promising applications in biomedicine (immobilizing biomolecules; capturing target molecules; for drug delivery; for wound healing), biotechnology, and bioseparation segments.

2. Results

2.1. Starch Oxidation

Purified starch from pea pod powder was enzymatically oxidized by using fungal laccase and the mediator TEMPO in mild reaction conditions and at a variable molar ratio (see Table 1), as described in Section 4.2.

Table 1. Reaction conditions for the TEMPO-mediated laccase oxidation of PS in water.

Sample	TEMPO (mg)	Laccase [1] (mg)
A	1	4
B	1	40
C	10	40
D [2]	-	-

[1] Laccase was dissolved in 1 mL of water prior use. [2] Sample D was not enzymatically oxidized.

Trametes versicolor was chosen as a source of laccase because its carboxyl content was the largest compared to that of other enzymes [27] and because it is able to promote the oxidation of the mediator TEMPO in an unbuffered water medium. During oxidation, the mediator TEMPO is converted into an oxonium ion, able to selectively act on the primary hydroxyl groups present on pea pod starch (PS) chains, thus generating aldehyde groups. The chemical nature of PS derivatives was deeply investigated by mono- and two-dimensional NMR spectroscopy. Results were perfectly in line with the literature data, supporting experimentally the occurrence of the oxidation in low yield (10%) as observed for other polysaccharides, such as polygalactomannans [25] arabinoxylan and konjac glucomannans [10], for which a maximum of 12% of oxidation degree was reached. As a consequence, the resonances of the partially oxidized PS, in the proton spectrum of Figure 1, have small intensities overlapping with those of the native PS. The obtainment of aldehyde derivatives was confirmed by the appearance in the proton spectrum of characteristic resonances at 9.23 and 9.28 ppm in the ^{1}H spectrum of Figure 1. Moreover, ^{1}H chemical shifts of partially oxidized PS were assigned and are listed in Table S1 according to available literature data and two-dimensional experiments. Some peculiar signals in the proton spectrum were very close to those reported for acetylated starches [28,29] and oxidized polygalactomannans [24,25].

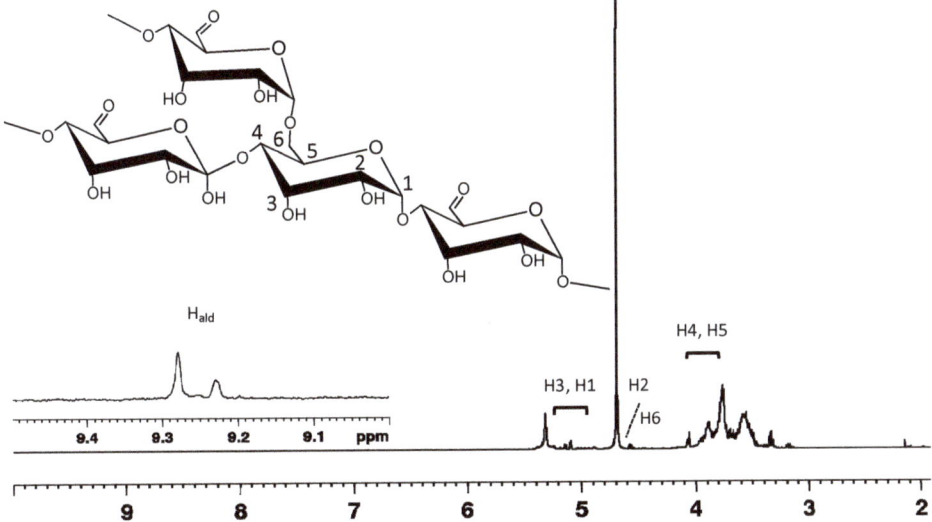

Figure 1. ^{1}H NMR spectrum of partially oxidized pea starch (sample C), recorded at 298 K, in D$_2$O (for simplicity, only the numbering scheme of the amylopectin derivative is illustrated; the assignment refers to partially oxidized starch).

In the ^{13}C spectrum of partially oxidized PS in Figure S3, the signals of produced acid residues are scarcely detectable because of the low yield of the oxidization reaction and especially the absence of NOE signal enhancement together with a long relaxation delay. In addition, the carbonyl signal expected in the 190–200 ppm region in the ^{13}C spectrum cannot be easily detected, thus indicating that the aldehyde groups are hydrated or forming hemiacetals with the hydroxyl groups [30]. Nevertheless, the formation of a carboxyl carbon derivative for the modified PS was confirmed by the HMBC spectrum in Figure 2; this is because of the major sensitivity of the experiment along the proton dimension. Analyzing in detail the carboxyl region in Figure 2 (at 170–190 ppm), it is possible to observe a cross peak at 177.9 ppm referring to a $^3J_{CH}$ correlation of a proton at 4.1 ppm with the carboxyl atom. This cross peak was assigned to the newly formed carboxyl group at the C6 position of the modified PS correlating through three bonds with the H4 proton. The enhanced technique also allowed easier detection of minor peaks attributable to the partially oxidized PS. Indeed, signals related to hemiacetalic derivatives were revealed from the HMBC analysis (at ca. 80–90 ppm), in agreement with literature data [25,30,31] and confirming the ^{13}C NMR data. These derivatives can be justified from the chemo-enzymatic oxidation mechanism that supports the creation of a crosslinked network between the newly formed carbonyl and free hydroxyl groups. These groups are able to form intra- and inter-chain hemiacetalic bonds that are finally responsible for the modified material behavior.

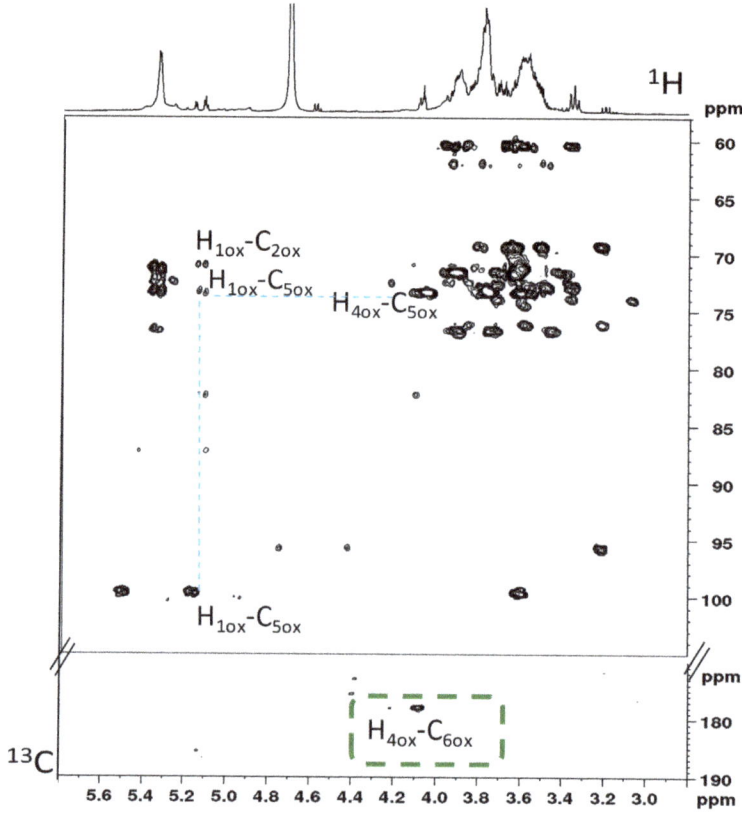

Figure 2. ^{1}H–^{13}C HMBC spectrum of partially oxidized pea pod starch (PS) from sample C in D$_2$O at 298 K. Some characteristic resonances are highlighted and refer to minor components from the oxidation process assigned with this technique.

Finally, the entire spin system was verified by 2D ^{1}H–^{1}H double quantum filtered-total correlation spectroscopy (TOCSY) experiment reported in Figure S4.

2.2. Cryogels

The final recovered cryogels from the modified PSs, obtained as illustrated on Section 4.2, showed different structures depending on the mediator TEMPO/laccase ratio in Table 1; therefore, samples A and B both showed fragile textures as fluffy and easy water dispersible matrices (sample B in Figure 3a); by contrast, sample C evidenced a compact and reinforced structure, as shown in Figure 3b.

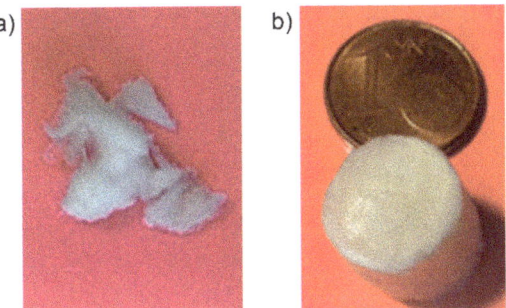

Figure 3. Cryogels from the modified PS as obtained from variable 2,2,6,6-tetramethyl-1-piperidinyl-1-oxy radical (TEMPO)/laccase ratio as shown in Table 1: (**a**) sample B; (**b**) sample C.

Cryogel Morphology

SEM analysis on sample C in Figure 4 shows a highly porous structure, with the dimension of pores appearing to be not homogeneous in the whole fragile fractured surface. Indeed, areas with both smaller and bigger pores are observed. Moreover, nanometric holes are visible within some walls.

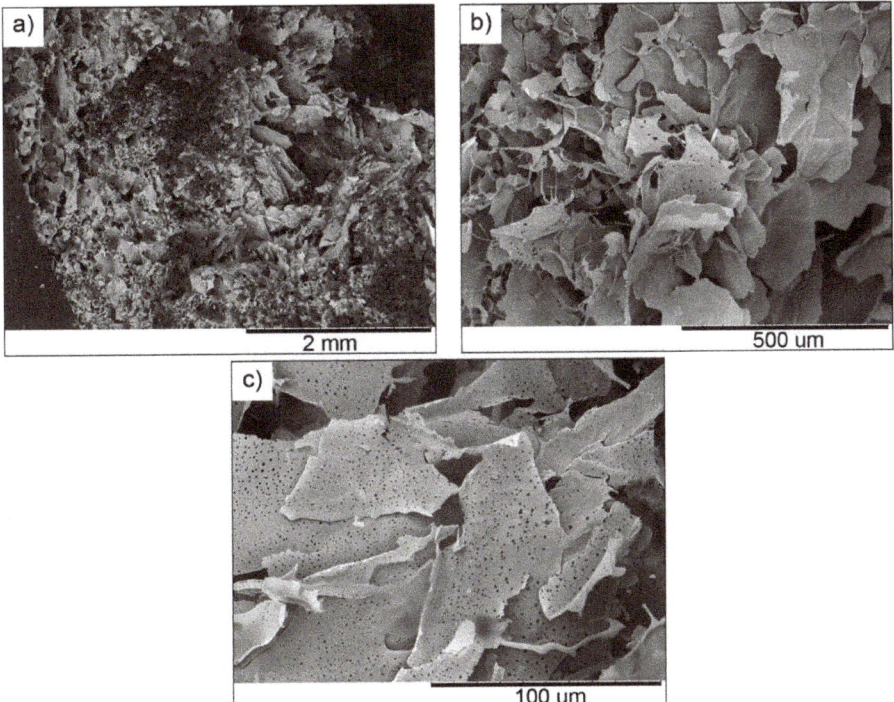

Figure 4. SEM images at different magnifications of the fragile fractured surface of sample C.

The morphological analysis carried at higher magnification by AFM in Figure 5 confirmed the presence of pores heterogeneously shaped and sized, of which the smallest ones range from approximately 200 nm to a few microns. Grain morphology of the flat areas (inlet of Figure 5b) was also evidenced.

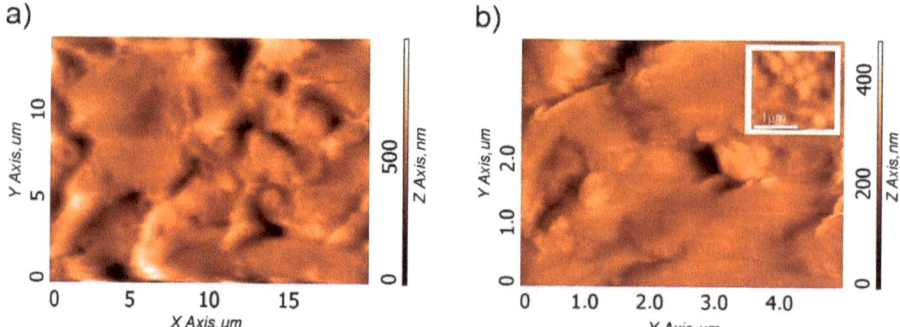

Figure 5. Atomic force microscopy (AFM) images of the sample C cryogel surface at: lower (**a**) and higher (**b**) magnifications. The inlet in (**b**) represents a magnification of the flat area.

This morphology with heterogeneously shaped pores is similar to that reported for superabsorbent aerogels obtained from cellulose nanofibrils [32,33] and hydrogels for tissue regeneration [34]. The presence of pores heterogeneous in shape and size together with nanometric pores in the walls could be useful for tuning the absorption/release of active molecules, such as caffeine.

3. Discussion

Cryogels as Carrier

The ability of the partially modified PS to act as a delivery system of active molecules was investigated by solution NMR spectroscopy, as this technique is not limited to specific classes of compounds or functional groups but can be extended to the determination of all hydrocarbon compounds and is very useful for the analysis of mixture. Moreover, together with the release profile, it is possible to observe when the cryogel starts to dissolve. Finally, it is a quantitative and non-disruptive technique.

To test the cryogels' ability to act as drug carrier, caffeine was chosen as model molecule because of the affinity of its functional groups with those of modified PS and because it is a well-known antioxidant and pro-oxidant and has reinforcing properties [35]. All samples in Table 1 were loaded with caffeine by immersing each of them into an Eppendorf tube containing caffeine in water, as illustrated in Section 4.3. (route (a)), and finally, samples A and B were discarded because of their fragile texture and easy water solubility; thus, cryogels from sample C conditions were used like carriers due to their compact and sTable Structure. Successively, the uploading capacity was evaluated for both samples. The main difference between the two loading methods is in the wet or dry use of the cryogels. For wet uses, the idea is to enhance the dissolution rate of poorly water-soluble drugs, thus increasing the therapeutic effects linked to drug availability. In the case of dry-loaded cryogels, wound healing applications are considered. This cryogel may be able to generate a wet gel at the wound site when an exudate is present, thus avoiding perilesional skin damages.

Firstly, for sponge cryogels from route (a), the release profiles of adsorbed caffeine were evaluated by collecting a series of proton NMR experiments acquired as detailed in Section 4.5. Direct quantification of released caffeine was done through a proportional comparison between the signal of the internal standard (TMS at $\delta = 0$ ppm) and a selected signal of caffeine (e.g., a methyl signal at $\delta = 3.32$ ppm,) considering that in a proton spectrum, the area of the signals is directly proportional to the number of protons present in the active volume of the sample [36]. Milligrams of released caffeine were determined by applying Equation (1) and then plotted vs. contact time in Figure 6 (considering cumulative milligrams over time). Data analysis for the sponge cryogel evidenced that the maximum of released caffeine was reached in the first 1560 min of elution, probably due to the quick release of caffeine from the surface of the PS material. Successively, for more prolonged contact time, the concentration goes down, and a more constant profile was reached probably because the caffeine entrapped in the core system was slowly released over time. After prolonged contact time, the cryogel starts to dissolve. Two stock solutions were analyzed to replicate data showing the same trend.

In the case of the dry-loaded cryogel from route (b), the procedure for the quantitative analysis of released caffeine was the same as described above. The plot of NMR data vs. contact time in Figure 6 evidenced no significant differences on the release profile for this material with respect to the sponge cryogel. The only valuable difference is attributable to the stability of this material that is more fragile and difficult to handle. In addition, in this case, two stock solutions were analyzed to replicate data showing the same trend.

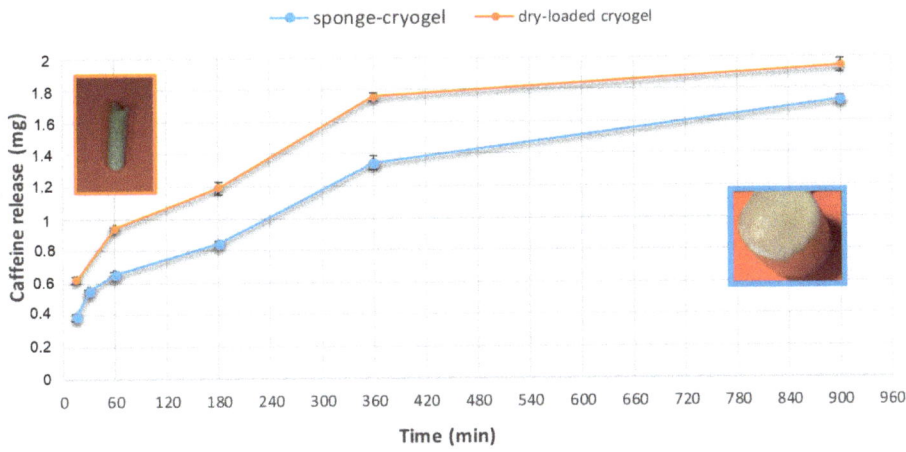

Figure 6. Percentage/mg medium values of the cumulative caffeine release versus time (standard deviation bars are reported) for the sponge cryogel and dry-loaded sample.

These preliminary studies are encouraging and aspire to develop cryogels for specific applications. The sponge cryogels may contribute to the development of specific administration routes (topical, pulmonary, oral), thus shaping on demand, and on the "site" the drug availability. The dry-loaded cryogel will be useful for wound healing applications; it will mimic the natural tissue environment, and when loaded with antioxidant molecules, it can enhance antibiotic resistance during bacterial invasion [37].

4. Materials and Methods

4.1. Materials

Starch from pea pods (PS) in powder was generously provided by Dr. Marco Radice of Emsland Group and used after purification, carried out by dispersing it (10% w/w) in MilliQ water and ethanol in a 60/40 ratio by stirring at room temperature for 1 h. The material was recovered by filtration and then dispersed at 10% w/w in acetone and stirred for an additional hour at room temperature. After vacuum filtration, the material was dried at 50 °C overnight. The final yield was 94% (w/w).

Laccase from *Trametes versicolor* in powder form (0.5 U/mg as declared by Sigma-Aldrich), mediator TEMPO, caffeine, and all other chemicals were purchased from Sigma-Aldrich (Sigma-Aldrich, Darmstadt, Germany) and used as received. Deuterated water, (D_2O 99.9%), and tetramethylsilane (TMS) for NMR spectroscopy were purchased from CortecNet (CortecNet, Les Ulis France) and used as received.

4.2. Oxidation Process and Cryogel Preparation

Purified PS was dispersed in milliQ water and stirred for 1 h at room temperature and then left overnight without stirring. Successively, a suspension of PS (10 mg) in water (2 mL) was prepared and stirred for 30 min at 30 °C, and then the mediator TEMPO and laccase were added in a molar ratio as reported in Table 1. The reaction mixture was stirred for 4 h at 30 °C and then kept at room temperature overnight. Finally, the enzyme was inactivated by placing the reactor into a boiling bath for 15 min.

The so-obtained reaction mixture, slightly viscous, was kept frozen at 8–0 °C for 18 h in cylindrical reactors and then lyophilized at −55 °C for 24 h (0.03 mbar). Recovered samples after lyophilization were stored at room temperature. Syntheses were duplicated to verify the reaction reproducibility. Furthermore, to verify the possibility of generating cryogels from the not enzymatically oxidized PS, the freeze-drying procedure was applied to a suspension of PS (10 mg) in water (2 mL) (sample D in Table 1) obtaining no cryogel.

4.3. Caffeine Adsorption in the Cryogel Structure

The adsorption of caffeine in cryogel was carried out following two different procedures, as follows: (a) for the sponge cryogel, a slice of 15 mm in diameter (5 ÷ 6 mg), obtained from sample C (in Table 1), was immersed into an Eppendorf tube containing caffeine in water (5 mM) for 90 min, then washed with 500 µL of water, and weighted to determine the "uploading capacity"; (b) the cryogel from route (a), after being charged with caffeine in water, was re-lyophilized, giving rise to the dry-loaded cryogel. Both procedures utilized the cryogel obtained from sample C condition in Table 1 because it is more stable in water with respect to samples A and B.

4.4. Studies on Sorption/Desorption of Caffeine in the Cryogels

The sorption/desorption capability of the loaded cryogel from route (a) was evaluated by immersing it into 700 µL of fresh deuterated water at regular interval time (respectively for 15, 30, 60, 180, 240, and 900 min as contact time) before acquisition of the NMR data. For all recovered solutions, proton spectra were recorded in quantitative conditions to evaluate the amount of released caffeine over time, and then this parameter was plotted as function of time considering the cumulative amount.

The sorption/desorption capability for the dry-loaded cryogel from route (b) was determined as detailed above by immersing it into 700 µL of fresh deuterated water at regular interval time, and proton NMR experiments were conducted on each solution. Finally, data were evaluated over time. Data were duplicated in both cases.

The experimental scheme illustrating the sorption/desorption procedure in the cryogels is reported in Figure S1.

4.5. NMR Spectroscopy

Mono- and two-dimensional NMR experiments were recorded on a 500-MHz Bruker DMX spectrometer, operating at 11.7 T, equipped with a 5 mm probe and gradient unit on z, and thermostated at 298 K (Bruker Biospin GmbH, Rheinstetten, Karlsruhe, Germany). The samples were prepared by dissolving 5.0 mg of oxidized starch into 700 µL of D_2O at room temperature (The NMR data were acquired on modified PS before the lyophilization process, and no precipitate or solid materials was observed in the NMR tube.). As internal standard, 20 µL of a 0.7 mM TMS/water solution was added to each NMR solution before data acquisition.

Acquisition parameters for ^1H experiments of enzymatically oxidized pea starch: 90° pulse 9.75 µs; PL1−2.2 dB; relaxation delay, 20.0 s. Spectral width, 8400 Hz; number of transient, 1024.

^{13}C parameters: spectral width, 14 KHz, 90° pulse, 11.0 µs; PL1−1.3 dB with a delay of 10 s.

2D ^1H-^1H DQF-TOCSY (double quantum filtered-total correlation spectroscopy) was acquired with 256 experiments over 2 K data points and 256 scans each, with a mixing time of 0.09 s and a relaxation delay of 1.2 s.

The 2D ^{1}H-^{13}C g-HSQC experiments (gradient-heteronuclear single quantum coherence) were performed by applying a coupling constant $^1J_{CH}$ = 150 Hz; data matrix 2 K × 256; number of scans: 128.

The 2D ^{1}H-^{13}C g-HMBC experiments (gradient-heteronuclear multiple bond correlation) were performed by applying a delay of 50 ms for the evolution of long-range coupling; data matrix 2 K × 256; number of scans 128; D1 2.00 s. Data were zero filled and weighted with a sine bell function before Fourier transformation.

Quantitative acquisition parameters for ^{1}H spectra of caffeine solutions: 90° pulse, 9.75 µs; PL1–2.2 dB; relaxation delay, 40.0 s. Spectral width, 8400 Hz; number of transient, 1024. Data processing: exponential line broadening of 0.1 Hz was applied as resolution enhancement function; zero-filling to 32 K prior FT (TopSpin 4.0.6 software, Bruker Biospin GmbH, Rheinstetten, Karlsruhe, Germany). Spectra were referenced to the residual solvent signal of TMS at δ = 0 ppm, as internal standard.

For all experiments, spectra phasing and integration were performed manually, and the NMR spectra were processed using the Bruker TopSpin 4.0.6 software (Bruker Biospin GmbH, Rheinstetten, Karlsruhe, Germany).

Caffeine content was determined from the integral value in the proton spectrum by applying Equation (1) [36]:

$$[mM]c = Ic/Hc \, [mM]st \, Hst/Ist \qquad (1)$$

where [mM]c is the millimolar concentration of caffeine; [mM]st is the millimolar concentration of the standard solution of TMS; Ic, Ist, and Hc and Hst are the integral value and number of protons generating the signals of caffeine and TMS, respectively. The ^{1}H spectrum of caffeine with resonance assignment is reported in Figure S2.

4.6. Cryogel Morphology

The morphology and structure of the samples were assessed using scanning electron microscopy (SEM) performed on a Hitachi TM 3000 Benchtop SEM instrument (Tokyo, Japan) operating at 15 kV acceleration voltage. Observations were carried out on fragile fractures (in liquid nitrogen) of samples lyophilized and sputter-coated with gold.

Observations at higher magnification were carried out with a commercial AFM (NTMDT) model NTEGRA in tapping mode. For AFM measurements, the oxidized PS sample was fixed on a glass slide with a double tape.

5. Conclusions

Sustainable and renewable starch-based cryogels have been synthesized from enzymatically modified starch from pea pods, combined with conventional lyophilization. The nature of the functional groups derived from the oxidation reaction seems to play a crucial role in affecting the final behavior and properties of the synthesized materials. This work highlights the role of NMR spectroscopy as an analytical tool for material characterization and determination of the drug release profile of cryogels, allowing at the same time, to follow the material degradation process. The ability of the prepared cryogels to act as drug carriers might be useful in designing novel bio-inspired materials with promising application for wound healing and for specific administration routes in the pharmacological field. In the future, antimicrobial effects will be investigated to improve the performance of cryogels and to open the scenario on novel applications.

Supplementary Materials: The following are available online: Figure S1. Experimental scheme illustrating the procedure for sorption/desorption of caffeine. Figure S2. ^{1}H spectrum of caffeine with resonance assignment. Figure S3. ^{13}C NMR spectrum of oxidized PS (sample C), recorded at 298 K, in D$_2$O. Figure S4. TOCSY spectrum of oxidized PS (sample C), recorded at 298 K, in D$_2$O. Table S1. Peculiar chemical shifts for ^{1}H species of modified PS.

Author Contributions: Conceptualization, A.C.B.; methodology, A.C.B.; characterization, A.C.B., G.S., I.S., and L.C.; writing—original draft preparation, A.C.B. and L.C.; investigation, data analysis, writing—review and editing, A.C.B., G.S., and L.C. All authors have read and agreed to the published version of the manuscript.

Funding: This research received no external funding.

Acknowledgments: Authors are grateful to Alberto Giacometti Schieroni for technical support.

Conflicts of Interest: The authors declare no conflict of interest.

References

1. García-González, C.A.; Budtova, T.; Durães, L.; Erkey, C.; DelGaudio, P.; Gurikov, P.; Koebel, M.; Liebner, F.; Neagu, M.; Smirnova, I. An Opinion Paper on Aerogels for Biomedical and Environmental Applications. *Molecules* **2019**, *24*, 1815. [CrossRef] [PubMed]
2. Gavillon, R.; Budtova, T. Aerocellulose: New highly porous cellulose prepared from cellulose-NaOH aqueous solutions. *Biomacromolecules* **2008**, *9*, 269–277. [CrossRef] [PubMed]
3. Aaltonen, O.; Jauhiainen, O. The preparation of lignocellulosic aerogels from ionic liquid solution. *Carbohyd. Polym.* **2009**, *75*, 125–129. [CrossRef]
4. Aulin, C.; Netrval, J.; Wagberg, L.; Lindstrom, T. Aerogels from nanofibrillated cellulose with tunable oleophobicity. *Soft Matter* **2010**, *6*, 3298–3305. [CrossRef]
5. Heath, L.; Thielemans, W. Cellulose nanowhisker aerogels. *Green Chem.* **2010**, *12*, 1448–1453. [CrossRef]
6. Zhang, W.; Zhang, Y.; Lu, C.; Deng, Y. Aerogels from crosslinked cellulose nano/micro-fibrils and their fast shape recovery property in water. *J. Mater. Chem.* **2012**, *22*, 11642–11650. [CrossRef]
7. Mingjie, C.; Xueqin, Z.; Aiping, Z.; Chuanfu, L.; Runcang, S. Direct preparation of green and renewable aerogel materials from crude bagasse. *Cellulose* **2016**, *23*, 1325–1334.
8. Sila, D.N.; Van Buggenhout, S.; Duvetter, T.; Fraeye, I.; De Roeck, A.; Van Loey, A.; Hendrickx, M. Pectins in processed fruits and vegetables: Part II-Structure-function relationship. *Compr. Rev. Food Sci. Food Saf.* **2009**, *8*, 86–104. [CrossRef]
9. Rudaz, C.; Courson, R.; Bonnet, L.; Calas-Etienne, S.; Sallée, H.; Budtova, T. Aeropectin: Fully Biomass-Based Mechanically Strong and Thermal Superinsulating Aerogel. *Biomacromolecules* **2014**, *15*, 2188–2195. [CrossRef]
10. Parikka, K.; Nikkila, I.; Pitkanen, L.; Ghafar, A.; Sontag-Strohm, T.; Tenkanen, M. Laccase/TEMPO oxidation in the production of mechanically strong arabinoxylan and glucomannan aerogels. *Carbohyd. Polym.* **2017**, *175*, 377–386. [CrossRef]
11. Ponzini, E.; Natalello, A.; Usai, F.; Bechmann, M.; Peri, F.; Muller, N.; Grandori, R. Structural characterization of aerogels derived from enzymatically oxidized galactomannans of fenugreek, sesbania and guar gums. *Carbohyd. Polym.* **2019**, *207*, 510–520. [CrossRef] [PubMed]
12. Cerqueira, M.A.; Bourbon, A.I.; Pinheiro, A.C.; Martins, J.T.; Souza, B.W.; Teixeira, J.A.; Vicente, A.A. Galactomannans use in the development of edible films/coatings for food applications. *Trends Food Sci. Technol.* **2011**, *22*, 662–671. [CrossRef]
13. Druel, L.; Bardl, R.; Vorwerg, W.; Budtova, T. Starch aerogels: A member of the family of thermal superinsulating materials. *Biomacromolecules* **2017**, *18*, 4232–4239. [CrossRef] [PubMed]
14. Kenar, J.A.; Eller, F.J.; Felker, F.C.; Jackson, M.A.; Fanta, G.F. Starch aerogel beads obtained from inclusion complexes prepared from high amylose starch and sodium palmitate. *Green Chem.* **2014**, *16*, 1921–1930. [CrossRef]
15. Quraishi, S.; Martins, M.; Barros, A.A.; Gurikov, P.; Raman, S.P.; Smirnova, I.; Duarte, A.R.C.; Reis, R.L. Novel non-cytotoxic alginate–lignin hybrid aerogels as scaffolds for tissue engineering. *J. Supercrit. Fluids* **2015**, *105*, 1–8. [CrossRef]
16. Sescousse, R.; Gavillon, R.; Budtova, T. Aerocellulose from cellulose–ionic liquid solutions: Preparation, properties and comparison with cellulose–NaOH and cellulose–NMMO routes. *Carbohydr. Polym.* **2011**, *83*, 1766–1774. [CrossRef]
17. Buchtova, N.; Budtova, T. Cellulose aero-, cryo-and xerogels: Towards understanding of morphology control. *Cellulose* **2016**, *23*, 2585–2595. [CrossRef]
18. Bakhshpour, M.; Idil, N.; Perçin, I.; Denizli, A. Biomedical Applications of Polymeric Cryogels. *Appl. Sci.* **2019**, *9*, 553. [CrossRef]
19. Nayak, A.K.; Das, B. Introduction to polymeric gels. In *Polymeric Gels*; Woodhead Publishing: Cambridge, UK, 2018; Volume 6, pp. 3–27. [CrossRef]

20. Ghafar, A.; Gurikov, P.; Subrahmanyam, R.; Parikka, K.; Tenkanen, M.; Smirnova, I.; Mikkonen, K. Mesoporous guar galactomannan based biocomposite aerogels through enzymatic crosslinking. *Compos. A* **2017**, *94*, 93–103. [CrossRef]
21. Lavazza, M.; Formantici, C.; Langella, V.; Monti, D.; Pfeiffer, U.; Galante, Y.M. Oxidation of galactomannan by laccase plus TEMPO yields an elastic gel. *J. Biotechnol.* **2011**, *156*, 108–116. [CrossRef]
22. Leppanen, A.S.; Niittymaki, O.; Parikka, K.; Tenkanen, M.; Eklund, P.; Sjoholm, R.; Willfor, S. Metal-mediated allylation of enzymatically oxidized methyl α-D-galactopyranoside. *Carbohydr. Res.* **2010**, *345*, 2610–2615. [CrossRef]
23. Tester, R.F.; Karkalas, J.; Qi, X. Starch—Composition, fine structure and architecture. *J. Cereal Sci.* **2004**, *39*, 151–165. [CrossRef]
24. Parikka, K.; Tenkanen, M. Oxidation of methyl alpha-D-galactopyranoside by galactose oxidase: Products formed and optimization of reaction conditions for production of aldehyde. *Carbohydr. Res.* **2009**, *344*, 14–20. [CrossRef] [PubMed]
25. Merlini, L.; Boccia, A.C.; Mendichi, R.; Galante, Y.M. Enzymatic and chemical oxidation of polygalactomannans from the seeds of a few species of leguminous plants and characterization of the oxidized products. *J. Biotechnol.* **2015**, *198*, 31–43. [CrossRef] [PubMed]
26. Daly, J.W.; Butts-Lamb, P.; Padgett, W. Subclasses of adenosine receptors in the central nervous system: Interaction with caffeine and related methylxanthines. *Cell. Mol. Neurobiol.* **1983**, *3*, 69–80. [CrossRef]
27. Sindhu, M.; Adlercreutz, P. Mediator facilitated, laccase catalysed oxidation of granular potato starch and the physico-chemical characterisation of the oxidized products. *Bioresour. Technol.* **2009**, *100*, 3576–3584.
28. Chi, H.; Xu, K.; Wu, X.; Chen, Q.; Xue, D.; Song, C.; Zhang, W.; Wang, P. Effect of acetylation on the properties of corn starch. *Food Chem.* **2008**, *106*, 923–928. [CrossRef]
29. Gidley, M.J. Observations on N.M.R. spectra of starches in dimethyl sulfoxide, iodine-complexing, and solvation in water-di-methyl sulfoxide. *Carbohydr. Res.* **1985**, *139*, 85–93. [CrossRef]
30. Wu, X.; Ye, Y.; Chen, Y.; Ding, B.; Cui, J.; Jiang, B. Selective oxidation and determination of the substitution pattern of hydroxypropyl guar gum. *Carbohydr. Polym.* **2010**, *80*, 1178–1182. [CrossRef]
31. Kato, Y.; Matsuo, R.; Isogai, A. Oxidation process of water-soluble starch in TEMPO-mediated system. *Carbohydr. Polym.* **2003**, *51*, 69–75. [CrossRef]
32. Jimenez-Saelices, C.; Seantier, B.; Cathala, B.; Grohens, Y. Spray freeze-dried nanofibrillated cellulos eaerogels with thermal superinsulating properties. *Carbohydr. Polym.* **2017**, *157*, 105–112. [CrossRef] [PubMed]
33. Jianga, F.; Hsieh, Y. Amphiphilic superabsorbent cellulose nanofibril aerogels. *J. Mater. Chem. A* **2014**, *2*, 6337–6342. [CrossRef]
34. Stagnaro, P.; Schizzi, I.; Utzeri, R.; Marsano, E.; Castellano, M. Alginate-polymethacrylate hybrid hydrogels for potential osteochondral tissue regeneration. *Carbohydr. Polym.* **2018**, *185*, 56–62. [CrossRef] [PubMed]
35. Griffiths, R.R.; Woodson, P.P. Reinforcing properties of caffeine: Studies in humans and laboratory animals. *Pharmacol. Biochem. Behav.* **1988**, *29*, 419–427. [CrossRef]
36. Bharti, S.K.; Roy, R. Quantitative 1H NMR spectroscopy. *Trend Anal. Chem.* **2012**, *35*, 5–26. [CrossRef]
37. Han, L.; Li, P.; Tang, P.; Wang, X.; Zhou, T.; Wang, K.; Ren, F.; Guo, T.; Lu, X. Mussel-inspired cryogels for promoting wound regeneration through photobiostimulation, modulating inflammatory responses and suppressing bacterial invasion. *Nanoscale* **2019**, *11*, 15846–15861. [CrossRef]

Sample Availability: Samples of the compounds C are available from the authors.

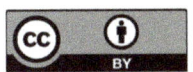

© 2020 by the authors. Licensee MDPI, Basel, Switzerland. This article is an open access article distributed under the terms and conditions of the Creative Commons Attribution (CC BY) license (http://creativecommons.org/licenses/by/4.0/).

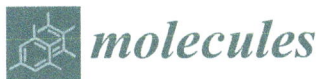

Article

Preparation and Characterization of Chitosan-Coated Pectin Aerogels: *Curcumin* Case Study

Milica Pantić, Gabrijela Horvat, Željko Knez and Zoran Novak *

Faculty of Chemistry and Chemical Engineering, University of Maribor, Smetanova 17, 2000 Maribor, Slovenia; milica.pantic1@um.si (M.P.); gabrijela.horvat@um.si (G.H.); zeljko.knez@um.si (Ž.K.)
* Correspondence: zoran.novak@um.si; Tel.: +386-2-2294-405; Fax: +386-2-2527-774

Academic Editors: Carlos A. García-González, Pasquale Del Gaudio and Ricardo Starbird
Received: 20 December 2019; Accepted: 5 March 2020; Published: 6 March 2020

Abstract: The following study describes the preparation of pectin aerogels and pectin aerogels coated with an external layer of chitosan. For the preparation of chitosan-coated pectin aerogels, a modified coating procedure was employed. Since pectin as well as pectin aerogels are highly water soluble, a function of chitosan coating is to slow down the dissolution of pectin and consequently the release of the active substances. Textural properties, surface morphologies, thermal properties, and functional groups of prepared aerogels were determined. Results indicated that the coating procedure affected the textural properties of pectin aerogels, resulting in smaller specific surface areas of 276 m^2/g, compared to 441 m^2/g. However, chitosan-coated pectin aerogels still retained favorable properties for carriers of active substances. The case study for prepared aerogels was conducted with curcumin. Prior to in-vitro release studies, swelling studies were performed. Curcumin's dissolution from both aerogels showed to be successful. Pectin aerogels released curcumin in 3 h showing a burst release profile. Chitosan-coated pectin aerogels prolonged curcumin release up to 24 h, thus showing a controlled release profile.

Keywords: curcumin; pectin aerogels; chitosan coating; burst release; controlled release

1. Introduction

Polysaccharides have gained increasing attention in biomedicine within the last decade. Due to their exquisite properties such as non-toxicity, biodegradability, and biocompatibility, they are listed as excellent candidates for use in various biomedical formulations.

Pectin is a linear polysaccharide mainly consisting of galacturonic acid units which are connected via α-(1-4) bonds. Gelling properties of pectin depend on the ratio of esterified and amidated acid groups, and particularly the type of pectin (low methoxyl pectin, high methoxyl pectin, or amidated pectin) [1]. Different gelation methods have been reported in the literature: ionotropic gelation with Ca^{2+} [2], ionotropic gelation with ethanolic solution of Ca^{2+} [3], emulsification in oil followed by coagulation in ethanol [4], and ethanol gelation [5]. Pectin aerogels are highly water soluble in the same way as pectin. They could be used for improving the dissolution and bioavailability of poorly water-soluble drugs [6].

Chitosan is a linear polysaccharide consisting of linked β-(1-4)-glucosamine units. It can be obtained by deacetylation of chitin from seafood industry waste, such as squid pens and crab shells. Gels can be formed either by irreversible covalent links with chemical cross-linkers, such as glutaraldehyde, or by various reversible links with ions and polyelectrolyte complexes. The latter are formed by dissolution of chitosan in an acidic medium, followed by precipitation in an alkaline solution, which is the simplest way of preparing chitosan gels [7]. Chitosan aerogels, in the literature usually referred to as scaffolds, are in most cases used for tissue engineering applications [8]. Unlike pectin, chitosan is soluble in an acidic medium, in lower pH ranges. This property is very important and opens up possibilities for new applications.

The drug release properties from water-soluble polysaccharides, such as pectin, suffer some problems. The main disadvantage is the burst release of active substances due to quick breakdown of gels in vitro. To improve the performance of water-soluble polysaccharides, chitosan coatings can be added to protect the core and prolong the release of active substances trapped inside. There are efforts in the literature to achieve these formulations and mentioned effect [9–13].

Curcumin is a yellow pigment present in the spice turmeric (*Curcuma longa*). It is associated with antioxidant, anti-inflammatory, anticancer, antiviral, and antibacterial activities, confirmed by more than 6000 citations and hundreds of clinical studies [14]. Curcumin, however, has poor absorption, biodistribution, metabolism, and bioavailability. There are suggestions to overcome these problems, by incorporating curcumin into formulations such as nanoparticles, liposomes, micelles, and phospholipid complexes [15–18].

The aim of this study was to improve the bioavailability of curcumin by attaching it to highly water-soluble pectin aerogels in the first step. Secondly, the curcumin release was optimized by adding a chitosan layer over the pectin core.

To the best of our knowledge, this is one of the first studies on the topic of chitosan coatings over pectin aerogels.

2. Results

2.1. Synthesis of Pectin Aerogels and Chitosan-Coated Pectin Aerogels

Figure 1 shows a schematic presentation of the modified coating method, applied for covering the pectin core with a chitosan layer. In the first step (a), 4% (w/w) pectin solution was prepared, poured into molds and covered with ethanol to obtain gels. Once the stable gel was obtained, tablet shape forms were cut (b) for further treatment. Step (c) refers to dipping pectin cores into 1.5% (w/w) chitosan solution in 0.2 M CH$_3$COOH. To attach chitosan to the pectin core, tablets were transferred to NaOH solution in ethanol (d), which triggered the gelation of chitosan. In the last step, before further processing, pectin gels coated with chitosan were washed out with ethanol (e).

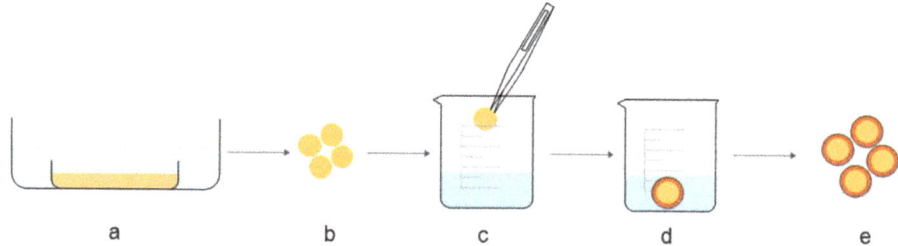

Figure 1. Schematic presentation of the coating procedure.

To prepare aerogels from gels, a supercritical drying technique was applied at 120 bar and 40 °C for 6 h. The aerogels obtained are presented in Figure 2. Chitosan-coated pectin aerogels (right side) are more massive with clearly changed shapes. Unlike the pectin aerogels (left side), which have a precise, tablet-shaped form, chitosan-coated pectin aerogels have less defined shapes. The average diameter-to-height ratio for pectin aerogels is 3, while for chitosan-coated pectin aerogels, it is 1.5.

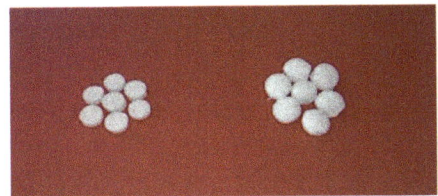

Figure 2. Pectin aerogels and chitosan-coated pectin aerogels.

2.2. Characterization of Pectin Aerogels and Chitosan-Coated Pectin Aerogels

2.2.1. Textural properties

Specific surface areas were measured using N_2 adsorption–desorption analysis. Furthermore, bulk and skeletal densities were determined, and porosity was calculated. All values are shown in Table 1.

Table 1. Specific surface areas, densities and porosities of pectin aerogels and chitosan-coated pectin aerogels.

	Pectin Aerogels	Chitosan-Coated Pectin Aerogels
Specific surface area, m^2/g	441 ± 6	276 ± 8
Bulk density, g/cm^3	0.084	0.098
Skeletal density, g/cm^3	2.1	1.9
Porosity, %	96.0 ± 0.05	94.8 ± 0.03

Specific surface area of chitosan-coated pectin aerogels is 276 m^2/g, which is significantly lower compared to pure pectin aerogels, which have a surface area of 441 m^2/g. It seems that the coating procedure affected the structure of pure pectin aerogels, resulting in smaller specific surface areas. However, the specific surface area of 276 m^2/g is still high enough for loading of the active substances (such as curcumin) and the potential as a drug carrier. Very high porosities of 96 ± 0.05% and 94.8 ± 0.03% undoubtedly shows aerogels nature of both pectin and chitosan-coated pectin materials.

The N_2 adsorption–desorption isotherms for both pectin aerogels and chitosan-coated pectin aerogels, presented in Figure 3 could be classified as type IV isotherms. From the types of isotherms, it can be concluded that the prepared aerogels are mesoporous materials.

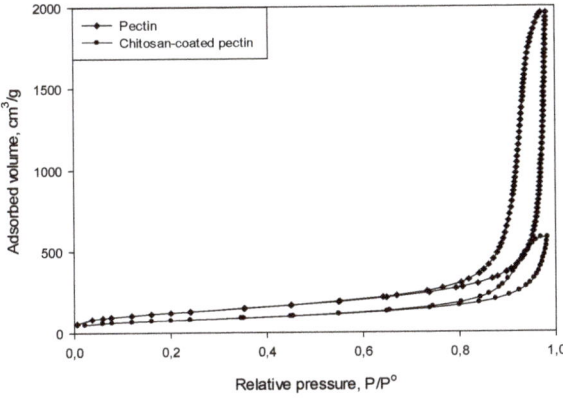

Figure 3. Adsorption–desorption isotherms for pectin aerogel and chitosan-coated pectin aerogels.

2.2.2. Scanning Electron Microscopy

Scanning electron microscopy (SEM) was employed for determining the surface morphology of prepared aerogels. The coating of pectin core with chitosan layer was confirmed by SEM image on a 100 μm scale. Figure 4a undoubtedly shows a two-layer aerogel. The upper layer represents a chitosan coating over a pectin core. Porous structure is visible in both layers. Furthermore, Figure 4b represents the outer part of the coating on a 1 μm scale, confirming the porous structure of the chitosan.

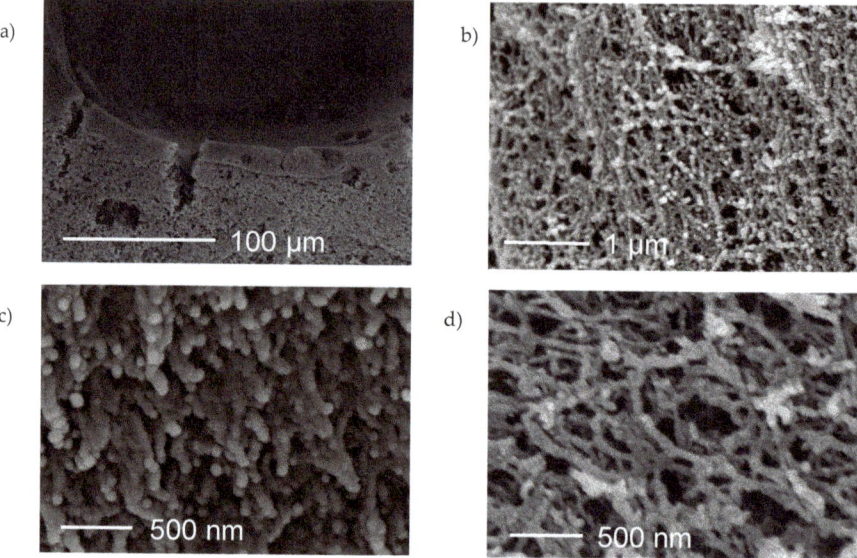

Figure 4. Scanning electron microscopy (SEM) images: (**a**) chitosan-coated pectin aerogels, the inner part (100 μm scale); (**b**) chitosan-coated pectin aerogels, the outer part (1 μm scale); (**c**) pectin aerogel (500 nm scale); and (**d**) chitosan-coated pectin aerogels (500 nm scale).

Figure 4c,d present the pore network of pectin aerogels and chitosan-coated pectin aerogels on a 500 nm scale. In both cases, the structure is highly porous, having a complex interconnected network of pores. The structure of pectin aerogels seems to be more compact compared to the structure of chitosan-coated pectin aerogels, which is expected since the specific surface area and porosity of pure pectin aerogels is higher.

2.2.3. Thermal Analysis

Thermogravimetry (TGA) and differential scanning calorimetry (DSC) were carried out simultaneously. The analyses were performed at air atmosphere at a temperature range from 30 to 600 °C, with a heating rate of 10 °C per minute.

Figure 5 shows DSC curves for pectin polysaccharide (powder), curcumin (powder), and pectin aerogel loaded with curcumin. Chitosan-coated pectin aerogels loaded with curcumin were not subjected to TGA/DSC analysis due to the size and weight limits.

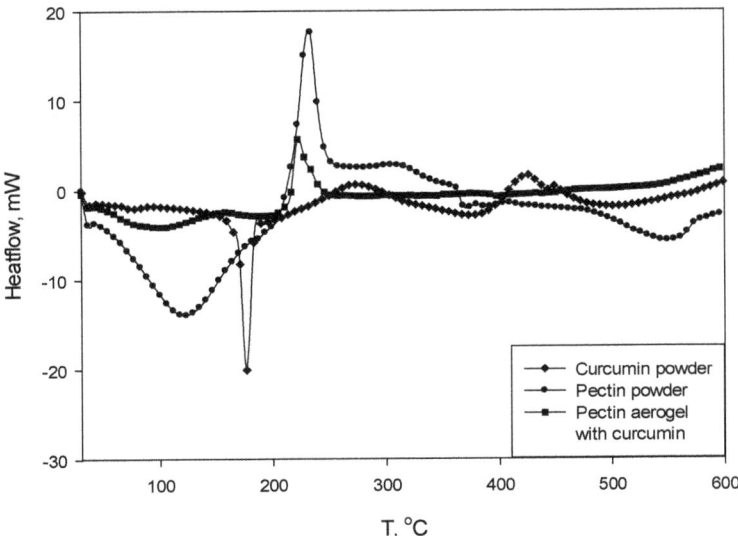

Figure 5. Differential scanning calorimetry (DSC) curves for curcumin powder, pectin powder and pectin aerogel loaded with curcumin.

The DSC curve for curcumin shows a clear peak at 178 °C, indicating the melting point of the substance. The curve for pectin shows an exothermic peak at 237 °C, indicating a degradation of this polysaccharide. As for pectin, the DSC curve for pectin aerogel loaded with curcumin has an exothermic degradation peak at 225 °C. In this case, the peak is shifted to the left, which means that the degradation occurs earlier. On the other hand, the melting peak of the curcumin is not visible on the pectin–curcumin curve.

Simultaneously with DSC, TGA was measured as presented in Figure 6.

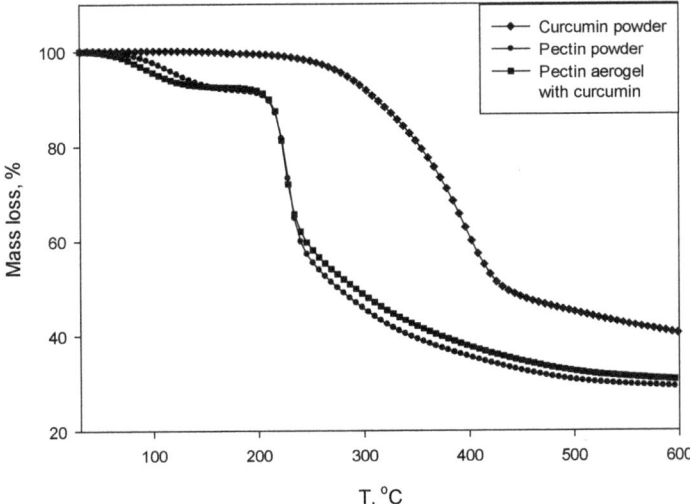

Figure 6. Thermogravimetry (TGA) curves for curcumin powder, pectin powder, and pectin aerogel loaded with curcumin.

The values read from TGA curves are given in Table 2. The thermal degradation of pectin polysaccharide as well pectin aerogel loaded with curcumin occurs in the two steps. The main decomposition (62%) occurs at higher temperatures, which is confirmed by DSC curves (exothermic degradation peaks at 237 and 225 °C). Decomposition of curcumin of 59% occurs in one step and corresponds to the melting of the substance.

Table 2. Mass degradation of curcumin powder, pectin powder, and pectin aerogel loaded with curcumin.

	Mass Degradation
Curcumin powder	1st step: 59%
Pectin powder	1st step: 8%
	2nd step: 62%
Pectin aerogel loaded with curcumin	1st step: 7%
	2nd step: 62%

2.2.4. Fourier Transform Infrared Spectroscopy

Figure 7 presents infrared (IR) spectra for curcumin powder, pectin aerogels loaded with curcumin, and chitosan-coated pectin aerogels also loaded with curcumin.

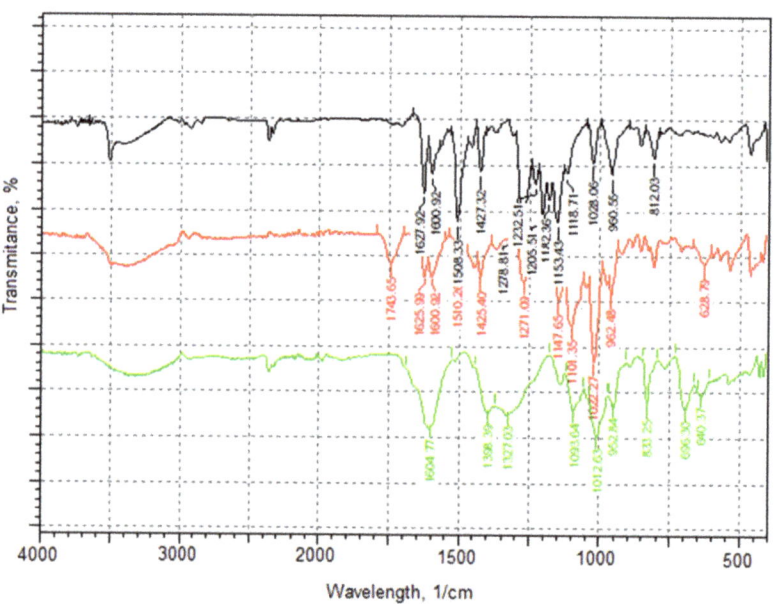

Figure 7. Infrared (IR) spectra: curcumin powder (black), pectin aerogel loaded with curcumin (red), and chitosan-coated pectin aerogel loaded with curcumin (green).

IR spectrum of curcumin clearly shows characteristic peaks [19]: 3500 cm^{-1} for phenolic O-H stretching, 1628 cm^{-1} aromatic moiety C=C stretching, and 1600 cm^{-1} benzene ring stretching vibrations identifying curcumin. Furthermore, the IR spectrum contains C=O and C=C vibrations at 1508 cm^{-1}, olefinic C-H bending vibrations at 1427 cm^{-1}, and aromatic C-O stretching vibrations at 1278 cm^{-1}.

The IR spectrum for pectin aerogels loaded with curcumin shows a characteristic peak at 1743 cm^{-1}, presenting esterified carboxyl groups. Peaks at 1625 cm^{-1} and 1600 cm^{-1} are clearly visible, confirming the presence of loaded curcumin.

Lastly, the IR spectrum of chitosan-coated pectin aerogels show characteristic peaks at 1604 cm^{-1} presenting N-H bending of the primary amine, 1398 cm^{-1} and 1327 cm^{-1} presenting CH$_2$ bending and CH$_3$ symmetrical deformations. These peaks are the characteristic signature of chitosan. Characteristic peaks for curcumin, however, are overlapping with peaks of chitosan; hence, they are not visible in the spectrum. The presence of curcumin was later confirmed by in-vitro release studies.

2.3. Swelling Studies

Swelling studies are more or less able to predict the behavior of aerogels during in-vitro release studies. The studies were performed for both pectin aerogels and chitosan-coated pectin aerogels without the presence of curcumin. Experiments were performed in simulated gastric fluid (SGF) at pH = 1.2, and simulated intestinal fluid (SIF) at pH = 6.8, in both cases for 24 h. The aerogels were afterwards compared to see the influence of the coating on their behavior in SGF/SIF.

Figure 8 presents the swelling behavior of both aerogels at SGF. It can be clearly seen that pectin aerogels and chitosan-coated pectin aerogels behave completely differently.

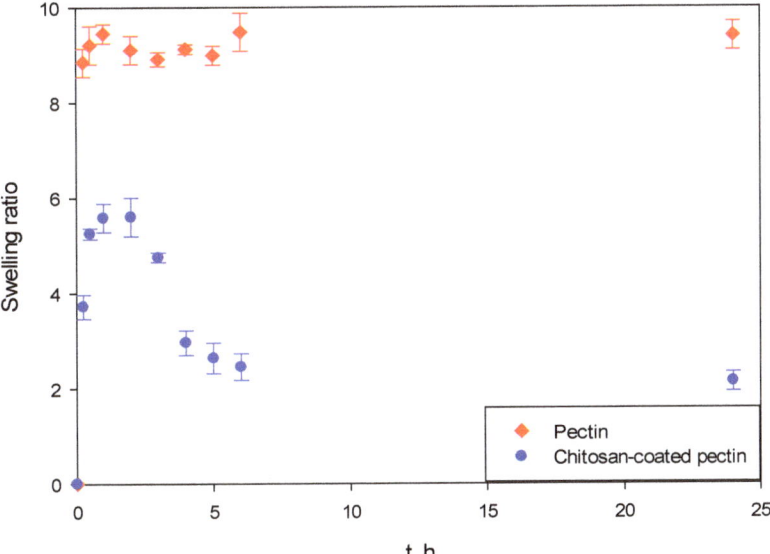

Figure 8. Swelling behavior of pectin aerogel and chitosan-coated pectin aerogel in SGF at pH = 1.2 for 24 h.

Both pectin aerogels as well as chitosan-coated pectin aerogels in contact with SGF immediately swelled. However, once pectin aerogels reached their maximal swelling ratio, they stayed unchanged for the next 24 h. This means that they are stable in the mentioned fluid. Chitosan-coated pectin aerogels reached their maximal swelling ratio after 2 h. Unlike pectin, they started to decompose after 2 h and continued decomposing over the next 4 h. Chitosan-coated pectin aerogels have an additional chitosan layer which is soluble at a lower pH. This means that the chitosan layer swells and afterwards decomposes. Once the chitosan layer decomposes after approximately 6 h, the pectin core stays stable in the SGF, in the same way as pectin aerogels.

In SIF, the behavior of aerogels again differs, as shown in Figure 9. Almost immediately after contact with SIF, pectin aerogels reach their maximal ratio. After 3 h, pectin aerogels completely decompose. On the other hand, the swelling ratio of chitosan-coated pectin aerogels increases slowly, reaching its maximal ratio after approximately 5 h. Afterwards, they stay stable in the mentioned fluid.

In this case, a chitosan layer over the pectin core prolongs the decomposition of the pectin core from 3 to 6 h. Once the pectin core is decomposed, the chitosan layer is stable in SIF, in the same way pectin is in SGF.

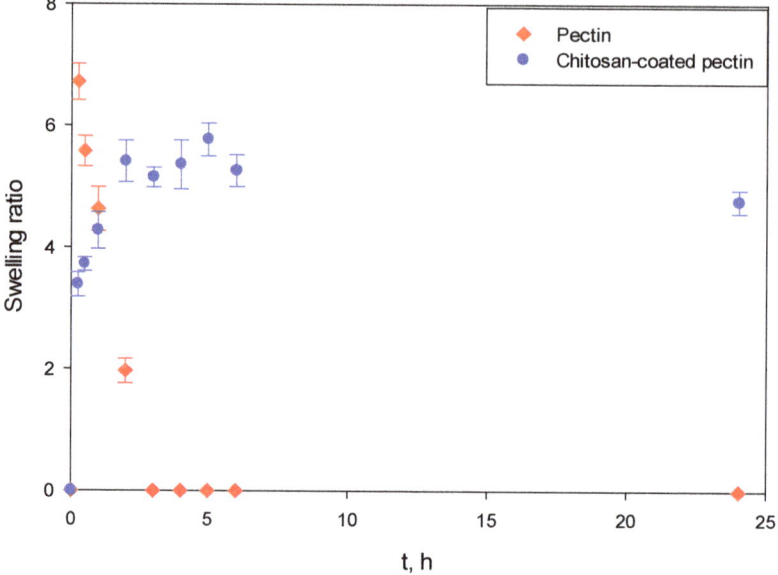

Figure 9. Swelling behavior of pectin aerogel and chitosan-coated pectin aerogels in SIF at pH = 6.8 for 24 h.

It is important to emphasize that swelling studies in SGF and SIF were performed independently. Entirely new aerogels were used for both SGF and SIF. The human body, however, functions differently. Once a drug is taken, it stays in the stomach up to 2 h, and then moves (if it does not dissolve) to the intestines for another 6 to 24 h, depending on bowel movements and their emptying.

Based on the aforementioned mechanism, drug release studies for both pectin aerogels and chitosan-coated pectin aerogels were performed first in SGF for 2 h and were afterwards transferred to SIF for an additional 22 h.

2.4. In-Vitro Curcumin Release Studies from Aerogels

To increase the bioavailability of curcumin, two types of aerogels were proposed as carriers: pectin aerogels and pectin aerogels coated with a layer of chitosan. The release of curcumin was tested through in-vitro release studies. Additionally, dissolution of curcumin powder was performed as a comparison.

As shown in Figure 10, the studies were performed for the first 2 h in SGF at pH = 1.2, and SIF at pH = 6.8 for the next 22 h. Weighted samples were immersed in SGF, after which they were immediately transferred to SIF. The experiments were monitored for 24 h.

In the first part of the study, both pectin aerogels and chitosan-coated pectin aerogels showed almost no release of curcumin in SGF at pH = 1.2. Both aerogels swell in this environment, but apparently not enough to release a significant amount of curcumin. These results are in good agreement with swelling studies, in which it was shown that both aerogels needed approximately 2 h to reach their maximal swelling ratio. In this case, this behavior of aerogels is highly desirable since the absorption of curcumin occurs in the intestine [14]; hence, there is no need for its release in the stomach.

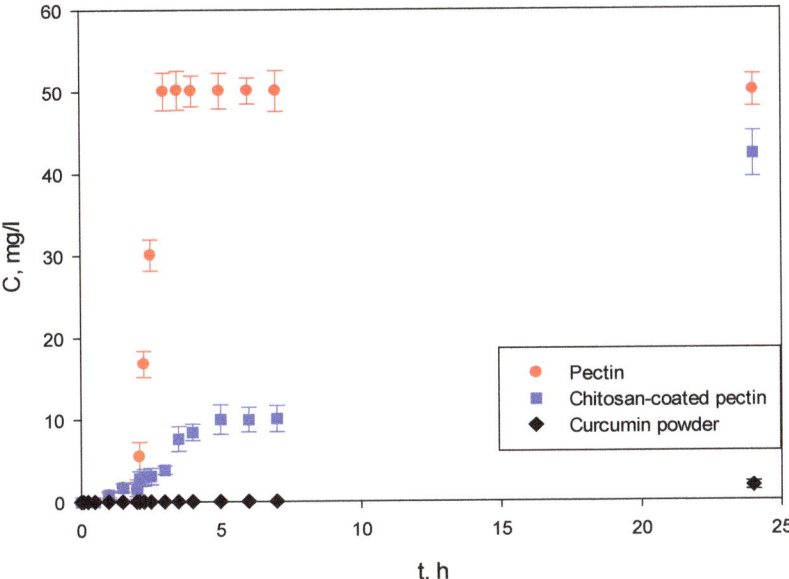

Figure 10. In-vitro curcumin release studies: 2 h in SGF followed by 22 h in SIF, 24 h overall.

When transferred to SIF, the release of curcumin from pectin aerogels is completely different from that of -chitosan-coated pectin aerogels. Pectin aerogels release all of their curcumin after just 1 h in SIF, of 3 h overall.

If the desired release is controlled release, which it is in most cases, then the release from pectin aerogels has to be slowed down, but not too much. Controlling drug diffusion from the dosage form is an excellent approach to maintaining therapeutic levels of the drug in the body. Controlled drug release in this particular case is important because of the poor adsorption of curcumin by the human body. It is crucial that a controlled amount of the drug reaches the body so that as much as possible can be adsorbed. If a large amount of the drug reaches the body at once, much of it will pass through without any adsorption at all.

Chitosan-coated pectin aerogels demonstrated slower release of curcumin, prolonged up to 24 h. As seen from Figure 10, curcumin was released for 24 h, leaving enough time for the substance to be adsorbed and metabolized by the body.

Lastly, curcumin powder was shown to be practically insoluble in body fluids, showing almost no dissolution after 24 h.

3. Discussion

Besides pure pectin aerogels, chitosan-coated pectin aerogels were prepared. The shape of latter slightly changed, resulting in a more massive appearance and less defined shapes.

N_2 adsorption–desorption analysis showed that chitosan-coated pectin aerogels had significantly reduced specific surface areas and porosity compared to pure pectin aerogels. Namely, the preparation procedure affected the pore network, reducing the specific surface areas of pure pectin aerogels from 441 m^2/g to 276 m^2/g. Transferring pectin cores to the NaOH solution apparently caused the shrinkage of pectin cores and some damages in the pore network. The adsorption capacity of pectin aerogels is higher compared to the adsorption capacity of chitosan-coated pectin aerogels, based on adsorption–desorption isotherms.

Scanning electron microscopy revealed porous structures for both pure pectin aerogels and chitosan-coated pectin aerogels, in both pectin core and chitosan layer. However, the structure of pectin aerogels showed to be more compact. SEM images are in good agreement with N_2 adsorption–desorption analysis, since pectin aerogels have higher specific surface areas. SEM images of chitosan-coated pectin aerogels show less compact structure, caused by the coating procedure and some damages to the pore network due to the shrinkage.

Thermal analysis consisted out of simultaneous thermogravimetry and differential scanning calorimetry to obtain TGA and DSC curves. The DSC curve of pectin aerogel loaded with curcumin compared to pectin polysaccharide showed a shifted peak, indicating the earlier degradation. A possible cause is the presence of curcumin. However, the melting peak of the curcumin is not visible on the pectin–curcumin curve. The overall mass of analyzed pectin aerogel loaded with curcumin is approximately 10 mg. This means that the mass of curcumin is quite low and could be simply covered or not detected in this case. TGA curves of pectin polysaccharide and pectin aerogels loaded with curcumin showed that the thermal degradation occurs in two steps.

Determined IR spectrum of pectin aerogels loaded with curcumin confirmed the presence of curcumin. The chemical structure of pectin, however, was not changed. This was verified by characteristic peaks for pectin that are still present in the spectrum. This means that the pectin aerogel serves as carrier, without chemical changes in the structure caused by the presence of active substances. In the case of chitosan-coated pectin aerogels, the characteristic peaks for curcumin are overlapping with characteristic peaks for chitosan. Even though it is not visible in the spectrum, the presence of curcumin was confirmed by further in-vitro release studies. In this case as well, the characteristic peaks for chitosan are present, again proving preserved chemical structure of polysaccharide.

Behavior of unloaded aerogels was tested in SGF at pH = 1.2 and SIF at pH = 6.8. At SGF, pectin aerogels showed to be stable. Contrary, chitosan-coated pectin aerogels started their decomposition after 2 h and finished the decomposition after 4 h. Actually, only the coating made of chitosan decomposed since the chitosan is soluble in acidic medium. Pectin core was, however, stable. This means that by using chitosan coating, pectin core is protected from the decomposition. Behavior in SIF fluids completely differs. While pectin aerogels completely decomposed after 3 h, chitosan-coated pectin aerogels are stable in neutral fluid. Chitosan coating was able to slow down and prolong the decomposition of pectin from 3 h up to 6 h. This behavior opens up the possibility for retaining the drug for a longer time period inside the core and, later on, the drug's retardation during release.

Release of curcumin from both pure pectin aerogels and chitosan-coated pectin aerogels was tested through in-vitro studies and compared with the dissolution of curcumin powder.

Release of curcumin in SGF was retained for both aerogels. However, when transferred to SIF, pectin aerogels show burst release within just 1 h (3 h overall). This result is in good agreement with the swelling studies, in which pectin aerogels were completely decomposed after just 3 h spent in SIF. During drug release studies, pectin aerogels swelled in SGF and decomposed and released curcumin after 1 h in SIF. The dissolution and bioavailability of curcumin is tremendously improved, compared to standard curcumin. The porous network structure of aerogels enabled the surrounding of the molecules of curcumin by molecules of water, thus providing the possibility of faster dissolution. Even though the dissolution of curcumin was significantly improved, the release was still a burst. In the case of chitosan-coated pectin aerogels, release of curcumin was prolonged up to 24 h. By covering pectin with a chitosan layer, the core and, consequently, the curcumin trapped inside are partially protected. This formulation slowly swells, and consequently slowly releases curcumin. By protecting the highly soluble pectin core with a chitosan layer, controlled release of curcumin was achieved. As expected, curcumin powder showed almost no dissolution for the tested period.

4. Materials and Methods

4.1. Materials

Polysaccharides, pectin from citrus (TCI Europe), and chitosan (Sigma Aldrich, medium molecular weight) were used for the synthesis of pectin aerogels and pectin aerogels coated with a layer of chitosan.

Ethanol absolute, C_2H_5OH (Merck, Darmstadt, Germany) and carbon dioxide, CO_2 (purity 99.5%, Messer, Ruše, Slovenia) were introduced for the solvent exchange during synthesis of gels and supercritical drying of prepared gels, respectively. Curcumin (purity ≥ 65%, Merck, Darmstadt, Germany) was used as an active substance for prepared aerogels. Chitosan was dissolved in acetic acid, CH_3COOH (purity ≥ 98%, Fisher Scientific, Pittsburgh, PA, USA). Hydrochloric acid, HCl (purity 37%, Merck, Darmstadt, Germany), potassium phosphate monobasic, KH_2PO_4 (purity ≥ 98%, Merck, Darmstadt, Germany) and sodium hydroxide, NaOH (purity ≥ 98%, Merck, Darmstadt, Germany) were employed for the preparation of simulated gastric (SGF) and simulated intestinal fluid (SIF) for swelling and drug release studies. SGF (HCl) with pH = 1.2 was prepared by diluting 8.3 mL of 37% HCl to 1000 mL with miliQ water. SIF (phosphate buffer solution) with pH = 6.8 was prepared by mixing 250 mL of 0.2 M KH_2PO_4 and 112 mL of 0.2 M NaOH and diluted to 1000 mL with miliQ water.

4.2. Methods

4.2.1. Synthesis of Pectin Aerogels

Pectin aerogels were prepared by ethanol-induced gelation, a method designed in our laboratory [20]. A weighed amount of pectin was dissolved in miliQ water to obtain a 4% (w/w) solution. The solution was strengthened by addition of a known amount of ethanol (not more than 10%). The hardened solution was transferred into molds and soaked in ethanol to obtain gels. The gels were cut into tablet form using a precise cutter with a diameter of 12.5 mm.

4.2.2. Synthesis of Chitosan-Coated Pectin Aerogels

For the preparation of pectin aerogels coated with a chitosan layer, a coating procedure was designed. Pectin core gels were prepared as described above. Chitosan solution, 1.5% (w/w), was prepared by dissolving a known amount of chitosan into 0.2 M CH_3COOH. Pectin core gels were soaked in a chitosan solution to bring the solution over the core. To attach the chitosan layer, soaked pectin cores were immediately transferred into 2 M NaOH. 2 M NaOH was prepared in ethanol. As pectin cores covered with chitosan solution were transferred into the NaOH solution, they immediately attached, since NaOH triggers the gelation of chitosan. After 20 min, the samples were transferred into ethanol to wash out the remaining NaOH.

4.2.3. Loading of Curcumin

The addition of curcumin was conducted using ethanol during the synthesis of pectin aerogels or chitosan-coated pectin aerogels. Since curcumin is highly soluble in ethanol (10 mg/mL), the molecules of the drug were easily diffusing inside the gel pore network. Once the curcumin was loaded, the samples were subjected to supercritical drying. Supercritical drying was conducted for 6 h at 120 bar and 40 °C, the conditions optimized for polysaccharides drying [21]. Since curcumin is poorly soluble in supercritical carbon dioxide (2×10^{-8} mole fraction for given drying conditions) [22], there was no risk of washing it out during drying.

4.3. Characterization

4.3.1. Scanning Electron Microscopy

A scanning electron microscope (Sirion 400 NC, FEI, Hillsboro, OR, USA) was used for determining the surface morphologies of the pectin aerogels and chitosan-coated pectin aerogels. The samples were fractioned and splatter-coated with gold particles prior to the analysis and then scanned at an accelerating voltage of 2–4 kV.

4.3.2. Thermal Analysis

Thermal analysis (thermogravimetry and differential scanning calorimetry) were carried out simultaneously using TGA/DSC1 apparatus (Mettler Toledo, Columbus, OH, USA). Samples were fractioned, weighed (not less than 10 mg) and placed into 100 µL aluminum crucibles. The analyses were performed at an air atmosphere in a temperature range from 30 to 600 °C, with a heating rate of 10 °C per minute.

4.3.3. Textural Properties

Specific surface areas (m^2/g) of synthetized aerogels were determined by gas N_2 adsorption-desorption analysis. The experiments were carried out at −196 °C using ASAP 2020MP (Micromeritics Instrument, Norcross, GA, USA). Prior to analysis, the samples were degassed under vacuum at 70 °C for 660 min until obtaining a stable 10 µm Hg pressure. BET (Brunauer–Emmett–Teller) method was employed for determining the specific surface area. Skeletal densities of aerogels were measured by gas pycnometer using AccuPyc II 1340 (Micromeritics Instrument, Norcross, GA, USA), while bulk densities were determined by simply measuring sample mass (weighting) and volume (dimensions). Finally, porosity was determined using Equation (1):

$$Porosity\ (\%) = 1 - \frac{\rho_{skeletal}}{\rho_{bulk}} \tag{1}$$

where $\rho_{skeletal}$ is skeletal density, while ρ_{bulk} is bulk density of aerogels.

4.3.4. Fourier Transform Infrared Spectroscopy

Fourier transform infrared spectroscopy using IRAffinity-1s (Shimadzu, Kyoto, Japan) was employed for characterization of pectin aerogels, chitosan-coated pectin aerogels, and curcumin. The collection of the absorption bands was used to confirm the identity of polysaccharides and curcumin and also for detection of curcumin loaded into aerogels. Aerogels were characterized by ATR-IR method. The samples were cut into halves and placed on the ATR detector. On the other hand, curcumin was ground into a fine powder and dispersed into a matrix made of potassium bromide (KBr). This is the most common method for solids.

4.4. Swelling studies

Swelling studies were performed as described elsewhere [6]. Briefly, pectin aerogels and chitosan-coated pectin aerogels (without curcumin) were weighed and immersed in 100 mL of either SGF at pH = 1.2 or SIF at pH = 6.8, conditions mimicking the conditions of the gastrointestinal tract. Samples were collected after selected time intervals, blot-dried with tissue paper for removing excess solution and weighed. All experiments were performed in triplicate.

The swelling ratio was calculated using Equation (2):

$$S_R = \frac{M_S - M_0}{M_0} \tag{2}$$

where M_S is the mass of the swollen aerogel after the selected period of time and M_0 is the initial mass of the sample.

4.5. In-Vitro Dissolution Tests

In-vitro dissolution tests for pectin aerogels and chitosan-coated pectin aerogels loaded with curcumin were performed using two dissolution media, SGF at pH = 1.2 and SIF at pH = 6.8, as described above. Aerogel samples were firstly placed in SGF for 2 h and immediately transferred to SIF for an additional 22 h.

In-vitro dissolution tests were performed following USP standards [23]. The experiments were carried out at 37 ± 0.5 °C on the Farmatester 3, USP II apparatus (Dema, Ilirska Bistrica, Slovenia). The volume of the dissolution medium was 900 mL, while the speed of rotation was set at 50 rpm. Aliquots of 2 mL for each sample were withdrawn at predetermined time periods and afterwards 2 mL of fresh dissolution medium was added to maintain a constant volume. Samples were subjected to a curcumin assay by a Cary 50 Probe UV spectrophotometer (Agilent Technologies, Santa Clara, CA, USA) at 429 nm. The concentration of curcumin was calculated using the calibration curves in SGF and SIF. All tests were performed in triplicate.

5. Conclusions

Two formulations for curcumin were presented in this study, for the purpose of improving the poor bioavailability of the substance. By attaching curcumin to water-soluble polysaccharide aerogels, the dissolution and consequently bioavailability was tremendously improved. While pure curcumin showed almost no dissolution after 24 h, the complete dissolution and release of curcumin from pectin aerogels was achieved after only 3 h and from pectin aerogels coated with an outer layer of chitosan after 24 h. A new coating procedure for pectin aerogels was developed for the purpose of optimizing the release of curcumin (and other active substances as well).

Both formulations proved to be useful for improving the problematic bioavailability of curcumin. On one hand, the pectin aerogels formulation showed burst release. On the other, pectin aerogels coated with chitosan showed controlled release of curcumin over 24 h and maintained a therapeutic dose of the substance.

Author Contributions: M.P. wrote the main manuscript text and planned and performed most of the experiments. G.H. helped with characterization of the materials and wrote part of the manuscript. Z.N. and Ž.K. supervised the findings of this work and helped shape the research, analysis and manuscript. All authors have read and agreed to the published version of the manuscript.

Funding: Special thanks to the Slovenian Research Agency (ARRS) for financial support of the research programme group P2–0046: Separation Processes and Production Design and research project L2-9199: Purification and Formulation of Chemicals Using Supercritical Fluids.

Conflicts of Interest: The authors declare no conflict of interest.

References

1. Ganesan, K.; Budtova, T.; Ratke, L.; Gurikov, P.; Baudron, V.; Preibisch, I.; Niemeyer, P.; Smirnova, I.; Milow, B. Review on the Production of Polysaccharide Aerogel Particles. *Materials* **2018**, *11*, 2144. [CrossRef] [PubMed]
2. Veronovski, A.; Tkalec, G.; Knez, Ž.; Novak, Z. Characterisation of biodegradable pectin aerogels and their potential use as drug carriers. *Carbohydr. Polym.* **2014**, *113*, 272–278. [CrossRef]
3. De Cicco, F.; Russo, P.; Reverchon, E.; García-González, C.A.; Aquino, R.P.; Del Gaudio, P. Prilling and supercritical drying: A successful duo to produce core-shell polysaccharide aerogel beads for wound healing. *Carbohydr. Polym.* **2016**, *147*, 482–489. [CrossRef] [PubMed]
4. García-González, C.A.; Carenza, E.; Zeng, M.; Smirnova, I.; Roig, A. Design of biocompatible magnetic pectin aerogel monoliths and microspheres. *RSC Adv.* **2012**, *2*, 9816–9823. [CrossRef]
5. Tkalec, G.; Knez, Ž.; Novak, Z. Fast production of high-methoxyl pectin aerogels for enhancing the bioavailability of low-soluble drugs. *J. Supercrit. Fluids* **2015**, *106*, 16–22. [CrossRef]
6. Horvat, G.; Pantić, M.; Knez, Ž.; Novak, Z. Encapsulation and drug release of poorly water soluble nifedipine from bio-carriers. *J. Non-Cryst. Solids* **2018**, *481*, 486–493. [CrossRef]
7. Quignard, F.; Valentin, R.; Renzo, F.D. Aerogel materials from marine polysaccharides. *New J. Chem.* **2008**, *32*, 1300–1310. [CrossRef]
8. Ahmed, S.; Ali, A.; Sheikh, J. A review on chitosan centred scaffolds and their applications in tissue engineering. *Int. J. Biol. Macromol.* **2018**, *116*, 849–862. [CrossRef]
9. Sun, X.; Shi, J.; Xu, X.; Cao, S. Chitosan coated alginate/poly(N-isopropylacrylamide) beads for dual responsive drug delivery. *Int. J. Biol. Macromol.* **2013**, *59*, 273–281. [CrossRef]

10. Nalini, T.; Basha, S.K.; Mohamed Sadiq, A.M.; Kumari, V.S.; Kaviyarasu, K. Development and characterization of alginate/chitosan nanoparticulate system for hydrophobic drug encapsulation. *J. Drug Deliv. Sci. Technol.* **2019**, *52*, 65–72. [CrossRef]
11. Dumont, M.; Villet, R.; Guirand, M.; Montembault, A.; Delair, T.; Lack, S.; Barikosky, M.; Crepet, A.; Alcouffe, P.; Laurent, F.; et al. Processing and antibacterial properties of chitosan-coated alginate fibers. *Carbohydr. Polym.* **2018**, *190*, 31–42. [CrossRef] [PubMed]
12. Rampino, A.; Borgogna, M.; Bellich, B.; Blasi, P.; Virgilio, F.; Cesàro, A. Chitosan-pectin hybrid nanoparticles prepared by coating and blending techniques. *Eur. J. Pharm. Sci.* **2016**, *84*, 37–45. [CrossRef]
13. Tamilvanan, S.; Karmegam, S. In vitro evaluation of chitosan coated- and uncoated-calcium alginate beads containing methyl salicylate-lactose physical mixture. *Pharm. Dev. Technol.* **2012**, *17*, 494–501. [CrossRef] [PubMed]
14. Prasad, S.; Tyagi, A.K.; Aggarwal, B.B. Recent Developments in Delivery, Bioavailability, Absorption and Metabolism of Curcumin: The Golden Pigment from Golden Spice. *Cancer Res. Treat. Off. J. Korean Cancer Assoc.* **2014**, *46*, 2–18. [CrossRef]
15. Aditya, N.P.; Chimote, G.; Gunalan, K.; Banerjee, R.; Patankar, S.; Madhusudhan, B. Curcuminoids-loaded liposomes in combination with arteether protects against Plasmodium berghei infection in mice. *Exp. Parasitol.* **2012**, *131*, 292–299. [CrossRef]
16. Gong, C.; Deng, S.; Wu, Q.; Xiang, M.; Wei, X.; Li, L.; Gao, X.; Wang, B.; Sun, L.; Chen, Y.; et al. Improving antiangiogenesis and anti-tumor activity of curcumin by biodegradable polymeric micelles. *Biomaterials* **2013**, *34*, 1413–1432. [CrossRef] [PubMed]
17. Agarwal, N.B.; Jain, S.; Nagpal, D.; Agarwal, N.K.; Mediratta, P.K.; Sharma, K.K. Liposomal formulation of curcumin attenuates seizures in different experimental models of epilepsy in mice. *Fundam. Clin. Pharmacol.* **2013**, *27*, 169–172. [CrossRef] [PubMed]
18. Kumar, S.S.D.; Surianarayanan, M.; Vijayaraghavan, R.; Mandal, A.B.; MacFarlane, D.R. Curcumin loaded poly(2-hydroxyethyl methacrylate) nanoparticles from gelled ionic liquid – In vitro cytotoxicity and anti-cancer activity in SKOV-3 cells. *Eur. J. Pharm. Sci.* **2014**, *51*, 34–44. [CrossRef]
19. Chen, X.; Zou, L.-Q.; Niu, J.; Liu, W.; Peng, S.-F.; Liu, C.-M. The Stability, Sustained Release and Cellular Antioxidant Activity of Curcumin Nanoliposomes. *Mol. Basel Switz.* **2015**, *20*, 14293–14311. [CrossRef]
20. Tkalec, G.; Knez, Ž.; Novak, Z. Formation of polysaccharide aerogels in ethanol. *RSC Adv.* **2015**, *5*, 77362–77371. [CrossRef]
21. Pantić, M.; Knez, Ž.; Novak, Z. Supercritical impregnation as a feasible technique for entrapment of fat-soluble vitamins into alginate aerogels. *J. Non-Cryst. Solids* **2016**, *432*, 519–526.
22. Zhan, S.; Li, S.; Zhao, Q.; Wang, W.; Wang, J. Measurement and Correlation of Curcumin Solubility in Supercritical Carbon Dioxide. *J. Chem. Eng. Data* **2017**, *62*, 1257–1263. [CrossRef]
23. U.S. Pharmacopeial Convention. Available online: http://www.usp.org/ (accessed on 21 July 2016).

Sample Availability: Samples of the compounds are not available from the authors.

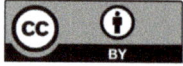

© 2020 by the authors. Licensee MDPI, Basel, Switzerland. This article is an open access article distributed under the terms and conditions of the Creative Commons Attribution (CC BY) license (http://creativecommons.org/licenses/by/4.0/).

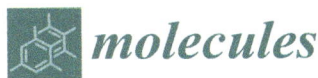

Review

Smart Porous Multi-Stimulus Polysaccharide-Based Biomaterials for Tissue Engineering

Fernando Alvarado-Hidalgo [1,2,*,†], Karla Ramírez-Sánchez [1,3,*,†] and Ricardo Starbird-Perez [1,*]

1. Centro de Investigación en Servicios Químicos y Microbiológicos, CEQIATEC, Escuela de Química, Instituto Tecnológico de Costa Rica, Cartago 159-7050, Costa Rica
2. Master Program in Medical Devices Engineering, Instituto Tecnológico de Costa Rica, Cartago 159-7050, Costa Rica
3. Centro de Investigación en Enfermedades Tropicales, CIET, Facultad de Microbiología, Universidad de Costa Rica, San José 11501-2060, Costa Rica
* Correspondence: a.alvarado@itcr.ac.cr (F.A.-H.); karamirez@itcr.ac.cr (K.R.-S.); rstarbird@itcr.ac.cr (R.S.-P.); Tel.: +506-2550-27-31 (R.S.-P.)
† These authors contributed equally to this work.

Academic Editor: T. Jean Daou
Received: 2 October 2020; Accepted: 5 November 2020; Published: 13 November 2020

Abstract: Recently, tissue engineering and regenerative medicine studies have evaluated smart biomaterials as implantable scaffolds and their interaction with cells for biomedical applications. Porous materials have been used in tissue engineering as synthetic extracellular matrices, promoting the attachment and migration of host cells to induce the in vitro regeneration of different tissues. Biomimetic 3D scaffold systems allow control over biophysical and biochemical cues, modulating the extracellular environment through mechanical, electrical, and biochemical stimulation of cells, driving their molecular reprogramming. In this review, first we outline the main advantages of using polysaccharides as raw materials for porous scaffolds, as well as the most common processing pathways to obtain the adequate textural properties, allowing the integration and attachment of cells. The second approach focuses on the tunable characteristics of the synthetic matrix, emphasizing the effect of their mechanical properties and the modification with conducting polymers in the cell response. The use and influence of polysaccharide-based porous materials as drug delivery systems for biochemical stimulation of cells is also described. Overall, engineered biomaterials are proposed as an effective strategy to improve in vitro tissue regeneration and future research directions of modified polysaccharide-based materials in the biomedical field are suggested.

Keywords: biomaterials; porous materials; biomimetic; multi-stimulation; tissue engineering; conductive polymers

1. Introduction

The number of publications related to the tissue engineering field has increased dramatically in recent years, referring to the potential regenerative methods and strategies for almost every tissue and organ of the human body. Progress has been reached by the integration of interdisciplinary research from cell biology, biomaterial sciences, and medical fields [1]. Specifically, tissue engineering involves the design and synthesis of three-dimensional (3D) matrices from biomaterials to provide a structural framework and to facilitate the attachment and migration of host cells, inducing a successful in vitro andin vivo regeneration of tissues [2–4]. Biomimetic 3D scaffolds may allow the control and application of a multi-stimulus to cells, including mechanical, electrical, and biochemical stimulations, in order to trigger specific responses, such as cell differentiation and tissue repair [5–8].

Tissue regeneration is naturally mediated by molecular processes, which direct gene expression to control renewal, restoration, and cell proliferation [9]. Nevertheless, normal regeneration is affected by aging, diseases, or accidents [10,11]. Thus, the increasing incidence of skin, muscle, and bone disorders, suffered by many people around the world, has prompted a critical need to develop engineered strategies to improve the replacement and regeneration of biological materials [11–13]. While many repair techniques have been proposed over recent decades, most of the surgical interventions have been directed toward the treatment of clinical symptoms but none have successfully repaired damaged tissues [14]. Consequently, in recent years, tissue engineering and regenerative medicine studies are focused on using the regenerative abilities of cells, in combination with engineered biomaterials, to create implantable scaffolds for tissue regeneration and reparation [1,10].

Porous materials from polysaccharides have been used as extracellular matrices (ECM) in tissue engineering in order to generate diverse types of cell lineages, promoting regeneration [15,16], for instance, in stem cells [17], osteoblasts [18], skeletal muscle cells [19], and endothelial cells [20]. In the biomedical field, aerogels from different sources have found applications as implantable devices, dressings for wound healing, synthetic bone grafts, carriers for different drugs, biosensing, and biomedical imaging [6,21].

Since they were first fabricated in 1932, aerogels have become the subject of great interest for different application fields [22]. Most common aerogel sources are from inorganic or petrochemical-based materials, such as those used to produce silica and graphene aerogels [23,24]. Recently, large efforts have been dedicated to produce aerogels using polysaccharides as raw materials. Relating them with inorganic starting materials and those derived from fossil oil, natural polysaccharides are more sustainable, green, non-toxic [25], biodegradable [26] and they have more abundant natural sources [27]. Several examples of engineering porous materials from polysaccharides have been developed. Starch and alginate aerogels [28,29], starch microspheres [30], and cellulose nanowhiskers [31] are among the different examples found in the literature. From a basic science perspective, the capacity to modulate the biomaterial properties to convey unique material characteristics allows their application in different fields, with biomedical being the most important, from our point of view.

Numerous strategies have been reported to obtain polysaccharide-based aerogels to guide functional restoration to the site of injury. Control of the size and porosity in the scaffold mediates cellular infiltration [32] and facilitates the transport of nutrients [33], oxygen [34], and waste products [35]. Porosity also regulates the vascularization by angiogenesis and cell attachment [30,36]. Mechanical properties of biomaterials, such as stiffness, structure, and topography, are also considered during ECM synthesis, mainly because they can alter the local tissue microenvironments through intracellular and intercellular signaling [7,9,37]. Besides, one of the most relevant applications of polysaccharide-based aerogels is the capability of releasing drugs as controlled delivery systems. The synthetic scaffold acts as a carrier for drug molecules, in order to release them specifically to target cells or tissues and improve their differentiation and regeneration [6,38,39]. Specifically, the combination of polysaccharide-based porous materials with biomolecules is known as a polymer bioconjugate and is a novel strategy used for the fixation of amino acids, nuclei acids, peptides, and carbohydrates to different polymers, in order to improve their application as therapeutics [40]. Alternatively, conductive polymers have been proposed in combination with aerogels as a system for electrical stimulation of cells and tissues in regenerative medicine [5,41].

Our review summarizes the current status of smart 3D scaffold systems based on polysaccharides regarding their production, properties, and potential applications in the biomedical field. Although those topics have been extensively reviewed in the past, our approach will focus on the potential development of biomimetic 3D scaffold systems including the physical, mechanical, electrical, and biochemical properties of modified polysaccharide-based aerogels and cryogels. Moreover, novel research directions of these smart materials, including strategies for the impregnation of drugs and their subsequent release from porous materials, and modification with conductive polymers were covered to be applied in the biomedical field.

2. Overview: Polysaccharide-Based Porous Materials

Aerogels are solid, lightweight, and high specific surface area materials with interconnected networks of particles obtained from a wet gel during a process where their liquid phase is removed and replaced with gas without the collapsing of the solid structure [6,22].

Through time, aerogels have been obtained by structuring both organic and inorganic materials. Silica [24,42,43], silica/pre-polymerized vinyl trimethoxy silane (VTMS) composites [44], and graphene-based aerogels [23,45] are among the most used inorganic materials reported for aerogel production. However, despite several relevant features found for inorganic aerogels, biopolymer-based aerogels have been the object of much research lately due to their mechanical properties [46], non-toxicity [25], and biocompatibility [21], all desirable properties in systems to be used in biomedical field [47].

Polysaccharide-based aerogels were reported first by Kistler [22], using cellulose, nitrocellulose, gelatin, agar, and egg albumin. More recent research has reported the obtention of aerogels from polysaccharides such as chitosan [48], chitosan/alginate [49], cellulose [50], starch [13,30,51–53], starch/κ-carrageenan (κC) [53], and pectin [27].

Considering that polysaccharides possess abundant natural sources from which they can be obtained [27], along with renewability and non-toxicity, they are excellent raw material candidates for aerogel processing regarding circular economy principles, relying on renewable raw material or energy sources [25,54].

2.1. Processing Strategies for Polysaccharide-Based Aerogels

Diverse strategies have been used to obtain polysaccharide-based aerogels. The sol-gel method is commonly reported as an initial step in the processing pathways for organic or inorganic materials [28]. In the sol-gel process, a hydrogel formation is induced by crosslinking of the base material. Once the hydrogel is formed, it is necessary to select the drying method to be used; materials obtained from supercritical drying are commonly known as aerogels, whereas materials dried by freeze drying (lyophilization) are known as cryogels [21]. Figure 1 illustrates the scheme for supercritical drying and freeze drying, the most widely used methods in processing porous materials [21].

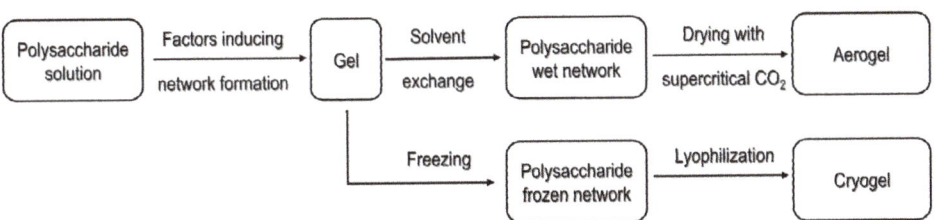

Figure 1. Pathway for porous materials produced by supercritical drying as well as freeze drying. Modified from [55] under Creative Commons attribution license.

2.1.1. Processing Using Supercritical Fluid Technology

The usage of supercritical fluid technology allows the material design with different composition, morphology, porosity, and linear architecture [56]. In addition, processing with supercritical fluids (SCFs) leads to a solvent-free end-product with high purity. This environmentally friendly feature has been noted by other studies. In fact, SCFs have been regarded as "the green solvents for the future" since they compress different ecological benefits, an emphasis is made on their low energy consumption [21,57].

Carbon dioxide (CO_2) is the most widely used supercritical fluid, in part due to the mild operating conditions, 7.38 MPa and 304 K [56]. Supercritical drying (SCD) avoids the formation of the vapor–liquid interface that occurs upon solvent evaporation. When evaporation of the solvent occurs, the capillary pressure gradient on the pore walls may reach up to 100–200 MPa [28]. Aerogels processed by means of SCD tend to show a mesoporous structure (pores of a 2–50 nm diameter) and thus require a templating technique for inducing the formation of macropores [56]. Finally, SCF technology has been applied not only to obtain porous materials but also as a strategy for the sterilization of polymeric scaffolds from aerogels [13].

2.1.2. Cryogels Obtained by Freeze Drying

Freeze drying (FD), or lyophilization, is a drying process in which the solvent or the medium of suspension is crystallized at low temperatures and is thereafter sublimated from the solid state directly into the vapor state [58]. It is reported as a simple, environmentally friendly and economic technique for producing highly porous cryogels with reduced shrinkage [21].

Significant advantages of using FD during cryogel synthesis are that the whole conversion of raw materials and the recycling of water without pollution or volatile organic compounds problems are achieved [59]. High safety derived from its straightforward operation is an important feature that has been remarked in the literature [27]. Nevertheless, one important drawback reported for freeze drying is that the process takes several hours to be completed [23]. In addition, freeze-dried materials tend to have larger macroporosity (pores >50 nm diameter) than SCD-processed materials [21].

Freeze drying requires freezing the hydrogels, transforming all the liquid that fills the interconnected 3D structure, to solid. Then, at low pressures, the sublimation of the solid solvent is promoted, avoiding the formation of the vapor–liquid interface [51,59]. The morphology of the porous structure is determined by the nucleation and ice crystal growth process of the gel solution [27], producing cryogel pores due to sublimation of the ice crystals [60]. Large ice crystals are obtained with low nucleation rates; this is reached by using small subcooling temperatures, as close to the equilibrium state as possible, between solution and ice crystals (0 °C) [58].

Two important steps are found for the crystallization process: nucleation and ice crystal growth [27]. Since pores are formed due to the sublimation of the ice crystals [60], the crystal morphology has a direct effect on the final pore morphology of the cryogel. The crystal morphology can be related to the freezing or and pre-freezing conditions (temperature and rate), additives, suspended solids [60], or the initial material concentration [27]. In addition, increasing the pressure at the freezing phase can shorten the cooling time and form small regular ice crystals [27].

Direct comparison between the porous materials obtained by SCD or by FD results in an important specific surface area decrement for the freeze-dried cryogels [51]. However, cryogels have shown porosity values equal to or higher than SCD aerogels, with an important macropore fraction that may be suitable for different applications where macroporosity is required. See detailed information in Table 1.

Table 1. Properties reported in different research studies for porous materials from biopolymers.

Raw Material	Fabrication Method	Specific Surface Area (m^2/g)	Porosity (%)	Reference
Corn starch	scCO$_2$	130–183	80–89	[13]
	scCO$_2$	102–274	N.R.	[61]
	scCO$_2$	221–234	85–90	[62]
	scCO$_2$	79–87	N.R.	[52]
	scCO$_2$	183–197	61–73	[51]
	FD	0.6–7.7	>80	[51]
	scCO$_2$	223–247	87	[53]
	scCO$_2$	313–362	N.R.	[63]
	scCO$_2$	254	N.R.	[64]
	scCO$_2$	370	N.R.	[65]
Wheat starch	scCO$_2$	52.6–57.9	N.R.	[66]
	scCO$_2$	34.7–60.9	91–93	[66]
Pea starch	scCO$_2$	204–230	84–92	[62]
	scCO$_2$	221	N.R.	[64]
Potato starch	scCO$_2$	42–70	N.R.	[67]
	scCO$_2$	85–88	N.R.	[64]
Starch/κ-carrageenan	scCO$_2$	194–231	78–85	[53]
κ-carrageenan	scCO$_2$	≈ 230	N.R.	[68]
Chitosan	scCO$_2$	>250	>96	[48]
Cellulose	scCO$_2$	287–303	92–96	[50]
	FD	297	96.4	[50]
	scCO$_2$	20–246	91–99	[69]
Alginate/chitosan	scCO$_2$	127.4–192.3	N.R.	[49]
Alginate composites	scCO$_2$	200–800	N.R.	[70]
Whey protein isolate	scCO$_2$	14–447	N.R.	[71]
	FD	<5	N.R.	[71]
Poly (ε-caprolactone)	scCO$_2$	N.R.	54–58.8	[72]

N.R.: Not reported; scCO$_2$: Supercritical CO$_2$; FD: Freeze Drying.

3. Polysaccharide-Based Porous Materials for Tissue Engineering

In recent years, tissue engineering and regenerative medicine studies have been based on the combination of specific types of cells and 3D porous scaffolds to induce a successful in vitro regeneration of diverse tissues [2–4].

The main efforts on engineered ECM in the biomedical field have been focused on the use and stimulation of pluripotent stem cells, which are special cells that have the ability to perpetuate themselves through a mechanism of self-renewal and to generate diverse types of cells through differentiation processes [15–17]. Nevertheless, osteoblasts [18], skeletal muscle cells [18], and endothelial cells [20] have been also studied.

3.1. Polysaccharide-Based Porous Materials as Extracellular Matrices

An extracellular matrix is an organized network composed by a mixture of cellular and non-cellular components. It plays an important role in tissue and organ morphogenesis, cell function, and structure maintenance. The biochemical and mechanical stimulus that cells receive from the matrix influences their growth, migration, differentiation, survival, and homeostasis [73].

Aerogels, as porous 3D matrices, possess a nanostructure that is able to mimic the extracellular matrix of the natural tissue, providing a favorable environment for the regeneration of tissues and organs [6,74]. Coupled with high porosity, low densities, and high inner surface areas, porous materials can provide appropriate morphology engineering, opening the possibility for their application as synthetic scaffolds for tissue engineering [52].

A scaffold acts as a template for new tissue formation [75] and its 3D structure guides the proliferation and colonization of cells, promoting tissue growth [56]. An ideal synthetic ECM should exhibit a highly open and uniform porosity, over 80%, with micro- and mesopores that enable cell attachment and macropores for proper vascularization [56]. The configuration of the scaffold topology is critical in controlling cellular function, it should match the endogenous topology of the cell membrane in order to enhance signaling and function [36].

Nowadays, regenerative medicine is focused on the evaluation of novel skeletal muscle regeneration strategies, which involve the prefabrication of muscle tissues in vitro by differentiation and maturing of muscle precursor cells on a scaffold, providing the required environment for myogenic differentiation of the cultured cells [76]. Researchers are studying the incorporation of products obtained from cellular metabolism in synthetic ECMs. These materials are mainly constituted of glycosaminoglycans, a group of polysaccharides that can modulate cell activity by mimicking aspects of the in vivo extracellular environment, providing important roles in cell signaling, proliferation, and differentiation through their ability to interact with ECM proteins and growth factors [77–81]. Hyaluronic acid, heparan sulfate, and heparin are the most used glycosaminoglycans in synthetic ECMs, mainly to direct the differentiation on mesenchymal stem cells (MSC) [82,83].

The synthesis of alginate hydrogels for platelet-rich plasma encapsulation as a coating for polylactic acid porous devices is another strategy used to improve cellular responses on synthetic ECM, the hydrogel system allows for better cellular integration and influences the vascularization into the membrane after skin implantation of the device, and the access to nutrients and growth factors was also improved with the engineered hydrogel. Platelet-rich plasma hydrogels could also support oxygenation of cells, avoiding hypoxia immediately post-transplantation [84,85]. In a similar study, calcium peroxide (CPO) was used during the synthesis of a gelatin methacryloyl bioprinted scaffold to achieve improved cellular oxygenation and increase fibroblast viability under hypoxia conditions [86].

The spatial arrangement, porosity, biocompatibility, and proper scale of the ECM are some of the most important features that must be adjusted for use in nervous tissue, skin, bone, and muscle [76]. Nevertheless, several other factors, such as mechanical properties and chemical modification of scaffolds, significantly influence cellular behavior [5,87]. For example, recent studies have shown that the cell nucleus works as a fast mechanical respondent in cell contractility events because of the three-dimensional extracellular matrix restriction environment, inducing deformation and the movement of cells through the activation of cytosolic phospholipase A_2 and arachidonic acid, which regulate myosin activity [88,89] (Figure 2).

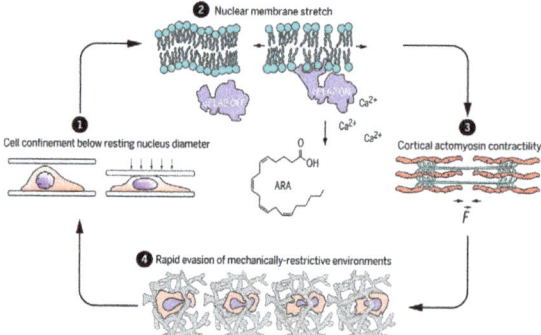

Figure 2. Schematic representation of nuclear deformation and stretching of the nuclear envelope after cell compression (1), which cause calcium release, phospholipase A_2 activation, and arachidonic acid production (2), for the regulation of actomyosin (3) and the increasing of cell migratory capacity through the 3D matrix (4). Reproduced from [89] under Science Copyright Clearance Center (CCC) license.

3.2. Influence of the Mechanical Properties of the Scaffold in Cells and Tissues Behavior

The main goal of tissue engineering and regenerative medicine is to create strategies for replacing defective tissue. The use of polymeric scaffolds as extracellular matrices tries to mimic the in vivo host conditions to restore or improve the regeneration of damaged tissues. An extracellular matrix requires not only pore size control to induce cell adhesion and the ingress of nutrients and oxygen but also the incorporation of signal molecules, such as growth and differentiation factors, as well as a proper matrix architecture and mechanical properties to keep the implanted cells alive [46,90–94].

The mechanical characteristics of a scaffold for in vitro or in vivo cell studies may ultimately impact how the hosted tissue responds to the scaffold [87]. In this regard, the architecture, chemistry, topography, and physical properties of the employed scaffold as an ECM influence the structure and function of the surrounding tissue. Cells are constantly subjected to physical forces from their microenvironment. Mechanical properties of the porous materials are indispensable to determine the viability of a tissue and play a crucial role in cellular phenotype and homeostasis [95]. There are several types of cells that respond to a mechanical stimulus. The mechanoresponsive cells include chondrocytes [88], cardiomyocytes [94], osteoblasts [96], muscle cells [97], endothelial cells [98], stem cells [7], and other tissue connective cells.

Atomic force microscopy (AFM) analysis, magnetic resonance elastography (MRE), shear rheometry, micropipette aspiration, and microindentation are some techniques commonly used to determine systematic cell responses, induced by mechanical properties of scaffold [95]. These methods cause the compression, bending, twisting, and stretching of the scaffold [99–101], inducing specific cellular responses.

Cells may sense physical cues, such as osmotic pressure, shear force, and compression loading, as well as architecture, rigidity, and other several properties of the ECM, through a process known as mechanotransduction [95]. Thus, mechanotransduction corresponds to the cell capacity to transform a mechanical stimulus into biochemical signals. There are surface proteins in cell membranes which detect a force differential and then amplify and propagate this mechanical signal to elicit a change in cell behavior [37,95].

Compression and shear stress, caused by the synthetic ECM in a cell culture, transfer mechanical stimulation to the cells and enhance their biochemical signaling. The upregulation of gene expression and the changes in cellular metabolism during mechanical stimulation are regulated by mechanically sensitive surface receptors on cell membranes. There are several proteins related with the mechanotransduction to biochemical events, integrins, specifically β1 and α5β1 integrins, are the best proteins studied so far [37].

Scaffold stiffness has been shown to have a significant impact on numerous cells and their fate, such as cell adhesion, cytoskeleton rearrangement, cell migration, stem cell differentiation, and muscle cell contractility [87]. The stiffness of an ECM in 2D cell cultures may influence the differentiation pattern of a same cell type; it has been reported that a soft matrix (0.1–1 kPa) promotes neurogenic differentiation, matrices with a medium stiffness (8–17 kPa) promote myogenic differentiation, and matrices with high stiffness (25–40 kPa) promote the osteogenic differentiation of mesenchymal stem cells [9]. Several authors have reported that the stiffness of a synthetic ECM induces mechanical stimulation of cells and the subsequent expression of cellular differentiation markers [93], tissue organization [97], causes the synthesis of extracellular matrix components [93], changes cell morphology, and improves their adhesion to synthetic scaffolds [93,98]. Additionally, the positive inotropic and chronotropic responses to both ion concentration (i.e., calcium, Ca^{2+}) and temperature after mechanical stimulation of cardiomyocytes are also reported [94].

Complexity of the mechanotransduction induced by integrins is multifaceted as the proteins can form 24 possible functional distinct dimers and each dimer forms diverse complexes with multiple intracellular adaptor proteins to dictate the interplay between biochemical and cytoskeletal elements to determine their contribution to cellular mechanoresponses [37,93]. Nevertheless, it is well known that efficient force transfer and associated cytoskeleton changes are correlated with focal adhesion formation, as defined by the recruitment of talin, vinculin, and α-actinin to the stimulated integrin; these focal adhesion proteins form the molecular bridge that physically interlinks integrins with actin microfilaments [9,92,102].

Cytoskeletal changes caused by mechanical stimulation of cells are influenced by several biochemical pathways. It has been reported that maturation of focal adhesions causes activation of focal adhesion kinase (FAK); the scaffold protein, associated with adhesion plaque, triggered the Rho-associated protein kinase cascade (ROCK), which enhanced cellular tension through engagement of actomyosin contractility [95,103]. ROCK protein involves several downstream signals, including extracellular signal-regulated kinases (ERKs) and the hippo pathway, which is related with yes-associated protein 1 (YAP1); both biochemical pathways translocate some activated proteins to the nucleus and associated with transcriptional factors to regulate cell proliferation, tissue growth, and differentiation, as well as cell migration [89,104,105]. The chronical cellular tension reinforces these downstream signaling pathways to potentiate the production of ECM and ECM remodeling proteins that stiffen the local microenvironment and reinforce mechanosignaling [95].

Experiments related with the mechanical stimulation of cells have been carried out since 1938, when Glücksmann studied endosteal cells from embryonic chick tibiae [106]. Cells were grown on substrates of explanted intercostal muscle, to which pairs of neighboring ribs were left attached [106]. After several days, cells were compressed when the ribs were drawn near toward one another as the muscle tissue degenerated. Table 2 summarizes the main strategies to induce mechanical stimulation of synthetic ECM and their effect in cultured cells.

The study of mechanical properties of extracellular matrices is important to ensure resistance of cultivated cells to in vivo stress were the matrix is used to replace damaged tissue [110,111]. Cellular responses depend on the magnitude and duration of the stimulus and high pressures may cause damage to the cell membrane and nucleus, followed by inflammatory reactions due to tissue breakdown in vivo [101]. Additionally, stiffness, roughness, and viscoelasticity are important in directing the immune response of cells. There are several T cell receptors that act as mechanical sensors, enabling the T cells to discriminate between a wide range of stiffness found in the body and respond accordingly [9]. Thus, hydrogels with higher stiffness stimulate the production of both pro- and anti-inflammatory cytokines, in contrast with low stiffness hydrogels, where the inflammatory response is suppressed and results in an overall lower foreign-body reaction in vivo [9]. The effect of the substrate mechanical properties on the in vitro response of macrophages has been also studied using poly(ethylene glycol) hydrogels (PEG) [87]. Results showed that stiffness did not impact the macrophage attachment; nevertheless, it elicited differences in their morphology.

The mechanical characteristics of scaffolds can be adjusted using adequate dynamic biomaterials in order to create matrices with an appropriate stiffness to direct specific cellular responses. Mechanical properties of synthetic scaffolds are also used to design stimulation protocols to induce the controlled release of responsive drugs potentially used for tissue regeneration.

3.3. Polysaccharide-Based Porous Materials as Scaffolds for Electrical Stimulation of Cells

Another research field of interest is focused on the preparation of electrical systems to induce specific cellular responses. Diverse tissues (e.g., nerve, muscle, and glandular) make use of endogenous electric fields (EF) to transmit electrical signals. The endogenously-generated EF exists in both the cytoplasm and extracellular space [112]. Ionic currents and EFs in living cells play critical roles in important biological processes as they generate electromotive force, maintain a required electric potential, and allow some cellular functions [113,114]. These bioelectric signals are generated by gap junctional connections and ion channels or pumps moving ions, mainly potassium (K^+) and chloride (Cl^-), across the membrane [113,115], and the regulation in cellular physiology is induced by pH gradients, specific ion flows, and changes in transmembrane potential [116].

Table 2. Used methods to induce mechanical stimulation of cells in synthetic extracellular matrices (ECM).

Raw Material	Mechanical Test	Result	Reference
Gelatin/nanohydroxiapatite cryogels	Compressive mechanical stimulation of cryogels for 14 days in a bioreactor containing 150 mL of cultured medium at 30% compression strain.	Mesenchymal stem cells were attached to the scaffold and a higher extent of osteogenic differentiation was obtained after compression.	[7]
Self-assembled peptide hydrogel (arginine, leucine, aspartic acid, and alanine)	The hydrogel containing cells was placed into a hand-control stretch device for 120 h.	Smooth muscle cells resulting in a tight adhesion in the porous structure and a lineal cell proliferation rate were reported.	[46]
Poly(lactic-co-glycolic acid) fiber coated with polypyrrole	The electrical stimulation of the matrix induced their volume modification, causing changes in the mechanical strain.	The direct dual electrical and mechanical stimulation of the pluripotent stem cells cultured in the scaffold caused a faster expression of cardiomyocytes genes, important for myocardial regeneration.	[107]
Collagen matrix reinforced with rings of electrospun silk fi-broin mat	Dynamic stimulation with pulsatile or laminar flow. Pulsatile flow was induced with a gear pump which supply a steady flow (75 mL/min) in series with a pulsatile manifold. Laminar flow was carried out of steady flow of 75 mL/min.	Chondrogenic differentiation of MSCs was observed in the presence of chondrogenic supplements in laminar flow cultures. Pulsatile flow resulted in preferential cellular orientation, as dictated by dynamic circumferential strain, and induced MSC contractile phenotype expression.	[108]
Silicon tubes with inner surfaces modified with collagen type I solutions	Cells cultured on collagen-coated silicon tubes were exposed for 24 hours to the shear stress created when culture medium passes through the tube.	Mechanical stimulation caused by shear stress on adipose-derived mesenchymal stem cells depicted significantly higher gene expression of osteoblasts and adipogenic lineages. Moreover, mechanical stimulus induced endothelial differentiation after the addition of VEGF on cultured medium.	[98]
Microcracked hydroxyapatite substrates	Bending the top surface of the cracked substrate in a piezoelectric actuator using a force of 50 N at 5 Hz for 150 s.	Flexoelectricity caused by mechanical stimulation on a hydroxyapatite substrate induced apoptotic responses on osteoblasts and osteocytes. Apoptosis was followed by proliferation of the cells adjacent to the crack, better attachment on the substrate, and an increased expression of osteocytes markers.	[109]

Currently, exogenous electrical stimulation of cells is a widely used method to improve their biological functions. Many authors have reported the use of nerve [117], bone [118], muscle [119], and neural stem cells [120], because their extensively recognized piezoelectric characteristics make them attractive for research on the role of exogenous electrical stimulation.

Coupling of an electromagnetic field with a live cell can occur via field interaction with charged molecules and proteins in the cell membrane [114]. The application of an electrical stimulus to induce cellular responses depends mainly on the level and nature of the electric potential or current applied, the frequency of the stimulus, and the type of cell studied [113]. It is reported that the application of the EF in a culture medium affects the migration [121], orientation [122], proliferation, and differentiation of cells [123,124]. Nevertheless, in most cases, it is used specifically to revive damaged or disabled tissues in the neuromuscular system as well as to accelerate the healing of injured musculoskeletal tissues, such as bone, ligament, and articular cartilage [112].

In this regard, biomaterials may receive considerable attention for their influence on cellular behaviors, ability to mimic biological functions, and, more recently, as electronic conductive systems with a potential use as tissue engineering scaffolds [5,125].

Some electroactive materials, such as conductive polymers (CPs) (e.g., poly(3,4-ethylenedioxythiophene) (PEDOT)), which are a special class of polymeric materials that present electric and ionic conductivity, are currently being studied in combination with aerogels or cryogels as a promising field in regenerative medicine (Figure 3). Nevertheless, in the past, research studies have extensively used this kind of polymer to create organic conductive interfaces, neuroprosthetic devices, neural probes, and controlled drug-delivery systems [5,41,126].

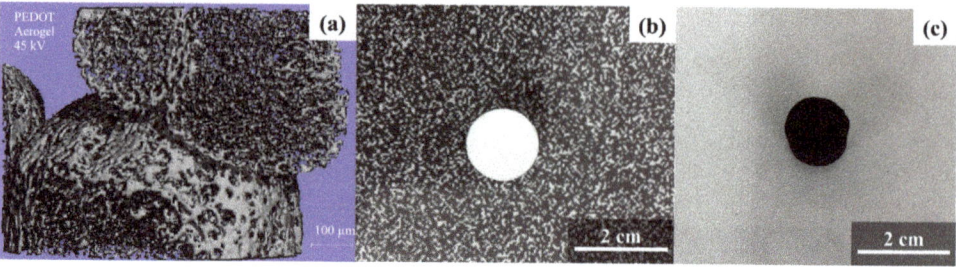

Figure 3. Porous material microtomography (micro-CT) image (**a**) and aerogel images before (**b**) and after conductive polymer (i.e., poly(3,4-ethylenedioxythiophene) (PEDOT)) modification (**c**). Reproduced from [52,53] under Elsevier Copyright Clearance Center (CCC) licenses.

Conductive polymers can be structured with porous systems using different techniques [127–129]. Starch and starch/κ-carrageenan aerogels have been used as templates for the obtention of nanoporous conductive materials [52,53]. In the biomedical field, conductive nanoporous materials have been applied not only as physical support but also as a medium to provide electrical stimulation of a cell culture. Electrical stimulation in neural cells has shown great potential for function restoring and wound healing [130].

On the other hand, the incorporation of anionic drugs and κ-carrageenan on the structure of starch porous materials is particularly interesting since both compounds may act as dopant agents for the conductive matrix, as it was shown recently [39,53,131]. Dexamethasone, a well-known glucocorticoid anionic drug, has recently been the object of research from an electrochemical point of view, regarding its doping properties on conductive matrices [132] and for its ability to be released by electrochemical stimulation from a PEDOT/κ-carrageenan film [39]. The above opens the possibility to create scaffolds from conductive porous materials and the incorporation of specific drugs in their structure to be applied as stimulation systems in tissue engineering.

3.4. Polysaccharide-Based Porous Materials as Drug-Delivery Systems

One of the main approaches and most relevant applications of biopolymer-based aerogels is their use as drug-delivery systems [6,38]. The application of these materials as controlled drug-release matrices has gained interest in the last years due to aerogel properties, such as its high surface area, high porosity, and biocompatibility [38]. Aerogels can act as a carrier for bioactive compounds, showing high loading capacity, enhanced stability upon storage, and accelerated drug release, if required [48]. Along with the high loading capacity, biopolymer-based aerogels also show an improved dissolution rate of poorly water-soluble drugs [6].

The biocompatibility of natural polymers along with the outstanding performance of aerogels as carriers for active compounds, such as drugs, have promoted the systems as scaffolds in body implants to accelerate tissue formation by providing a suitable porous structure that promotes cell colonization [62,133]. Diverse authors have also studied the incorporation of drugs and growth factors to promote the attachment, proliferation, and differentiation of cells, in order to provide both substitutes for damaged tissues and therapeutic schemes that reduce post-implantation inflammation and infections [12,133–135].

Controllable drug-release systems may be categorized as mechanical methods, which are mainly in vivo implantable pump delivery systems built from biocompatible nanomaterials [136,137], and as polymeric drug delivery systems. The last one makes use of biopolymers, in which the delivery of drugs is mainly dominated via diffusion and recently by electrochemical methods [137]. Hence, the incorporation of drugs within these kinds of porous scaffolds has been studied previously for osteogenic differentiation, bone repair activity, and the stimulation of neural tissues [126,133].

3.4.1. Diffusive Phenomena on the Controlled Release of Drugs on Polysaccharide-Based Aerogels

Different methods for drug impregnation or loading can be found in literature regarding porous materials from polysaccharides. Supercritical technology employing scCO$_2$ has been defined as the most innovative technique for producing polymer/drug composite systems for pharmaceutical applications [138]. By means of supercritical fluid technology, the impregnation of aerogel particles with drugs such as ketoprofen was achieved [62]. This process consists of placing aerogel particles and ketoprofen in a closed autoclave under agitation; the ketoprofen was dissolved in scCO$_2$ and adsorbed in the aerogel matrix [62]. The same procedure was reproduced for obtaining poly(ε-Caprolactone) (PCL) scaffolds loaded with ketoprofen [72] and for alginate-based aerogel microparticles for mucosal drug-delivery [38]. In addition, maize starch aerogels and calcium alginate aerogels were impregnated with different non-steroidal anti-inflammatory drugs, such as nimesulide, ketoprofen, and diclefenac sodium [138].

Supercritical CO$_2$ was also applied in the impregnation of starch and sodium alginate aerogels with five different active compounds, namely loratadine, ibuprofen, rifabutin, dihydroquercetin, and artemisinin, showing enhanced releasing times as well as double bioavailability in some drug–aerogel systems [139]. In addition, this research concludes that the affinity between the aerogel and the active substance must be high so that the active compound loading will be high enough to provide an increase in the dissolution rate and bioavailability [139].

Another method for loading aerogel particles was reported by mixing the active compound (Vancomycin) with a chitosan solution in different weight ratios, thus obtaining vancomycin-loaded chitosan aerogel particles, which are proposed as a system for fast local administration of the antibiotic for wound dressings [48]. A similar procedure was performed by [67], where mesoporous starch aerogels were loaded with celecoxib by adsorption during the solvent exchange steps.

Three steps are considered for the diffusion model: first, the film diffusion; the second step is the slowest, thus controlling the kinetics of the phenomenon, and it is called intraparticle diffusion; finally, the last step is the adsorbate release on adsorbent active sites [140]. Several works have been published regarding the release of drugs by means of diffusion phenomena [38,48,62,71,72,139,141]. The first mechanism when a drug-loaded polymeric material meets an aqueous solution is the filling of the pores near the surface; then, drug diffusion is initiated by the dissolution of the solute in the water-filled pores and the continuous diffusion in water [142]. Through time, the polymeric network starts swelling, inducing several structural changes that are affected by the cross-linking density and the degree of crystallinity of the 3D network. From the swelling of the polymer, a new diffusion starts through the swelled polymer structure [142]. By analyzing the release profile of drugs, conclusions can be obtained on whether the kinetics follow a Fickian or non-Fickian diffusion profile [143,144].

Innovative drug delivery systems are not only studied to improve cellular responses in different tissues but as a strategy that develops platforms and nano-scale devices for selective delivery of therapeutic small drug molecules to the cells or tissues of interest, for the maintenance of appropriate doses, and to improve individual therapy. To meet this demand, many drugs have been reformulated in new drug delivery systems to provide enhanced efficiency and more beneficial therapies [136,137].

3.4.2. Controlled Drug Release by Electrical Stimulation Employing Conductive Porous Materials

In order to prevent the negative effects resulting from exposure to high dosages of drugs, local electronically-controlled release of pharmaceutical compounds from implantable devices appears as a promising option [145]. Drugs anchored inside the conductive materials have been reported using supercritical technology and electropolymerization [126,146].

Electrochemical methods involve the use of conductive polymers, which are electrochemically oxidized during the polymerization processes, generating charge carriers, and, thus, allowing ionic drugs' impregnation based on electrostatic interactions [147]. There are two main electrochemical methods to induce the immobilization of drugs. In the first one, an ionic drug (preferably anionic) acts as a doping agent and its anchoring proceeds simultaneously with the process of matrix formation, commonly named one-step immobilization or *in situ* immobilization [146,148,149]. Drug fixation is the result of the ion-exchange processes during polymer oxidation. Ionic drugs can serve as counter-ions for the positively charged centers in the growing polymer chain [149]. Anti-cancer drugs, anti-inflammatory compounds, and hormones have been fixed on conductive materials using one-step immobilization, mainly for the development of neural devices [150–152].

The second method corresponds to the two-step or *ex situ* immobilization. The incorporation of the drug is carried out after the synthesis of the matrix, through ion exchange processes taking place at their surface. First, the polymer film is synthesized from a solution consisting of the monomer and a small ionic molecule as doping agent, without the drug. The obtained film is later reduced and oxidized by an electrical stimulus [148,149]. Reduction induces the removal of the dopant from the film; meanwhile, the drug, which acts as the second doping agent, is incorporated during the process of matrix oxidation [149]. This approach allows to prevent the interference of drugs during the growth of polymer matrix and their subsequent release does not have much impact on their physicochemical properties [148,149].

Related with the above, some strategies of drug fixation on conductive polymers using two different doping agents have been reported [39,149,153]. The anti-inflammatory drugs dexamethasone and κ-carrageenan were anchored simultaneously during PEDOT film formation, using *in situ* immobilization. After film oxidation, κC was maintained on the matrix, granting the film greater stability and integrity even after drug release [39].

Drug delivery is caused by electrochemical stimulation of the conductive matrix, which induces the oxidation and/or reduction of the film. By applying a negative potential, the polymeric matrix is reduced and the cationic charge of the polymer backbone is neutralized, causing the release of the anionic drug by electrostatic mechanisms [148]. In a similar procedure, applying negative and positive cyclic potentials induces the reduction and oxidation of the polymeric film, respectively; meanwhile, the matrix experiments expansion and contraction, which force the release of the drug. Although cyclic stimulation allows a greater amount of drug release in comparison with other methods, some authors have reported that the application of the stimulus may cause delamination, cracks, and breakdowns of the matrix, mainly in one-step immobilization systems [126,154,155].

The controlled release of drugs using electrical stimulation from conductive polymer films [39,126,151] opens the door for a different approach regarding the application of polysaccharide aerogels on drug delivery. Since these materials can be coated with an electrically conductive material while incorporating active compounds, those composites may be used in the controlled release of bioactive molecules by electrical stimulation [156,157]. These biochemical release systems are the main focus of several research groups and further investigations should follow this path in order to promote smart scaffolds that merge mechanical, electrical, and biochemical stimulation processes, mimicking the in vivo ECM conditions, in order to promote specific cell behavior, as shown in Figure 4.

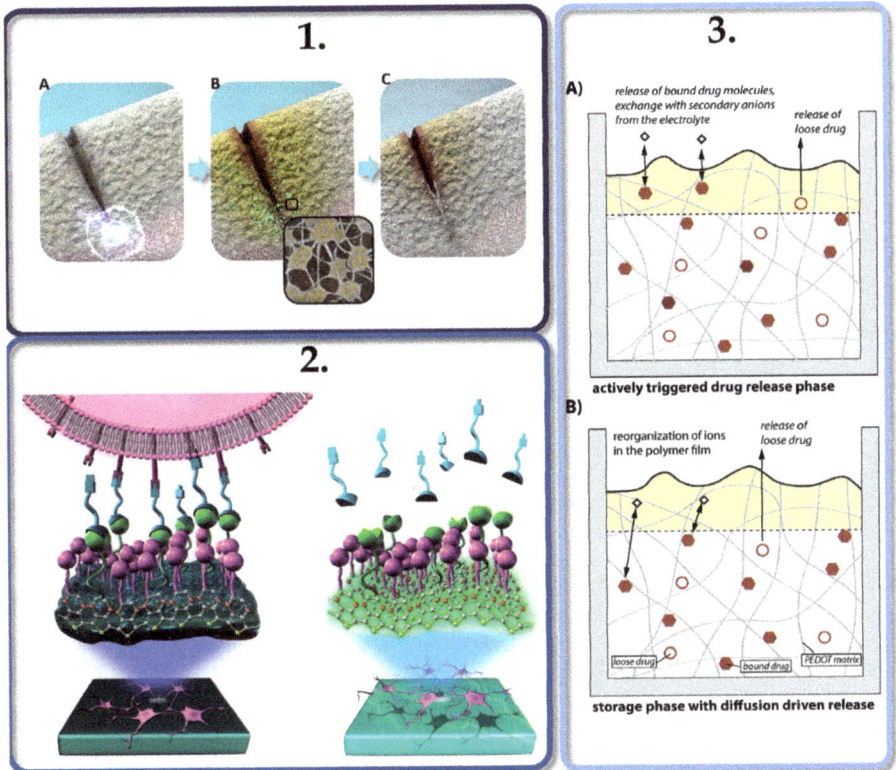

Figure 4. (1) Flexoelectricity induced by mechanical stimulation (**A**) plays an important role in bone repair and remodeling by inducing osteoblasts migration (**B**) and mineralization (**C**). Reproduced from [109] under Creative Commons Attribution License. (**2**) Electrical communication and redox-triggered interaction between neurons and (PEDOT) matrices functionalized with hydroquinone electroswitches and phosphorylcholine zwitterions. (**3**) Schematic representation of the active drug-delivery triggered by an electrical stimulus (**A**) and passive drug-release induced by diffusion processes from a conductive polymeric matrix (**B**). Reproduced from [151,158] under Elsevier Copyright Clearance Center (CCC) licenses.

4. Conclusions

The current status of biomimetic scaffold systems based on polysaccharides has been reviewed regarding multi-stimulation, mechanical, electrical, and biochemical, in order to trigger specific responses in cells during growth and differentiation, specifically in the biomedical field. Some details of their production and properties have been summarized, including modification with conductive polymers and strategies for controlled drug release from porous materials, such as aerogels. Therefore, future studies of modified polysaccharide-based aerogels for tissue engineering could consider promoting physical, mechanical, electrical, and biochemical multi-stimulation with the aim to mimic in vivo conditions.

Author Contributions: Conceptualization, F.A.-H. and K.R.-S.; methodology, F.A.-H. and K.R.-S.; validation, F.A.-H., K.R.-S. and R.S.-P.; formal analysis, F.A.-H., K.R.-S. and R.S.-P.; investigation, F.A.-H., K.R.-S. and R.S.-P.; resources, R.S.-P.; data curation, F.A.-H., K.R.-S. and R.S.-P.; writing, original draft preparation, F.A.-H. and K.R.-S.; writing, review and editing, F.A.-H., K.R.-S. and R.S.-P.; visualization, F.A.-H., K.R.-S. and R.S.-P.; supervision, R.S.-P.; project administration R.S.-P.; funding acquisition, R.S.-P. All authors have read and agreed to the published version of the manuscript.

Funding: This research was funded by Vicerrectoría de Investigación from Instituto Tecnológico de Costa Rica (VIE-ITCR), grant number 5402-1360-4401 and the Ministerio de Ciencia, Tecnología y Telecomunicaciones de Costa Rica (MICITT), grant number FI-038B-19.

Acknowledgments: The authors would like to thank the Centro de Investigación y Extensión en Materiales (CIEMTEC) and the Centro de Investigación en Biotecnología (CIB) from Instituto Tecnológico de Costa Rica. Aerogels COST action (CA18125). F.A.-H would like to thank Carlos A. García-González for his mentoring on aerogel processing and characterization.

Conflicts of Interest: The authors declare no conflict of interest.

References

1. Dhandayuthapani, B.; Yoshida, Y.; Maekawa, T.; Kumar, D.S. Polymeric scaffolds in tissue engineering application: A review. *Int. J. Polym. Sci.* **2011**, *2011*, 290602. [CrossRef]
2. Stratton, S.; Shelke, N.B.; Hoshino, K.; Rudraiah, S.; Kumbar, S.G. Bioactive polymeric scaffolds for tissue engineering. *Bioact. Mater.* **2016**, *1*, 93–108. [CrossRef] [PubMed]
3. Santoro, M.; Shah, S.R.; Walker, J.L.; Mikos, A.G. Poly(lactic acid) nanofibrous scaffolds for tissue engineering. *Adv. Drug Deliv. Rev.* **2016**, *107*, 206–212. [CrossRef] [PubMed]
4. Jo, H.; Sim, M.; Kim, S.; Yang, S.; Yoo, Y.; Park, J.-H.; Yoon, T.H.; Kim, M.-G.; Lee, J.Y. Electrically conductive graphene/polyacrylamide hydrogels produced by mild chemical reduction for enhanced myoblast growth and differentiation. *Acta Biomater.* **2017**, *48*, 100–109. [CrossRef] [PubMed]
5. Aznar-Cervantes, S.; Pagán, A.; Martínez, J.G.; Bernabeu-Esclapez, A.; Otero, T.F.; Meseguer-Olmo, L.; Paredes, J.I.; Cenis, J.L. Electrospun silk fibroin scaffolds coated with reduced graphene promote neurite outgrowth of PC-12 cells under electrical stimulation. *Mater. Sci. Eng. C* **2017**, *79*, 315–325. [CrossRef] [PubMed]
6. García-González, C.A.; Budtova, T.; Duraes, L.; Erkey, C.; Del Gaudio, P.; Gurikov, P.; Koebel, M.; Liebner, F.; Neagu, M.; Smirnova, I. An opinion paper on aerogels for biomedical and environmental applications. *Molecules* **2019**, *24*, 1815. [CrossRef] [PubMed]
7. Shalumon, K.T.; Liao, H.; Kuo, C.; Wong, C.; Li, C.; Mini, P.A.; Chen, J. Rational design of gelatin/nanohydroxyapatite cryogel scaffolds for bone regeneration by introducing chemical and physical cues to enhance osteogenesis of bone marrow mesenchymal stem cells. *Mater. Sci. Eng. C* **2019**, *104*, 109855. [CrossRef]
8. Afanasenkau, D.; Kalinina, D.; Lyakhovetskii, V.; Tondera, C.; Gorsky, O.; Moosavi, S.; Pavlova, N.; Merkulyeva, N.; Kalueff, A.V.; Minev, I.R.; et al. Rapid prototyping of soft bioelectronic implants for use as neuromuscular interfaces. *Nat. Biomed. Eng.* **2020**, *4*, 1010–1022. [CrossRef] [PubMed]
9. Gaharwar, A.K.; Singh, I.; Khademhosseini, A. Engineered biomaterials for in situ tissue regeneration. *Nat. Rev. Mater.* **2020**, *5*, 686–705. [CrossRef]
10. Jahromi, M.; Razavi, S.; Bakhtiari, A. The advances in nerve tissue engineering: From fabrication of nerve conduit to in vivo nerve regeneration assays. *J. Tissue Eng. Regen. Med.* **2019**, *13*, 2077–2100. [CrossRef]
11. Lin, H.; Sohn, J.; Shen, H.; Langhans, M.T.; Tuan, R.S. Bone marrow mesenchymal stem cells: Aging and tissue engineering applications to enhance bone healing. *Biomaterials* **2019**, *203*, 96–110. [CrossRef]
12. Paun, I.A.; Zamfirescu, M.; Luculescu, C.R.; Acasandrei, A.M.; Mustaciosu, C.C.; Mihailescu, M.; Dinescu, M. Electrically responsive microreservoires for controllable delivery of dexamethasone in bone tissue engineering. *Appl. Surf. Sci.* **2017**, *392*, 321–331. [CrossRef]
13. Santos-Rosales, V.; Ardao, I.; Alvarez-Lorenzo, C.; Ribeiro, N.; Oliveira, A.L.; García-González, C.A. Sterile and dual-porous aerogels scaffolds obtained through a multistep supercritical CO_2-based approach. *Molecules* **2019**, *24*, 871. [CrossRef] [PubMed]
14. Francis Suh, J.K.; Matthew, H.W.T. Application of chitosan-based polysaccharide biomaterials in cartilage tissue engineering: A review. *Biomaterials* **2000**, *21*, 2589–2598. [CrossRef]
15. Hamidouche, Z.; Haÿ, E.; Vaudin, P.; Charbord, P.; Schüle, R.; Marie, P.J.; Fromigué, O. FHL2 mediates dexamethasone-induced mesenchymal cell differentiation into osteoblasts by activating Wnt/β-catenin signaling-dependent Runx2 expression. *FASEB J.* **2008**, *22*, 3813–3822. [CrossRef] [PubMed]
16. Reya, T.; Morrison, S.J.; Clarke, M.; Weissman, I. Stem cells, cancer, and cancer stem cells. *Nature* **2001**, *414*, 105–111. [CrossRef]

17. Sammons, J.; Ahmed, N.; Hassan, H.T. The role of BMP-6, IL-6, and BMP-4 in mesenchymal stem cell-dependent bone development: Effects on osteoblastic differentiation induced by parathyroid hormone and vitamin D3. *Stem Cells Dev.* **2004**, *280*, 273–280. [CrossRef]
18. Wojak-Ćwik, I.M.; Rumian, Ł.; Krok-Borkowicz, M.; Hess, R.; Bernhardt, R.; Dobrzyński, P.; Möller, S.; Schnabelrauch, M.; Hintze, V.; Scharnweber, D.; et al. Synergistic effect of bimodal pore distribution and artificial extracellular matrices in polymeric scaffolds on osteogenic differentiation of human mesenchymal stem cells. *Mater. Sci. Eng. C* **2019**, *97*, 12–22. [CrossRef] [PubMed]
19. Cheema, U.; Yang, S.Y.; Mudera, V.; Goldspink, G.G.; Brown, R.A. 3-D in vitro model of early skeletal muscle development. *Cell Motil. Cytoskelet.* **2003**, *54*, 226–236. [CrossRef]
20. He, H.; Sofman, M.; Wang, A.J.S.; Ahrens, C.C.; Wang, W.; Griffith, L.G.; Hammond, P.T. Engineering helical modular polypeptide-based hydrogels as synthetic extracellular matrices for cell culture. *Biomacromolecules* **2020**, *21*, 566–580. [CrossRef]
21. El-Naggar, M.E.; Othman, S.I.; Allam, A.A.; Morsy, O.M. Synthesis, drying process and medical application of polysaccharide-based aerogels. *Int. J. Biol. Macromol.* **2020**, *145*, 1115–1128. [CrossRef]
22. Kistler, S.S. Coherent expanded aerogels. *J. Phys. Chem.* **1932**, *36*, 52–64. [CrossRef]
23. Korkmaz, S.; Kariper, A. Graphene and graphene oxide based aerogels: Synthesis, characteristics and supercapacitor applications. *J. Energy Storage* **2020**, *27*, 101038. [CrossRef]
24. Shewale, P.M.; Rao, A.V.; Gurav, J.L.; Rao, A.P. Synthesis and characterization of low density and hydrophobic silica aerogels dried at ambient pressure using sodium silicate precursor. *J. Porous Mater.* **2009**, *16*, 101–108. [CrossRef]
25. Zhu, F. Starch based aerogels: Production, properties and applications. *Trends Food Sci. Technol.* **2019**, *89*, 1–10. [CrossRef]
26. Ulery, B.D.; Nair, L.S.; Laurencin, C.T. Biomedical applications of biodegradable polymers. *J. Polym. Sci. Part B Polym. Phys.* **2011**, *49*, 832–864. [CrossRef]
27. Wang, Y.; Su, Y.; Wang, W.; Fang, Y.; Riffat, S.B.; Jiang, F. The advances of polysaccharide-based aerogels: Preparation and potential application. *Carbohydr. Polym.* **2019**, *226*, 115242. [CrossRef]
28. García-González, C.A.; Alnaief, M.; Smirnova, I. Polysaccharide-based aerogels-promising biodegradable carriers for drug delivery systems. *Carbohydr. Polym.* **2011**, *86*, 1425–1438. [CrossRef]
29. Martins, M.; Barros, A.A.; Quraishi, S.; Gurikov, P.; Raman, S.P.; Smirnova, I.; Duarte, A.R.C.; Reis, R.L. Preparation of macroporous alginate-based aerogels for biomedical applications. *J. Supercrit. Fluids* **2015**, *106*, 152–159. [CrossRef]
30. García-González, C.A.; Jin, M.; Gerth, J.; Alvarez-Lorenzo, C.; Smirnova, I. Polysaccharide-based aerogel microspheres for oral drug delivery. *Carbohydr. Polym.* **2015**, *117*, 797–806. [CrossRef]
31. Rosa, M.F.; Medeiros, E.S.; Malmonge, J.A.; Gregorski, K.S.; Wood, D.F.; Mattoso, L.H.C.; Glenn, G.; Orts, W.J.; Imam, S.H. Cellulose nanowhiskers from coconut husk fibers: Effect of preparation conditions on their thermal and morphological behavior. *Carbohydr. Polym.* **2010**, *81*, 83–92. [CrossRef]
32. Sussman, E.M.; Halpin, M.C.; Muster, J.; Moon, R.T.; Ratner, B.D. Porous implants modulate healing and induce shifts in local macrophage polarization in the foreign body reaction. *Ann. Biomed. Eng.* **2014**, *42*, 1508–1516. [CrossRef]
33. Loh, Q.; Choong, C. Three-dimensional scaffolds for tissue engineering applications: Role of porosity and pore size. *Tissue Eng. Part B Rev.* **2013**, *19*, 485–502. [CrossRef]
34. Takahashi, Y.; Tabata, Y. Effect of the fiber diameter and porosity of non-woven PET fabrics on the osteogenic differentiation of mesenchymal stem cells. *J. Biomater. Sci. Polym. Ed.* **2012**, *15*, 37–41. [CrossRef] [PubMed]
35. Pramanik, S.; Pingguan-Murphy, B.; Abu Osman, N.A. Progress of key strategies in development of electrospun scaffolds: Bone tissue. *Sci. Technol. Adv. Mater.* **2012**, *13*, 43002. [CrossRef] [PubMed]
36. Viswanathan, P.; Ondeck, M.G.; Chirasatitsin, S.; Ngamkham, K.; Reilly, G.C.; Engler, A.J.; Battaglia, G. 3D surface topology guides stem cell adhesion and differentiation. *Biomaterials* **2015**, *52*, 140–147. [CrossRef]
37. Shuaib, A.; Motan, D.; Bhattacharya, P.; McNabb, A.; Skerry, T.M.; Lacroix, D. Heterogeneity in the mechanical properties of integrins determines mechanotransduction dynamics in bone osteoblasts. *Sci. Rep.* **2019**, *9*, 13113. [CrossRef]
38. Gonçalves, V.S.S.; Gurikov, P.; Poejo, J.; Matias, A.A.; Heinrich, S.; Duarte, C.M.M.; Smirnova, I. Alginate-based hybrid aerogel microparticles for mucosal drug delivery. *Eur. J. Pharm. Biopharm.* **2016**, *107*, 160–170. [CrossRef]

39. Ramírez-Sánchez, K.; Ledezma-Espinoza, A.; Sánchez-Kopper, A.; Avendaño-Soto, E.; Prado, M.; Starbird Perez, R. Polysaccharide κ-carrageenan as doping agent in conductive coatings for electrochemical controlled release of dexamethasone at therapeutic doses. *Molecules* **2020**, *25*, 2139. [CrossRef]
40. Chen, C.; Yuen, D.; Ng, W.; Weil, T. Progress in polymer science polymer bioconjugates: Modern design concepts toward precision hybrid materials. *Prog. Polym. Sci.* **2020**, *105*, 101241. [CrossRef]
41. Pires, F.; Ferreira, Q.; Rodrigues, C.A.V.; Morgado, J.; Ferreira, F.C. Neural stem cell differentiation by electrical stimulation using a cross-linked PEDOT substrate: Expanding the use of biocompatible conjugated conductive polymers for neural tissue engineering. *BBA-Gen. Subj.* **2015**, *1850*, 1158–1168. [CrossRef] [PubMed]
42. Smirnova, I.; Mamic, J.; Arlt, W. Adsorption of drugs on silica aerogels. *Langmuir* **2003**, *19*, 8521–8525. [CrossRef]
43. Durães, L.; Hajar, M.; Vareda, J.P.; Lamy-Mendes, A.; Portugal, A. Exploring the versatile surface chemistry of silica aerogels for multipurpose application. *MRS Adv.* **2017**, *2*, 3511–3519. [CrossRef]
44. Rezaei, S.; Jalali, A.; Zolali, A.M.; Alshrah, M.; Karamikamkar, S.; Park, C.B. Robust, ultra-insulative and transparent polyethylene-based hybrid silica aerogel with a novel non-particulate structure. *J. Colloid Interface Sci.* **2019**, *548*, 206–216. [CrossRef]
45. Ziegler, C.; Wolf, A.; Liu, W.; Herrmann, A.K.; Gaponik, N.; Eychmüller, A. Modern inorganic aerogels. *Angew. Chem. Int. Ed.* **2017**, *56*, 13200–13221. [CrossRef]
46. Nagai, Y.; Yokoi, H.; Kaihara, K.; Naruse, K. The mechanical stimulation of cells in 3D culture within a self-assembling peptide hydrogel. *Biomaterials* **2012**, *33*, 1044–1051. [CrossRef]
47. García-González, C.A.; Carenza, E.; Zeng, M.; Smirnova, I.; Roig, A. Design of biocompatible magnetic pectin aerogel monoliths and microspheres. *RSC Adv.* **2012**, *2*, 9816–9823. [CrossRef]
48. López-Iglesias, C.; Barros, J.; Ardao, I.; Monteiro, F.J.; Alvarez-Lorenzo, C.; Gómez-Amoza, J.L.; García-González, C.A. Vancomycin-loaded chitosan aerogel particles for chronic wound applications. *Carbohydr. Polym.* **2019**, *204*, 223–231. [CrossRef]
49. Baldino, L.; Cardea, S.; Scognamiglio, M.; Reverchon, E. A new tool to produce alginate-based aerogels for medical applications, by supercritical gel drying. *J. Supercrit. Fluids* **2019**, *146*, 152–158. [CrossRef]
50. Ganesan, K.; Dennstedt, A.; Barowski, A.; Ratke, L. Design of aerogels, cryogels and xerogels of cellulose with hierarchical porous structures. *Mater. Des.* **2016**, *92*, 345–355. [CrossRef]
51. Baudron, V.; Gurikov, P.; Smirnova, I.; Whitehouse, S. Porous starch materials via supercritical-and freeze-drying. *Gels* **2019**, *5*, 12. [CrossRef]
52. Starbird, R.; García-González, C.A.; Smirnova, I.; Krautschneider, W.H.; Bauhofer, W. Synthesis of an organic conductive porous material using starch aerogels as template for chronic invasive electrodes. *Mater. Sci. Eng. C* **2014**, *37*, 177–183. [CrossRef]
53. Zamora-Sequeira, R.; Ardao, I.; Starbird, R.; García-González, C.A. Conductive nanostructured materials based on poly-(3,4-ethylenedioxythiophene) (PEDOT) and starch/κ-carrageenan for biomedical applications. *Carbohydr. Polym.* **2018**, *189*, 304–312. [CrossRef] [PubMed]
54. Avraamidou, S.; Baratsas, S.G.; Tian, Y.; Pistikopoulos, E.N. Circular economy—A challenge and an opportunity for Process Systems Engineering. *Comput. Chem. Eng.* **2020**, *133*, 106629. [CrossRef]
55. Ganesan, K.; Budtova, T.; Ratke, L.; Gurikov, P.; Baudron, V.; Preibisch, I.; Niemeyer, P.; Smirnova, I.; Milow, B. Review on the production of polysaccharide aerogel particles. *Materials* **2018**, *11*, 2144. [CrossRef]
56. García-González, C.A.; Concheiro, A.; Alvarez-Lorenzo, C. Processing of materials for regenerative medicine using supercritical fluid technology. *Bioconjug. Chem.* **2015**, *26*, 1159–1171. [CrossRef]
57. Knez, Ž.; Pantić, M.; Cör, D.; Novak, Z.; Knez Hrnčič, M. Are supercritical fluids solvents for the future? *Chem. Eng. Process. Process Intensif.* **2019**, *141*, 107532. [CrossRef]
58. Wilhelm Oetjen, G. *Freeze Drying*; Wiley-VCH Verlag GmbH & Co. KGaA: Weinheim, Germany, 1999; ISBN 3-527-29571-2.
59. Liao, W.; Zhao, H.B.; Liu, Z.; Xu, S.; Wang, Y.Z. On controlling aerogel microstructure by freeze casting. *Compos. Part B Eng.* **2019**, *173*, 107036. [CrossRef]
60. Ni, X.; Ke, F.; Xiao, M.; Wu, K.; Kuang, Y.; Corke, H.; Jiang, F. The control of ice crystal growth and effect on porous structure of konjac glucomannan-based aerogels. *Int. J. Biol. Macromol.* **2016**, *92*, 1130–1135. [CrossRef]

61. García-gonzález, C.A.; Camino-rey, M.C.; Alnaief, M.; Zetzl, C.; Smirnova, I. Supercritical drying of aerogels using CO_2: Effect of extraction time on the end material textural properties. *J. Supercrit. Fluids* **2012**, *66*, 297–306. [CrossRef]
62. García-González, C.A.; Smirnova, I. Use of supercritical fluid technology for the production of tailor-made aerogel particles for delivery systems. *J. Supercrit. Fluids* **2013**, *79*, 152–158. [CrossRef]
63. Kenar, J.A.; Eller, F.J.; Felker, F.C.; Jackson, A.; Fanta, G.F. Starch aerogel beads obtained from inclusion complexes prepared from high amylose starch and sodium palmitate. *Green Chem.* **2014**, *16*, 1921–1930. [CrossRef]
64. Druel, L.; Bardl, R.; Vorwerg, W.; Budtova, T. Starch aerogels: A member of the family of thermal super-insulating materials. *Biomacromolecules* **2017**, *18*, 4232–4239. [CrossRef]
65. Zhang, Y.; Zhu, J.; Ren, H.; Bi, Y.; Shi, X.; Wang, B.; Zhang, L. A novel starch-enhanced melamine-formaldehyde aerogel with low volume shrinkage and high toughness. *J. Porous Mater.* **2017**, *24*, 1303–1307. [CrossRef]
66. Ubeyitogullari, A.; Brahma, S.; Rose, D.J.; Ciftci, O. In vitro digestibility of nanoporous wheat starch aerogels. *J. Agric. Food Chem.* **2018**, *66*, 9490–9497. [CrossRef]
67. Mohammadi, A.; Moghaddas, J. Mesoporous tablet-shaped potato starch aerogels for loading and release of the poorly water-soluble drug celecoxib. *Chin. J. Chem. Eng.* **2020**, *28*, 1778–1787. [CrossRef]
68. Ganesan, K.; Ratke, L. Facile preparation of monolithic κ-carrageenan aerogels. *Soft Matter* **2014**, *10*, 3218–3224. [CrossRef]
69. Nedelec, J.-M.; Pircher, N.; Strauß, C.; Carbajal, L.; Kasper, C.; Rosenau, T.; Fischhuber, D.; Liebner, F. Preparation and reinforcement of dual-porous biocompatible cellulose scaffolds for tissue engineering. *Macromol. Mater. Eng.* **2015**, *300*, 911–924.
70. Raman, S.P.; Gurikov, P.; Smirnova, I. Hybrid alginate based aerogels by carbon dioxide induced gelation: Novel technique for multiple applications. *J. Supercrit. Fluids* **2015**, *106*, 23–33. [CrossRef]
71. Betz, M.; García-González, C.A.; Subrahmanyam, R.P.; Smirnova, I.; Kulozik, U. Preparation of novel whey protein-based aerogels as drug carriers for life science applications. *J. Supercrit. Fluids* **2012**, *72*, 111–119. [CrossRef]
72. Goimil, L.; Braga, M.E.M.; Dias, A.M.A.; Gómez-Amoza, J.L.; Concheiro, A.; Alvarez-Lorenzo, C.; De Sousa, H.C.; García-González, C.A. Supercritical processing of starch aerogels and aerogel-loaded poly(ε-caprolactone) scaffolds for sustained release of ketoprofen for bone regeneration. *J. CO_2 Util.* **2017**, *18*, 237–249. [CrossRef]
73. Theocharis, A.D.; Skandalis, S.S.; Gialeli, C.; Karamanos, N.K. Extracellular matrix structure. *Adv. Drug Deliv. Rev.* **2016**, *97*, 4–27. [CrossRef]
74. Brien, F.J.O. Biomaterials & scaffolds every day thousands of surgical procedures are performed to replace. *Mater. Today* **2011**, *14*, 88–95.
75. Gleeson, J.P.; Brien, F.J.O. Composite scaffolds for orthopaedic regenerative medicine. In *Advances in Composite Materials for Medicine and Nanotechnology*; InTech Open Access: Rijeka, Croatia, 2011; Volume 10, pp. 39–59.
76. Chen, H.; Zhong, J.; Wang, J.; Huang, R.; Qiao, X.; Wang, H.; Tan, Z. Enhanced growth and differentiation of myoblast cells grown on E-jet 3D printed platforms. *Int. J. Nanomed.* **2019**, *14*, 937–950. [CrossRef]
77. Miroslaw, L.; Capila, I.; Kaundinya, G. Mass spectrometric methods for the analysis of heparin and heparan sulfate. *Glycosaminoglycans Methods Mol. Biol.* **2014**, *1229*, 119–128.
78. Park, J.S.; Lim, H.J.; Yi, S.W.; Park, K.H. Stem cell differentiation-related protein-loaded PLGA microspheres as a novel platform micro-typed scaffold for chondrogenesis. *Biomed. Mater.* **2016**, *11*, 55003. [CrossRef]
79. Simann, M.; Schneider, V.; Le Blanc, S.; Dotterweich, J.; Zehe, V.; Krug, M.; Jakob, F.; Schilling, T.; Schütze, N. Heparin affects human bone marrow stromal cell fate: Promoting osteogenic and reducing adipogenic differentiation and conversion. *Bone* **2015**, *78*, 102–113. [CrossRef] [PubMed]
80. Solakyildirim, K. Recent advances in glycosaminoglycan analysis by various mass spectrometry techniques. *Anal. Bioanal. Chem.* **2019**, *411*, 3731–3741. [CrossRef]
81. Uygun, B.E.; Stojsih, S.E.; Matthew, H.W.T. Effects of immobilized glycosaminoglycans on the proliferation and differentiation of mesenchymal stem cells. *Tissue Eng. Part A* **2009**, *15*, 3499–3512. [CrossRef]
82. Benoit, D.S.W.; Durney, A.R.; Anseth, K.S. The effect of heparin-functionalized PEG hydrogels on three-dimensional human mesenchymal stem cell osteogenic differentiation. *Biomaterials* **2007**, *28*, 66–77. [CrossRef]

83. Seto, S.P.; Casas, M.E.; Temenoff, J.S. Differentiation of mesenchymal stem cells in heparin-containing hydrogels via coculture with osteoblasts. *Cell Tissue Res.* **2012**, *347*, 589–601. [CrossRef]
84. Farina, M.; Chua, C.Y.X.; Ballerini, A.; Thekkedath, U.; Alexander, J.F.; Rhudy, J.R.; Torchio, G.; Fraga, D.; Pathak, R.R.; Villanueva, M.; et al. Transcutaneously refillable, 3D-printed biopolymeric encapsulation system for the transplantation of endocrine cells. *Biomaterials* **2018**, *177*, 125–138. [CrossRef] [PubMed]
85. Paez-Mayorga, J.; Capuani, S.; Farina, M.; Lotito, M.L.; Niles, J.A.; Salazar, H.F.; Rhudy, J.; Esnaola, L.; Chua, C.Y.X.; Taraballi, F.; et al. Enhanced in vivo vascularization of 3D-printed cell encapsulation device using platelet-rich plasma and mesenchymal stem cells. *Adv. Healthc. Mater.* **2020**, *2000670*, 1–11. [CrossRef]
86. Erdem, A.; Darabi, M.A.; Nasiri, R.; Sangabathuni, S.; Ertas, Y.N.; Alem, H.; Hosseini, V.; Shamloo, A.; Nasr, A.S.; Ahadian, S.; et al. 3D bioprinting of oxygenated cell-laden gelatin methacryloyl constructs. *Adv. Healthc. Mater.* **2020**, *9*, e1901794. [CrossRef]
87. Blakney, A.K.; Swartzlander, M.D.; Bryant, S.J. The effects of substrate stiffness on the in vitro activation of macrophages and in vivo host response to poly (ethylene glycol)-based hydrogels. *Soc. Biomater.* **2012**, *100*, 1375–1386.
88. Venturini, V.; Pezano, F.; Frederic, C.; Hakkinen, H.-M.; Jiménez-delgado, S.; Colomer-rosell, M.; Marro, M.; Tolosa-ramon, Q.; Paz-lópez, S.; Valverde, M.A.; et al. The nucleus measures shape changes for cellular proprioception to control dynamic cell behavior. *Science* **2020**, *370*, 2644. [CrossRef]
89. Lomakin, A.; Cattin, C.; Cuvelier, D.; Alraies, Z.; Molina, M.; Nader, G.P.; Srivastava, N.; Saez, P.; Garcia-Arcos, J.M.; Zhitnyak, I.Y.; et al. The nucleus acts as a ruler tailoring cell responses to spatial constraints. *Science* **2020**, *370*, 2894. [CrossRef]
90. Fahy, N.; Alini, M.; Stoddart, M.J. Mechanical stimulation of mesenchymal stem cells: Implications for cartilage tissue engineering. *J. Orthop. Res.* **2018**, *36*, 52–63. [CrossRef]
91. Mao, A.S.; Mooney, D.J. Regenerative medicine: Current therapies and future directions. *Proc. Natl. Acad. Sci. USA* **2015**, *112*, 14452–14459. [CrossRef]
92. Pedersen, J.; Swartz, M. Mechanobiology in the third dimension. *Ann. Biomed. Eng.* **2005**, *33*, 1469–1490. [CrossRef] [PubMed]
93. Terraciano, V.; Hwang, N.; Moroni, L.; Park, H.B.; Zhang, Z.; Mizrahi, J.; Seliktar, D.; Elisseeff, J. Differential response of adult and embryonic mesenchymal progenitor cells to mechanical compression in hydrogels. *Stem Cells* **2007**, *25*, 2730–2738. [CrossRef]
94. Zhang, W.; Kong, C.W.; Tong, M.H.; Chooi, W.H.; Huang, N.; Li, R.A.; Chan, B.P. Maturation of human embryonic stem cell-derived cardiomyocytes (hESC-CMs) in 3D collagen matrix: Effects of niche cell supplementation and mechanical stimulation. *Acta Biomater.* **2017**, *49*, 204–217. [CrossRef]
95. Barnes, J.M.; Przybyla, L.; Weaver, V.M. Tissue mechanics regulate brain development, homeostasis and disease. *J. Cell Sci.* **2017**, *130*, 71–82. [CrossRef]
96. Liu, C.; Cui, X.; Ackermann, T.M.; Flamini, V.; Chen, W.; Castillo, A.B. Osteoblast-derived paracrine factors regulate angiogenesis in response to mechanical stimulation. *Integr. Biol.* **2016**, *8*, 785–794. [CrossRef]
97. Bono, N.; Pezzoli, D.; Levesque, L.; Loy, C.; Candiani, G.; Fiore, G.B.; Mantovani, D. Unraveling the role of mechanical stimulation on smooth muscle cells: A comparative study between 2D and 3D models. *Biotechnol. Bioeng.* **2016**, *113*, 2254–2263. [CrossRef]
98. Hasanzadeh, E.; Amoabediny, G.; Haghighipour, N.; Gholami, N.; Mohammadnejad, J.; Shojaei, S.; Salehi-Nik, N. The stability evaluation of mesenchymal stem cells differentiation toward endothelial cells by chemical and mechanical stimulation. *Vitr. Cell. Dev. Biol.—Anim.* **2017**, *53*, 818–826. [CrossRef]
99. Gaub, B.M.; Mu, D.J. Mechanical stimulation of piezo1 receptors depends on extracellular matrix proteins and directionality of force. *Nano Lett.* **2017**, *17*, 2064–2072. [CrossRef]
100. Godau, B. Determining the Effect of Structure and Function on 3D Bioprinted Hydrogel Scaffolds for Applications in Tissue Engineering. Bachelor´s Thesis, University of Victoria, Victoria, BC, Canada, 2019.
101. Peeters, E.A.G. Monitoring the biomechanical response of individual cells under compression: A new compression device. *Med. Biol. Eng. Comput.* **2003**, *41*, 498–503. [CrossRef]
102. Wang, N.; Butler, J.P.; Ingber, D.E. Mechanotransduction across the cell surface and through the cytoskeleton. *Science* **1993**, *260*, 1124–1128. [CrossRef] [PubMed]

103. Maldonado, H.; Calderon, C.; Burgos-Bravo, F.; Kobler, O.; Zuschratter, W.; Ramirez, O.; Härtel, S.; Schneider, P.; Quest, A.F.G.; Herrera-Molina, R.; et al. Astrocyte-to-neuron communication through integrin-engaged Thy-1/CBP/Csk/Src complex triggers neurite retraction via the RhoA/ROCK pathway. *Biochim. Biophys. Acta—Mol. Cell Res.* **2017**, *1864*, 243–254. [CrossRef]
104. Lee, H.J.; Diaz, M.F.; Price, K.M.; Ozuna, J.A.; Zhang, S.; Sevick-Muraca, E.M.; Hagan, J.P.; Wenzel, P.L. Fluid shear stress activates YAP1 to promote cancer cell motility. *Nat. Commun.* **2017**, *8*, 14122. [CrossRef]
105. Chen, X.; Zhang, S.; Wang, Z.; Wang, F.; Cao, X.; Wu, Q.; Zhao, C.; Ma, H.; Ye, F.; Wang, H.; et al. Supervillin promotes epithelial- mesenchymal transition and metastasis of hepatocellular carcinoma in hypoxia via activation of the RhoA/ROCK-ERK/p38 pathway. *J. Exp. Clin. Cancer Res.* **2018**, *37*, 1–16. [CrossRef] [PubMed]
106. Glücksmann, A. Studies on bone mechanics in vitro. I. Influence of pressure on orientation of structure. *Anat. Rec.* **1938**, *72*, 97–113. [CrossRef]
107. Gelmi, A.; Cieslar-Pobuda, A.; de Muinck, E.; Los, M.; Rafat, M.; Jager, E.W.H. Direct Mechanical stimulation of stem cells: A beating electromechanically active scaffold for cardiac tissue engineering. *Adv. Healthc. Mater.* **2016**, *5*, 1471–1480. [CrossRef]
108. Ghezzi, C.E.; Marelli, B.; Donelli, I.; Alessandrino, A.; Freddi, G.; Nazhat, S.N. The role of physiological mechanical cues on mesenchymal stem cell differentiation in an airway tract-like dense collagen-silk fibroin construct. *Biomaterials* **2014**, *35*, 6236–6247. [CrossRef]
109. Núñez-Toldrà, R.; Vasquez-Sancho, F.; Barroca, N.; Catalan, G. Investigation of the cellular response to bone fractures: Evidence for flexoelectricity. *Sci. Rep.* **2020**, *10*, 254. [CrossRef]
110. Ding, Q.; Xu, X.; Yue, Y.; Mei, C.; Huang, C.; Jiang, S.; Wu, Q.; Han, J. Nanocellulose-mediated electroconductive viscoelasticity, stretchability, and biocompatibility toward multifunctional applications. *ACS Appl. Mater. Interfaces* **2018**, *10*, 27987–28002. [CrossRef]
111. Huerta, R.R.; Silva, E.K.; Ekaette, I.; El-bialy, T.; Saldaña, M.D.A. High-intensity ultrasound-assisted formation of cellulose nanofiber scaffold with low and high lignin content and their cytocompatibility with gingival fibroblast cells. *Ultrason. Sonochem.* **2019**, *64*, 104759. [CrossRef]
112. Thrivikraman, G.; Boda, S.K.; Basu, B. Unraveling the mechanistic effects of electric field stimulation towards directing stem cell fate and function: A tissue engineering perspective. *Biomaterials* **2017**, *150*, 60–86. [CrossRef]
113. Jaatinen, L. The Effect of an Applied Electric Current on Cell Proliferation, Viability, Morphology, Adhesion, and Stem Cell Differentiation. Ph.D. Thesis, Tampere University of Technology, Tampere, Finland, 2017.
114. Taghian, T.; Narmoneva, D.A.; Kogan, A.B. Modulation of cell function by electric field: A high-resolution analysis. *J. R. Soc. Interface* **2015**, *12*, 21–25. [CrossRef]
115. Wang, L.; Liu, Y.; Jin, H.; Steinacker, J. Electrical stimulation induced Hsp70 response in C2C12 cells. *Exerc. Immunol. Rev.* **2010**, *16*, 86–97.
116. Ghasemi-mobarakeh, L.; Prabhakaran, M.P.; Morshed, M. Application of conductive polymers, scaffolds and electrical stimulation for nerve tissue engineering. *J. Tissue Eng. Regen. Med.* **2011**, *5*, 17–35. [CrossRef]
117. Sherrell, P.C.; Thompson, B.C.; Wassei, J.K.; Gelmi, A.A.; Higgins, M.J.; Kaner, R.B.; Wallace, G.G. Maintaining cytocompatibility of biopolymers through a graphene layer for electrical stimulation of nerve cells. *Adv. Funct. Mater.* **2014**, *24*, 769–776. [CrossRef]
118. Aleem, I.S.; Aleem, I.; Evaniew, N.; Busse, J.W.; Yaszemski, M.; Agarwal, A.; Einhorn, T.; Bhandari, M. Efficacy of electrical stimulators for bone healing: A meta-analysis of randomized sham-controlled trials. *Sci. Rep.* **2016**, *6*, 31724. [CrossRef] [PubMed]
119. Lou, J.W.H.; Bergquist, A.J.; Aldayel, A.; Czitron, J.; Collins, D.F. Interleaved neuromuscular electrical stimulation reduces muscle fatigue. *Muscle Nerve* **2017**, *55*, 179–189. [CrossRef] [PubMed]
120. Zhu, W.; Ye, T.; Lee, S.J.; Cui, H.; Miao, S.; Zhou, X.; Shuai, D.; Zhang, L.G. Enhanced neural stem cell functions in conductive annealed carbon nanofibrous scaffolds with electrical stimulation. *Nanomed. Nanotechnol. Biol. Med.* **2018**, *14*, 2485–2494. [CrossRef]
121. Yuan, X.; Arkonac, D.E.; Chao, P.G.; Vunjak-novakovic, G. Electrical stimulation enhances cell migration and integrative repair in the meniscus. *Sci. Rep.* **2014**, *4*, 3674. [CrossRef]
122. Tai, G.; Reid, B.; Cao, L.; Zhao, M. Electrotaxis and wound healing: Experimental methods to study electric fields as a directional signal for cell migration. *Methods Mol. Biol.* **2009**, *571*, 77–97.

123. Bajaj, P.; Bobby, R.; Millet, L.; Wei, C.; Zorlutuna, P.; Baoe, G.; Bashir, R. Patterning the differentiation of C2C12 skeletal myoblasts. *Integr. Biol.* **2011**, *3*, 897–909. [CrossRef]
124. Guo, W.; Zhang, X.; Yu, X.; Wang, S.; Qiu, J.; Tang, W.; Li, L.; Liu, H.; Wang, Z.L. Self-powered electrical stimulation for enhancing neural differentiation of mesenchymal stem cells on graphene–Poly(3,4-ethylenedioxythiophene) hybrid microfibers. *ASC Nano* **2016**, *10*, 5086–5095. [CrossRef]
125. Wang, J.; Tian, L.; Chen, N.; Ramakrishna, S.; Mo, X. The cellular response of nerve cells on poly-L-lysine coated PLGA-MWCNTs aligned nanofibers under electrical stimulation. *Mater. Sci. Eng. C* **2018**, *91*, 715–726. [CrossRef]
126. Boehler, C.; Kleber, C.; Martini, N.; Xie, Y.; Dryg, I.; Stieglitz, T.; Hofmann, U.G.; Asplund, M. Actively controlled release of Dexamethasone from neural microelectrodes in a chronic in vivo study. *Biomaterials* **2017**, *129*, 176–187. [CrossRef]
127. Hao, H.B.; Yuan, L.; Fu, Z.B.; Wang, C.Y.; Yang, X.; Zhu, J.; Qu, J.; Chen, H.; Schiraldi, D. Biomass-based mechanically-strong and electrically-conductive polymer aerogels and their application for supercapacitors. *ACS Appl. Mater. Interfaces* **2016**, *8*, 9917–9924.
128. You, I.; Jeong, U. Electromechanical decoupling by porous aerogel conducting polymer. *Matter* **2019**, *1*, 24–25. [CrossRef]
129. Zhang, X.; Chang, D.; Liu, J.; Luo, Y. Conducting polymer aerogels from supercritical CO_2 drying PEDOT-PSS hydrogels. *J. Mater. Chem.* **2010**, *20*, 5080–5085. [CrossRef]
130. Bertucci, C.; Koppes, R.; Dumont, C.; Koppes, A. Neural responses to electrical stimulation in 2D and 3D in vitro environments. *Brain Res. Bull.* **2019**, *152*, 265–284. [CrossRef]
131. Hernández-Suarez, P.; Ramírez, K.; Alvarado, F.; Avendaño, E.; Starbird, R. Electrochemical characterization of poly(3,4-ethylenedioxythiophene)/κ-carrageenan as a biocompatible conductive coat for biologic applications. *MRS Commun.* **2018**, *9*, 218–223. [CrossRef]
132. Ryan, E.M.; Breslin, C.B. Formation of polypyrrole with dexamethasone as a dopant: Its cation and anion exchange properties. *J. Electroanal. Chem.* **2018**, *824*, 188–194. [CrossRef]
133. Goimil, L.; Santos-Rosales, V.; Delgado, A.; Évora, C.; Reyes, R.; Lozano-Pérez, A.A.; Aznar-Cervantes, S.D.; Cenis, J.L.; Gómez-Amoza, J.L.; Concheiro, A.; et al. ScCO_2-foamed silk fibroin aerogel/poly(ε-caprolactone) scaffolds containing dexamethasone for bone regeneration. *J. CO_2 Util.* **2019**, *31*, 51–64. [CrossRef]
134. Costa, P.F.; Puga, A.M.; Díaz-Gomez, L.; Concheiro, A.; Busch, D.H.; Alvarez-Lorenzo, C. Additive manufacturing of scaffolds with dexamethasone controlled release for enhanced bone regeneration. *Int. J. Pharm.* **2015**, *496*, 541–550. [CrossRef]
135. Liu, Q.; Cen, L.; Zhou, H.; Yin, S.; Liu, G.; Liu, W.; Cao, Y.; Cui, L. The role of the extracellular signal-related kinase signaling pathway in osteogenic differentiation of human adipose-derived stem cells and in adipogenic transition initiated by dexamethasone. *Tissue Eng. Part A* **2009**, *15*, 3487–3497. [CrossRef] [PubMed]
136. Danckwerts, M.; Fassihi, A. Implantable controlled release drug delivery system: A review. *Drug Dev. Ind. Pharm.* **1991**, *7*, 1465–1502. [CrossRef]
137. Ding, C.; Li, Z. A review of drug release mechanisms from nanocarrier systems. *Mater. Sci. Eng. C* **2017**, *76*, 1440–1453. [CrossRef]
138. Franco, P.; Marco, I. De supercritical CO_2 adsorption of non-steroidal anti-inflammatory drugs into biopolymer aerogels. *J. CO_2 Util.* **2020**, *36*, 40–53. [CrossRef]
139. Lovskaya, D.D.; Lebedev, A.E.; Menshutina, N.V. Aerogels as drug delivery systems: In vitro and in vivo evaluations. *J. Supercrit. Fluids* **2015**, *106*, 5–11. [CrossRef]
140. De Marco, I.; Reverchon, E. Starch aerogel loaded with poorly water-soluble vitamins through supercritical CO_2 adsorption. *Chem. Eng. Res. Des.* **2017**, *119*, 221–230. [CrossRef]
141. García-González, C.A.; Uy, J.J.; Alnaief, M.; Smirnova, I. Preparation of tailor-made starch-based aerogel microspheres by the emulsion-gelation method. *Carbohydr. Polym.* **2012**, *88*, 1378–1386. [CrossRef]
142. Korsmeyer, R.W.; Gurny, R.; Doelker, E.; Buri, P.; Peppas, N.A. Mechanisms of solute release from porous hydrophilic polymers. *Int. J. Pharm.* **1983**, *15*, 25–35. [CrossRef]
143. Ritger, P.L.; Peppas, N.A. A simple equation for description of solute release II. Fickian and anomalous release from swellable devices. *J. Control. Release* **1987**, *5*, 37–42. [CrossRef]
144. Ritger, P.L.; Peppas, N.A. A simple equation for description of solute release I. Fickian and non-fickian release from non-swellable devices in the form of slabs, spheres, cylinders or discs. *J. Control. Release* **1987**, *5*, 23–36. [CrossRef]

145. Krukiewicz, K. Tailorable drug capacity of dexamethasone-loaded conducting polymer matrix. *IOP Conf. Ser. Mater. Sci. Eng.* **2018**, *369*, 12202. [CrossRef]
146. Löffler, S.; Seyock, S.; Nybom, R.; Jacobson, G.B.; Richter-Dahlfors, A. Electrochemically triggered release of acetylcholine from scCO$_2$ impregnated conductive polymer films evokes intracellular Ca^{2+} signaling in neurotypic SH-SY5Y cells. *J. Control. Release* **2016**, *243*, 283–290. [CrossRef]
147. Balint, R.; Cassidy, N.J.; Cartmell, S.H. Conductive polymers: Towards a smart biomaterial for tissue engineering. *Acta Biomater.* **2014**, *10*, 2341–2353. [CrossRef]
148. Alshammary, B.; Walsh, F.C.; Herrasti, P.; Ponce de Leon, C. Electrodeposited conductive polymers for controlled drug release: Polypyrrole. *J. Solid State Electrochem.* **2016**, *20*, 839–859. [CrossRef]
149. Krukiewicz, K.; Gniazdowska, B.; Jarosz, T.; Herman, A.P.; Boncel, S.; Turczyn, R. Effect of immobilization and release of ciprofloxacin and quercetin on electrochemical properties of poly(3,4-ethylenedioxypyrrole) matrix. *Synth. Met.* **2019**, *249*, 52–62. [CrossRef]
150. Alizadeh, N.; Shamaeli, E. Electrochemically controlled release of anticancer drug methotrexate using nanostructured polypyrrole modified with cetylpyridinium: Release kinetics investigation. *Electrochim. Acta* **2014**, *130*, 488–496. [CrossRef]
151. Boehler, C.; Oberueber, F.; Asplund, M. Tuning drug delivery from conducting polymer films for accurately controlled release of charged molecules. *J. Control. Release* **2019**, *304*, 173–180. [CrossRef]
152. Svirskis, D.; Sharma, M.; Yu, Y.; Garg, S. Electrically switchable polypyrrole film for the tunable release of progesterone. *Ther. Deliv.* **2013**, *4*, 307–313. [CrossRef]
153. Kim, B.D.; Richardson-burns, S.M.; Hendricks, J.L.; Sequera, C.; Martin, D.C. Effect of immobilized nerve growth factor on conductive polymers: Electrical properties and cellular response. *Adv. Funct. Mater.* **2007**, *17*, 79–86. [CrossRef]
154. Leprince, L.; Dogimont, A.; Magnin, D.; Demoustier-Champagne, S. Dexamethasone electrically controlled release from polypyrrole-coated nanostructured electrodes. *J. Mater. Sci. Mater. Med.* **2010**, *21*, 925–930. [CrossRef]
155. Stevenson, G.; Moulton, S.E.; Innis, P.C.; Wallace, G.G. Polyterthiophene as an electrostimulated controlled drug release material of therapeutic levels of dexamethasone. *Synth. Met.* **2010**, *160*, 1107–1114. [CrossRef]
156. Qu, J.; Liang, Y.; Shi, M.; Guo, B.; Gao, Y.; Yin, Z. Biocompatible conductive hydrogels based on dextran and aniline trimer as electro-responsive drug delivery system for localized drug release. *Int. J. Biol. Macromol.* **2019**, *140*, 255–264. [CrossRef]
157. Qu, J.; Zhao, X.; Ma, P.X.; Guo, B. Injectable antibacterial conductive hydrogels with dual response to an electric field and pH for localized "smart" drug release. *Acta Biomater.* **2018**, *72*, 55–69. [CrossRef]
158. Lin, H.; Zhu, B.; Wu, Y.; Sekine, J.; Nakao, A.; Luo, S. Dynamic poly(3,4 ethylenedioxythiophene)s integrate low impedance with redox-switchable biofunction. *Adv. Funct. Mater.* **2018**, *28*, 1703890. [CrossRef]

Publisher's Note: MDPI stays neutral with regard to jurisdictional claims in published maps and institutional affiliations.

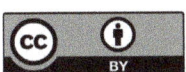

© 2020 by the authors. Licensee MDPI, Basel, Switzerland. This article is an open access article distributed under the terms and conditions of the Creative Commons Attribution (CC BY) license (http://creativecommons.org/licenses/by/4.0/).

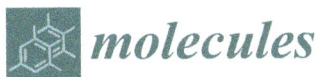

Article

Polysaccharide κ-Carrageenan as Doping Agent in Conductive Coatings for Electrochemical Controlled Release of Dexamethasone at Therapeutic Doses

Karla Ramírez Sánchez [1,2,*], Aura Ledezma-Espinoza [1], Andrés Sánchez-Kopper [1], Esteban Avendaño-Soto [3,4], Mónica Prado [2] and Ricardo Starbird Perez [1,*]

1. Centro de Investigación y de Servicios Químicos y Microbiológicos (CEQIATEC), School of Chemistry, Instituto Tecnológico de Costa Rica, 159-7050 Cartago, Costa Rica; aledezma@itcr.ac.cr (A.L.-E.); ansanchez@itcr.ac.cr (A.S.-K.)
2. Centro de Investigación en Enfermedades Tropicales (CIET), Faculty of Microbiology, Universidad de Costa Rica, 11501-2060 San José, Costa Rica; monica.pradoporras@ucr.ac.cr
3. Centro de Investigación en Ciencia e Ingeniería de Materiales (CICIMA), Universidad de Costa Rica, 11501-2060 San José, Costa Rica; esteban.avendanosoto@ucr.ac.cr
4. School of Physics, Universidad de Costa Rica, 11501-2060 San José, Costa Rica
* Correspondence: karamirez@itcr.ac.cr (K.R.S.); rstarbird@itcr.ac.cr (R.S.P.); Tel.: +506-25502731 (R.S.P.)

Academic Editor: Mitsuhiro Ebara
Received: 13 April 2020; Accepted: 30 April 2020; Published: 3 May 2020

Abstract: Smart conductive materials are developed in regenerative medicine to promote a controlled release profile of charged bioactive agents in the vicinity of implants. The incorporation and the active electrochemical release of the charged compounds into the organic conductive coating is achieved due to its intrinsic electrical properties. The anti-inflammatory drug dexamethasone was added during the polymerization, and its subsequent release at therapeutic doses was reached by electrical stimulation. In this work, a Poly (3,4-ethylenedioxythiophene): κ-carrageenan: dexamethasone film was prepared, and κ-carrageenan was incorporated to keep the electrochemical and physical stability of the electroactive matrix. The presence of κ-carrageenan and dexamethasone in the conductive film was confirmed by μ-Raman spectroscopy and their effect in the topographic was studied using profilometry. The dexamethasone release process was evaluated by cyclic voltammetry and High-Resolution mass spectrometry. In conclusion, κ-carrageenan as a doping agent improves the electrical properties of the conductive layer allowing the release of dexamethasone at therapeutic levels by electrochemical stimulation, providing a stable system to be used in organic bioelectronics systems.

Keywords: polysaccharide; κ-carrageenan; dexamethasone; electrochemical active deliver system; doping agent; charged molecule; conductive polymers

1. Introduction

Conductive polymers are a new generation of smart materials extensively used in organic bioelectronics, mostly in the development of neural implants, biosensors, and active controlled release systems [1–4]. Poly (3,4-ethylenedioxythiophene) (PEDOT) is a conductive polymer synthetized from 3,4-ethylenedioxythiophene (EDOT), used as a coating in diverse types of sensors due to its biocompatibility, conductivity, processing versatility, and stability [5,6]. Moreover, PEDOT is reported as a promising material for the immobilization of enzymes and other biologically active molecules [2,7,8]. The incorporation of charged molecules into the PEDOT backbone is described through an electrostatic mechanism due to the formation of charge carriers and the doping process during the electropolymerization process [9]. The subsequent release of the charged compounds was reported to be dependent on the polymer thickness and charge applied during the electrochemical stimulus [10–13].

Diverse implants and scaffolds are developed in regenerative medicine to serve as extracellular matrices for cell colonization [14–16]. Many of them are loaded with bioactive agents to improve the therapeutic efficacy and safety of the drugs, playing important roles in treatment of several chronic diseases, damaged tissues, and providing a potential stimulation of different types of cells [17–19].

Although diverse engineering groups established different types of implants for a broad range of applications, those implants can elicit body responses involving inflammatory processes, which may result in the formation of glial scars due to neural devices specifically [12,13,20,21]. One strategy to avoid immune responses consists of releasing an anti-inflammatory biomolecule (i.e., dexamethasone) in the vicinity of the implant [11,13,22,23]. Dexamethasone (Dx) is a synthetic glucocorticoid that reduces inflammation in the central nervous system, acting through glucocorticoid receptors found in most neurons and glial cells. Due to being locally delivered, the specificity and efficiency of dexamethasone means that only small amounts of the drug are required [13,22,24–28].

κ-Carrageenan (κC) is a sulfonated polysaccharide recently used in aqueous micellar dispersions for the polymerization of EDOT, since it provides an appropriate environment for the monomer dispersion while acting as a doping agent in the conductive layer [29–31]. According to the previous work, the electrochemical properties of PEDOT are retained when κC is used as a doping agent [29,30], avoiding a potential delamination during the reduction-oxidation process needed during the active delivering process. Biocompatibility of PEDOT:κC composite has been demonstrated in previous studies [2,29].

In this work, we induce the loading of dexamethasone phosphate during the deposition of the electroactive composite onto a bare gold electrode by changing the amount of drug in the dispersion prior the polymerization. κC was incorporated to maintain the electrochemical stability and biocompatibility of the PEDOT matrix and the subsequent drug release using electrical stimulation. The presence of κC and Dx inside the conductive film was confirmed by μ-Raman spectroscopy and their effect in the topography was studied using profilometry. Dexamethasone release was evaluated by cyclic voltammetry and High-Resolution (HR) mass spectrometry. Therapeutic doses of dexamethasone were achieved during the electrical stimulation of the bioelectronic device.

2. Results and Discussion

2.1. Evaluation of the Stability and Size of the Dispersion Systems

The dispersions used to electrodeposit the monomer and the Dx on the electrode were evaluated by their ζ-potential values and particle size distribution in order to determine its stability in aqueous medium. ζ-potential data was obtained for the six prepared dispersions, and they are shown in Table 1. It is possible to observe that EDOT:κC:Dx has an appropriate stability (−48.70 mV), which is dominated for the κC micellar system (−43.30 mV). Values of ζ-potential over −30 mV are considered stable assuming that an electrostatic charge is the main stabilization mechanism and the colloidal system is in the range of hundreds [32,33]. The anionic nature of the κC and Dx avoids aggregation due to the negative values obtained in the ζ-potential analysis, which are comparable with previously reported results for these molecules [30,34,35]. A stable dispersion prevents aggregation or deposition of the particles that carried the monomer during the electrochemical deposition. Additionally, the stable system may allow a homogeneous dispersion of κC and dexamethasone in the electrodeposited film as seen by Raman spectroscopy.

Table 1. ζ-potential values of dispersions used in the fixation of the drug on the electrode.

System	ζ-potential (mV)	SD (mV)
Dx	−69.40	1.14
κC	−43.30	3.31
κC:Dx	−42.63	1.67
EDOT:Dx	−70.83	1.09
κC:EDOT	−48.46	1.70
EDOT:κC:Dx	−48.70	1.21

Particle size measurements of the main three dispersions were performed to determine the dimension of their aggregates after the sonication process. Figure 1a shows the size distribution for the κC 0.2% w/v solution, it is possible to observe a single population for the surfactant. Some authors have reported previously that κC solutions are polydisperse (two or more populations), because it increases the gel behavior due to its polysaccharide nature [36,37]. Nevertheless, they emphasized that the main signal for the κC aggregates has an average size in the range of 800 to 1000 nm [37], which agrees with our results. The intensive sonication process before the measures and the low concentration of κC used in the analysis may explain why only one population were observed in the κC size distribution, similar to a previous report [30].

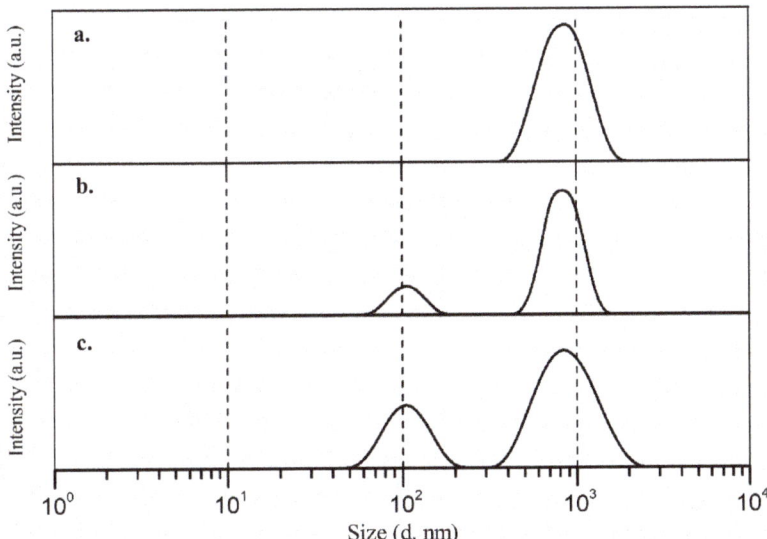

Figure 1. Size distribution (d. nm) of (**a**) κC; (**b**) κC:Dx; and (**c**) EDOT:κC:Dx dispersions, measured by dynamic light scattering (DLS) method.

On the other hand, once the Dx was added to the dispersion, a polydisperse behavior was found in the κC:Dx system and two populations were detected (Figure 1b,c). Dexamethasone solutions are characterized by a single population with a particle size average of 100 nm [38] and was consistent with our results. Eventually, it is possible to observe that the stability of the system has remained when the monomer was added (Figure 1c). The stability of the dispersions depends mainly on the used surfactant and it has an important influence in the physical and electrochemical properties of the electrodeposited films [39].

2.2. Analysis of the Topography and Composition of PEDOT:κC:Dx Coating by μ-Raman Spectroscopy and Profilometry Methods

The PEDOT:κC:Dx composite was obtained from a EDOT:κC:Dx dispersion by electrochemical deposition under galvanostatic conditions (Figure S1), as it was established in a previous work [2,30]. Then, the topography of the PEDOT:κC:Dx coating was characterized before (S_a: 0.270 ± 0.005 μm, surface area: 1361 mm^2, negative volume 0.1562 mm^3, and volume 1.695 mm^3) and after (S_a: 0.250 ± 0.005 μm, surface area: 1337 mm^2, negative volume 0.1707 mm^3, and volume 1.690 mm^3) releasing the Dx from the conductive coating. The roughness data of both surfaces did not show significant differences between them (see Figure 2a,b). The volume ratio between peaks and valleys describes the symmetry in the surface topography. A negative value is indicative of more distinct valleys and positive of more distinct peaks about the average plane. Our samples were dominated by peaks and low negative volume (around ten times) and those values are consistent with a previous report for PEDOT:κC coatings [30]. It is suggested that rough surfaces in comparison with smooth surfaces improve cell attachment due to the formation of specific surface-cell contacts by increasing the expression of different integrins subunits [40,41]. Although, diverse authors have reported that surface roughness values higher than 0.5 μm are desirable to ensure the maximum attachment and proliferation of cells, large rough surfaces also stimulate more anti-inflammatory responses because the activation of M2 macrophages and the subsequent release of anti-inflammatory cytokines [42]. The PEDOT:κC:Dx surface roughness value and the lack of their significative variation during the delivery of dexamethasone may indicate the reliability of electroactive composite for cell culture studies, since no additional mechanism may be seemed due to the topography changes.

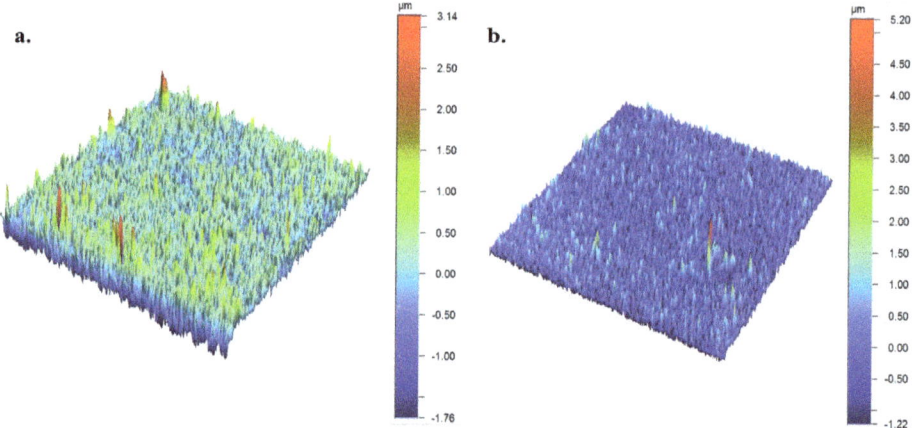

Figure 2. Profilometry images obtained for PEDOT:κC:Dx films (**a**) before and (**b**) after 160 cycles of cyclic voltammetry in a 0.10 M ammonium acetate solution.

The qualitative composition of the conductive film was determined using confocal μ-Raman spectroscopy before (Figure 3a,c) and after (Figure 3b,d) 160 sweeps of electrical stimulation in a 4 μm^2 area and 5 μm depth inside the composite. The analysis was performed in order to determine the presence of PEDOT, dexamethasone, and κ-carrageenan inside the electroactive composite. The signal was obtained and plotted in a 2D image that allows the association of the signal (counts) to the presence of the corresponding functional groups for each component.

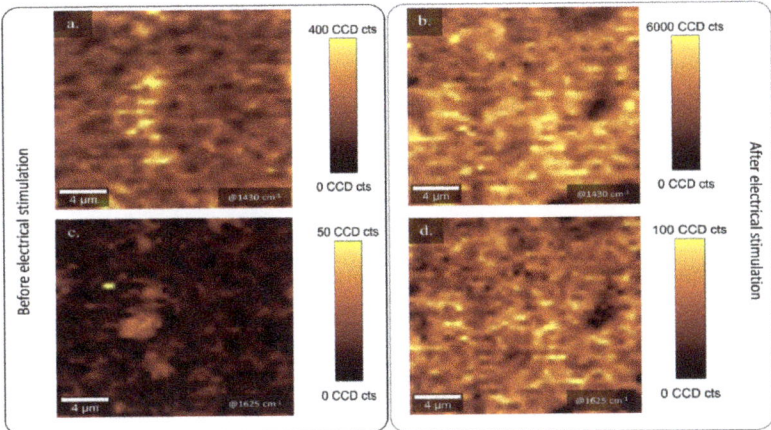

Figure 3. 2D confocal Raman map of the 1430 cm^{-1} band (**a**) before release process and (**b**) after 160 release cycles. Raman mapping of the 1625 cm^{-1} band intensity (**c**) before release process and (**d**) after 160 release cycles at 0.5 µm depth inside the conductive layer. The yellow areas are related to the presence of PEDOT and κC/Dx, respectively.

PEDOT shows a strong signal in the spectral range of 1421–1442 cm^{-1}, associated to the thiophene symmetric C$_\alpha$ = C$_\beta$ stretching [2,30,43] and its oxidation state. The corresponding signal was obtained from the composite before and after 160 cycles of electrical stimulation (Figure S2) and it was mapped at 1430 ± 25 cm^{-1} (Figure 3a,b), where bright yellow dots corresponded to presence of PEDOT. A homogeneous distribution of the conductive polymer was detected in both samples.

Additionally, a relative intense band at 1625 ± 30 cm^{-1} was detected, corroborating the qualitative existence of Dx and κC in the conductive film (Figure 3c,d). This signal, in the 2D, is distributed through the conductive matrix. The result is similar to previous studies [13,26], which reported the characteristic spectral signals of dexamethasone in the ranges of 3200–3500 cm^{-1}, 2850–3000 cm^{-1}, and near to 1650 cm^{-1}, as is verified in Figure S3, corresponding to hydroxyl, methyl, and carbonyl groups, respectively. Dexamethasone and κC act as doping agents, so there is a consistent association of the respective signal for both molecules and the PEDOT band. The identification of the band at 1625 cm^{-1} overlapping with PEDOT signal, confirmed the presence of the doping agent before and even after electrochemical stimulation, as is shown in Figure S2a,b, respectively. Adding κC in the formulation provides a proper doping agent during the release of the Dx, reducing the degradation by overoxidation and eventually delamination as is shown in Figure S4 [30].

2.3. Dexamethasone Release Experiments from the PEDOT:κC:Dx Coating

Drug loading into the conducting polymers films is based on the fact that these kinds of polymers are electrically oxidized during the polymerization processes, generating charge carriers [9,44,45]. The doping agent (e.g., Dx and κC) is incorporated to the oxidized polymer [46] to maintain charge neutrality. In this work, dexamethasone 21 phosphate and κC are used as doping agents, the presence of sulfate and phosphate groups imparts negative charges in the polysaccharide and the drug, respectively.

The electrochemical controlled release studies from PEDOT:κC:Dx coating were performed within a potential range of −600 to 1000 mV to evaluate intrinsic redox processes of the film [13,35,45]. Figure 4 shows the characteristic oxidation and reduction potential signal ranges at 0 to 500 mV and −100 to −400 mV, respectively, after a different number of voltammetry scans. According to some authors, the voltammetric behavior of dexamethasone shows a reduction signal at the potential of −350 mV [13,45], which indicates the release of the drug from a stimulated electrode. The corresponding CV signals are shown in Figure 4, this signal gradually decreased according to the sweep number, disappearing completely after 160 cycles of electrical stimulation. Electrochemical reduction of a conducting polymer results in the migration of small doping molecules from the conducting composite to maintain the electro neutrality of the matrix [44,46]. Thus, the application of alternating positive and negative potentials during cyclic voltammetry analysis caused the release of the Dx from the PEDOT coating.

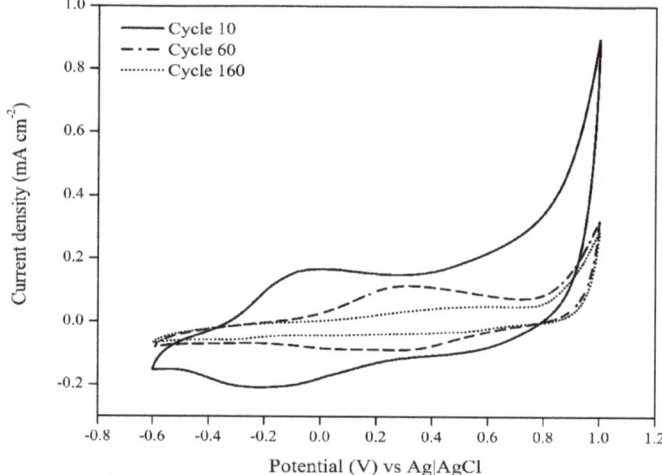

Figure 4. Cyclic voltammograms for the PEDOT:κC:Dx recorded at 25 mV·s^{-1} after 10, 60, and 160 cycles of electrical stimulation in ammonium acetate 0.10 M.

Spontaneous release of the dopant from the PEDOT structure is an instant process, but the Dx release is slow, since it is driven by diffusion from the inner film to the surface. κC is a large molecule, this type of dopant is more attached into the polymer coating and it is not leached out during the electrical stimulation, granting to the polymer greater electrochemical stability [13,46,47], as confirmed by Raman spectroscopy.

The release profile of the Dx was investigated under passive conditions (unstimulated) and active electrically stimulation using an ammonium acetate 0.10 M solution as supporting electrolyte. The surface area of the electrode is associated with promoting larger amounts of passive drug release according to the second Fick's law of diffusion [48,49], yet, in our case, the electrode surface and total area are maintained virtually constant. The quantification of Dx from the PEDOT:κC:Dx modified electrodes was achieved using HR-mass spectrometry (Figure 5).

The active release profile was performed with a total of 76 CV sweeps in five release events, taking around 300 min to be completed. Accordingly, the passive release profile from unstimulated electrodes were evaluated over the same period of 300 min.

Figure 5a shows the passive release profile of Dx as a function of square root of time according to the Higuchi model for the drug release from a polymer film [27,50], where pure Fickian diffusion is the dominant phenomena [48]. The low diffusion value, in the beginning of the process, may depend on the slow penetration of supportive electrolyte into the polymeric film [49]. The pattern changed after 80 min and a higher diffusion value reflects the diffusivity of the passive Dx release process. The three systems (1 mM, 5 mM, and 10 mM) showed analogous Fickian diffusion behavior.

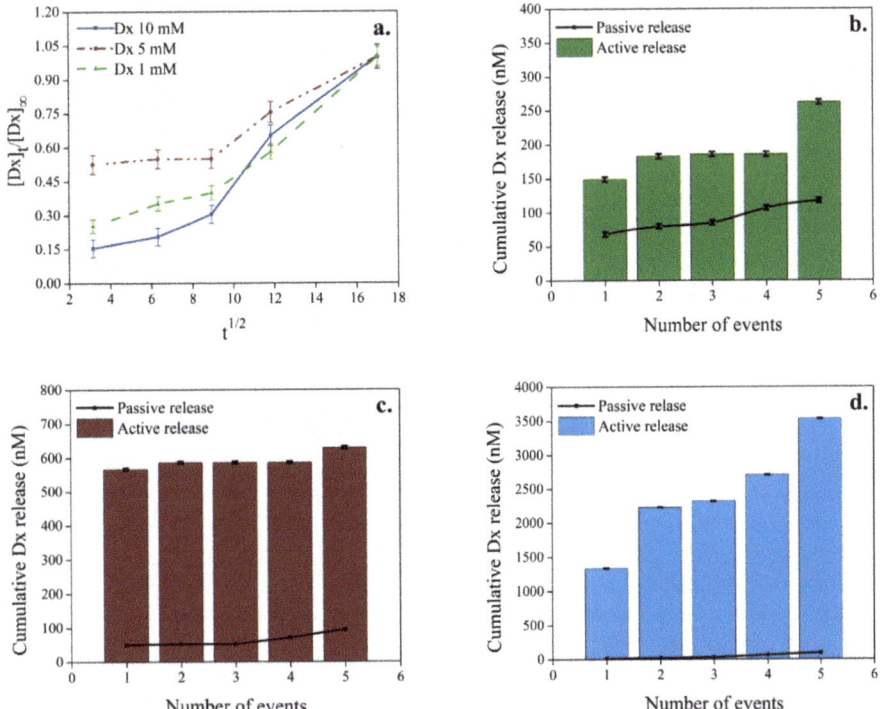

Figure 5. (**a**) The passive release profile of Dx as a function of square root of time, over 300 min from unstimulated electrodes. The active electrically controlled delivery process by stimulation events (columns) compared to the passive release profile (line) using: (**b**) 1 mM, (**c**) 5 mM, and (**d**) 10 mM of Dx in the initial formulation.

On the other hand, Figure 5b–d showed a remarkable dependency of the released Dx concentration during the electrical stimulated events (bars) compared to a passive unstimulated electrode (line). Some authors have studied controlled drug release systems using conductive polymers such as polypyrrole and PEDOT, where the anionic molecule is used as doping agent and their subsequent release is mainly determined via diffusion [11,13,44,45,51]. Nevertheless, for a controllable release system, it is desirable to have a high active release and low diffusion relationship [11,12], as shown by our system (see Figure 5). For instance, the initial concentration of 10 mM released in the passive process ca. 2% of the delivered Dx in stimulated process. This is probably associated with the use of κC as second doping in the matrix, which grants the film stability and integrity during stimulation cycles [30,46].

The therapeutic dosages of Dx in mesenchymal stem cell cultures are effective at levels of 100–1000 nM to promote their differentiation to osteoblast or in order to be used during anti-inflammatory treatment [52–54]. In this work, the accumulative concentration of the released Dx using 1 mM and 5 mM initial formulations (Figure 5b,c) were 300 nM (0.66 µg·cm^{-2}) and 600 nM (1.60 µg·cm^{-2}), respectively. Even though, these values are at therapeutically relevant levels, they are in part determined by the Dx amount release via diffusion.

Instead, when 10 mM of the drug was poured in the initial formulation, a total of 3700 nM (8.89 µg·cm^{-2}) of cumulative Dx was detected. This concentration range far in excess of the quantity of dexamethasone released from similar systems using an identical initial concentration of the drug for the coating preparation, for which values are even lower than 5.03 µg·cm^{-2} [11,12,51]. Such concentrations surpass the amount of the drug needed in cell cultures and it is not recommended to apply in biological systems. Nonetheless, using a specific electrochemical stimulation profile may be allowed to provide an adequate quantity of the drug for different biological applications.

3. Materials and Methods

3.1. Materials

Monomer 3,4-ethylenedioxythiophene (EDOT, 97.0% purity), κ-carrageenan (κC, ACS reagent), potassium chloride (KCl, >99.0% purity), dexamethasone 21-phosphate disodium salt (Dx, 98.0% purity), ammonium acetate ($NH_4CH_3CO_2$, 98.0% purity), ultrapure water MS quality, and MS methanol were purchased from Sigma Aldrich (San José, Costa Rica). All chemical reagents were used without further purification.

3.2. Synthesis and Preparation of the Modified PEDOT:κC:Dx Electrode

Electrodes (20.49 ± 0.02 mm^2) were fabricated by the deposition of gold on a polyimide substrate (see Figure S4) and they were passivated using a shadow mask to leave a specific exposed area to the electrode [55]. Prior to the polymer deposition, all electrodes were electrochemically cleaned applying cyclic voltammetry (CV) sweeps from a range of −600 to 900 mV with 100 $mV \cdot s^{-1}$ scan rate, in KCl 0.2 M [56], using an Autolab Potentiostat supplied by Metrohm (PGSTAT-302N, AUTOLAB, Utrecht, The Netherlands).

The surfactant dispersion was prepared according to a previous work [30], briefly: κC (0.2% w/v) and KCl (0.2 M) were added to deionized water previously heated at 50 °C. The samples were sonicated using 140 Joules in a Sonifier QSonica (Q700, Ultrasonic Corporation, Danbury, CT, USA), before and after adding the monomer EDOT (10 mM) and Dx at three different concentrations: 1 mM, 5 mM, and 10 mM.

The solution was electropolymerized on the electrode surface using galvanostatic conditions in the Autolab Potentiostat. The gold electrode (see Figure S4) is used as working electrode, platinum as counter electrode, and Ag|AgCl (KCl 3.0 M) works as reference electrode. The electrical polymerization was carried out with a constant current of 102.45 microamperes (current density: 0.5 $mA \cdot cm^{-2}$) using a potential limit of 1400 mV during 360 s (ca. 180 $mC \cdot cm^{-2}$ of charge density). Following the PEDOT:κC:Dx deposition, the electrodes were intensively rinsed with deionized water and stored at 4 °C before their use.

3.3. Evaluation of the Stability and Size of the Dispersion Systems

The characterization of the particle size and ζ-potential was performed using six dispersions, prepared in deionized water, namely: (1) κC 0.2% w/v; (2) Dx 10 mM; (3) EDOT 10 mM:κC 0.2% w/v; (4) EDOT 10 mM:Dx 10 mM; (5) κC 0.2% w/v:Dx 10 mM; and (6) EDOT 10 mM:κC 0.2% w/v:Dx 10 mM. Measurements were performed in a Zetasizer instrument (Nano ZS, Malvern Panalytical Ltd., Worcestershire, UK) at 25 °C and 173° angle. All the measurements were done by triplicate. Finally, dispersions were sonicated using a high-power ultrasonic bath (Bransonic®, Merck corporation, San José, Costa Rica) for 6 min to promote their homogenization. Two more formulations of EDOT:κC:Dx were prepared to reach lower dexamethasone concentrations into the conductive layer.

3.4. Analysis of the Topography and Composition of PEDOT:κC:Dx Coating by Profilometry and μ-Raman Spectroscopy Methods

The electrode topography was studied by profilometry analysis (Bruker, model: Dektak TX Advance, AZ, USA) and the arithmetical mean roughness of the surface (Sa) was calculated to describe the topography of the materials by using a 2 μm tip radius and a force of 1 mg in a 300 × 300 $μm^2$ and a scan area rate of 2.5 $μm \cdot s^{-1}$.

Raman spectroscopy analysis was carried out using a confocal µ-Raman microscope (Alpha300 R WITec, GmbH, Ulm, Germany) with a 532nm excitation laser, exposure time of 0.5 s, and 105 accumulations. The Raman stack scan was obtained using an integration time of 4 s in 4 µm^2 of area, 200 measurements per line were recorded for a total of 20 lines in each stack. Oversampling was used to improve the image quality, which was done in case of the cross-sectional scan. The scan depth was fixed at 5 µm and a total of 10 stack scans were achieved. The intensity of the relative wavenumber at 1435 cm^{-1} and 1625 cm^{-1} were extracted from each acquired spectrum, corresponding to PEDOT [2] and Dx/κC [44,57], respectively and plotted as 2D image. The intensity counts are related to the presence of the functional group and it is presented as bright yellow areas.

3.5. Dexamethasone Release Experiments from the PEDOT:κC:Dx Film

The Dx release from the modified electrode was carried out in a continuous flow cell using cyclic voltammetry (CV) sweeps with a three electrodes system (PEDOT:κC:Dx, Ag|AgCl and a gold film as working, reference, and counter electrodes, respectively). The active release of the drug was performed in 1 mL of fresh ammonium acetate solution (0.10 M) pH 7.2 [58], by scanning of CV from −600 to 1000 mV with a 25 mV·s^{-1} scan rate, over a period of 300 min (5 samples total) at room temperature.

The second release event, without electrical stimulation, was performed in order to analyze and to quantify the passive drug release process. For the experiment, 1.0 mL of 0.10 M ammonium acetate was injected through the cell containing the electrodes, a total of five samples were collected during 300 min of analysis.

Dexamethasone phosphate concentration, in the samples for the active and passive release events, was determined using a Xevo G2-XS quadrupole time of flight (Q-tof) mass spectrometer (Waters Corporation, Wilmslow, UK) coupled with an Acquity UPLC H-Class. For the analysis, a 10-µL injection of the sample was separated with an Acquity UPLC® C18 column (2.1 mm × 50.0 mm). The mobile phase consisted of a solution of water:formic acid 0.05% *v/v* and methanol:formic acid 0.05% *v/v* and they were supplied under not isocratic conditions with a constant flow of 0.3 mL·min^{-1} (Table S1).

The mass spectrometer was configured according to the parameters in a previous work [59], with the modifications shown in supplementary information S1. Quantification was carried out using Multiple Reaction Monitoring (MRM) acquisition method with the optimized transition of 471.1584 *m/z* for the precursor ion and 78.9585 *m/z* for the product ion, with a collision energy of 35 eV. Concentration in each sample was calculated using the Software MassLynx™ (V4.1, Waters Corporation, Wilmslow, UK) and an external calibration curve between 0.5 ppb to 5000 ppb of dexamethasone phosphate (R^2 = 0.9965).

4. Conclusions

We have successfully delivered therapeutic doses of dexamethasone by an electroactive controlled system, adjusting the initial formulation and the electrical stimulated events. Moreover, using κ-carrageenan as dispersant during the polymerization and as a doping agent in the composite, we avoided delamination and changes in the film roughness. The chemical composition inside the conductive film was confirmed by 2D Raman and electrochemical signal in the cyclic voltammetry analysis. Concentrations of dexamethasone in the range of 100 to 1000 nM were obtained using a lower amount of dexamethasone in the initial formulation. Those concentrations are recommended to induce differentiation in mesenchymal cell cultures and in anti-inflammatory responses. Therefore, an adequate formulation along with a proper active electrochemical stimulation profile allowed the delivery of therapeutic doses of charged molecules without significant changes in our film roughness. Our approach may be useful in the development of diverse strategies and implant systems in the regenerative medicine field.

Supplementary Materials: The following is available online, Figure S1: Galvanostatic curve of the electro-polymerization process from an EDOT:κC:Dx dispersion onto a bare gold electrode. Figure S2. Raman spectra of the PEDOT:κC:Dx coating (a.) before dexamethasone release process (Inset: PEDOT:κC:Dx electrode surface) and (b.) after 160 release cycles (Inset: PEDOT:κC:Dx electrode surface). Figure S3. μ-Raman spectral measurement of the dexamethasone 21-phosphate disodium salt. Figure S4. Deposited PEDOT:κC:Dx electrode after 160 cycles of electrical stimulation (left) and gold electrode without passivation as reference (right). Table S1: Gradient elution method for the mobile phase using during dexamethasone analysis. Solvents were water: 0.05% formic acid (A) and methanol: 0.05% formic acid (B). and S1: Configuration of the mass spectrometer during dexamethasone quantification.

Author Contributions: Conceptualization, K.R.S.; M.P., and R.S.P.; methodology, K.R.S.; A.L.-E.; A.S.-K.; E.A.-S., and R.S.P.; software, K.R.S.; A.L.-E.; A.S.-K.; E.A.-S., and R.S.P. validation, K.R.S.; A.L.-E.; A.S.-K., and R.S.P; formal analysis, R.S.P.; investigation, K.R.S. and R.S.P.; resources, E.A.-S. and R.S.P.; data curation, K.R.S.; A.L.-E., and A.S.-K.; writing—original draft preparation, K.R.S. and R.S.P.; writing—review and editing, K.R.S.; A.L.-E.; A.S.-K.; E.A.-S.; M.P., and R.S.P; visualization, K.R.S. and R.S.P.; supervision, M.P. and R.S.P.; project administration, K.R.S. and R.S.P.; funding acquisition, E.A.-S. and R.S.P. All authors have read and agree to the published version of the manuscript.

Funding: This research was funded by Costa Rica Institute of Technology (ITCR), project number: 5402-1360-4401.

Acknowledgments: Costa Rica Institute of Technology (ITCR), project number: 5402-1360-4401. Part of this work was carried out in the frame of the COST-Action "Advanced Engineering of Aerogels for Environment and Life Sciences" (AERoGELS, ref. CA18125) funded by the European Commission. The authors would like to thank to Steven Hidalgo and Jazmín Umaña for their participation in the electrode fabrication process. RGSF-RIP.

Conflicts of Interest: The authors declare no conflict of interest.

References

1. Ozkan, B.C.; Soganci, T.; Turhan, H.; Ak, M. Investigation of rGO and chitosan effects on optical and electrical properties of the conductive polymers for advanced applications. *Electrochim. Acta* **2019**, *295*, 1044–1051. [CrossRef]
2. Ramírez-Sánchez, K.; Alvarado-Hidalgo, F.; Zamora-Sequeira, R.; Sáenz-Arce, G.; Rojas-Carrillo, O.; Avedaño-Soto, E.; Ruepert, C.; Mena-Torres, F.; Starbird-Pérez, R. Biosensor based on the directly enzyme immobilization into a gold nanotriangles/conductive polymer biocompatible coat for electrochemical detection of Chlorpyrifos in water. *Med. Devices Sens.* **2019**, *2*, 1–18.
3. Mantione, D.; del Agua, I.; Sanchez-Sanchez, A.; Mecerreyes, D. Poly(3,4-ethylenedioxythiophene) (PEDOT) derivatives: Innovative conductive polymers for bioelectronics. *Polymers (Basel)* **2017**, *9*, 354. [CrossRef] [PubMed]
4. Ghorbani Zamani, F.; Moulahoum, H.; Ak, M.; Odaci Demirkol, D.; Timur, S. Current trends in the development of conducting polymers-based biosensors. *TrAC Trends Anal. Chem.* **2019**, *118*, 264–276. [CrossRef]
5. Khan, S.; Ul-Islam, M.; Ullah, M.W.; Israr, M.; Jang, J.H.; Park, J.K. Nano-gold assisted highly conducting and biocompatible bacterial cellulose-PEDOT:PSS films for biology-device interface applications. *Int. J. Biol. Macromol.* **2018**, *107*, 865–873. [CrossRef]
6. Lu, B.; Yuk, H.; Lin, S.; Jian, N.; Qu, K.; Xu, J.; Zhao, X. Pure PEDOT:PSS hydrogels. *Nat. Commun.* **2019**, *10*, 1–10. [CrossRef]
7. Kahoush, M.; Behary, N.; Cayla, A.; Mutel, B.; Guan, J.; Nierstrasz, V. Influence of remote plasma on PEDOT:PSS-coated carbon felt for improved activity of glucose oxidase. *J. Appl. Polym. Sci.* **2020**, *137*, 1–11. [CrossRef]
8. Luo, S.C.; Ali, E.M.; Tansil, N.C.; Yu, H.H.; Gao, S.; Kantchev, E.A.B.; Ying, J.Y. Poly(3,4-ethylenedioxythiophene) (PEDOT) nanobiointerfaces: Thin, ultrasmooth, and functionalized PEDOT films with in vitro and in vivo biocompatibility. *Langmuir* **2008**, *24*, 8071–8077. [CrossRef]
9. Starbird, R.; Bauhofer, W.; Meza-Cuevas, M.; Krautschneider, W.H. Effect of experimental factors on the properties of PEDOT-NaPSS galvanostatically deposited from an aqueous micellar media for invasive electrodes. In Proceedings of the 5th 2012 Biomedical Engineering International Conference, Ubon Ratchathani, Thailand, 5–7 December 2012; pp. 1–5.
10. Li, Y.; Neoh, K.G.; Kang, E.T. Controlled release of heparin from polypyrrole-poly (vinyl alcohol) assembly by electrical stimulation. *J. Biomed. Mater. Res. Part A* **2005**, *72*, 171–180. [CrossRef]

11. Boehler, C.; Oberueber, F.; Asplund, M. Tuning drug delivery from conducting polymer films for accurately controlled release of charged molecules. *J. Control. Release* **2019**, *304*, 173–180. [CrossRef]
12. Boehler, C.; Kleber, C.; Martini, N.; Xie, Y.; Dryg, I.; Stieglitz, T.; Hofmann, U.G.; Asplund, M. Actively controlled release of dexamethasone from neural microelectrodes in a chronic in vivo study. *Biomaterials* **2017**, *129*, 176–187. [CrossRef] [PubMed]
13. Wadhwa, R.; Lagenaur, C.F.; Cui, X.T. Electrochemically controlled release of dexamethasone from conducting polymer polypyrrole coated electrode. *J. Control. Release* **2006**, *110*, 531–541. [CrossRef] [PubMed]
14. Wang, W.; Yeung, K.W.K. Bone grafts and biomaterials substitutes for bone defect repair: A review. *Bioact. Mater.* **2017**, *2*, 224–247. [CrossRef] [PubMed]
15. Wang, Z.; Zhang, T.; Xie, S.; Liu, X.; Li, H.; Linhardt, R.J.; Chi, L. Sequencing the oligosaccharide pool in the low molecular weight heparin dalteparin with offline HPLC and ESI–MS/MS. *Carbohydr. Polym.* **2018**, *183*, 81–90. [CrossRef] [PubMed]
16. Mao, A.S.; Mooney, D.J. Regenerative medicine: Current therapies and future directions. *Proc. Natl. Acad. Sci. USA* **2015**, *112*, 14452–14459. [CrossRef]
17. Benoit, D.S.W.; Durney, A.R.; Anseth, K.S. The effect of heparin-functionalized PEG hydrogels on three-dimensional human mesenchymal stem cell osteogenic differentiation. *Biomaterials* **2007**, *28*, 66–77. [CrossRef]
18. He, Q.; Shi, J. Mesoporous silica nanoparticle based nano drug delivery systems: Synthesis, controlled drug release and delivery, pharmacokinetics and biocompatibility. *J. Mater. Chem.* **2011**, *21*, 5845–5855. [CrossRef]
19. Kumar, C.S.S.R.; Mohammad, F. Magnetic nanomaterials for hyperthermia-based therapy and controlled drug delivery. *Adv. Drug Deliv. Rev.* **2011**, *63*, 789–808. [CrossRef]
20. Vishwakarma, A.; Bhise, N.S.; Evangelista, M.B.; Rouwkema, J.; Dokmeci, M.R.; Ghaemmaghami, A.M.; Vrana, N.E.; Khademhosseini, A. Engineering immunomodulatory biomaterials to tune the inflammatory response. *Trends Biotechnol.* **2016**, *34*, 470–482. [CrossRef]
21. Thevenot, P.T.; Nair, A.M.; Shen, J.; Lotfi, P.; Ko, C.Y.; Tang, L. The effect of incorporation of SDF-1α into PLGA scaffolds on stem cell recruitment and the inflammatory response. *Biomaterials* **2010**, *31*, 3997–4008. [CrossRef]
22. Goimil, L.; Jaeger, P.; Ardao, I.; Gómez-Amoza, J.L.; Concheiro, A.; Alvarez-Lorenzo, C.; García-González, C.A. Preparation and stability of dexamethasone-loaded polymeric scaffolds for bone regeneration processed by compressed CO_2 foaming. *J. CO2 Util.* **2018**, *24*, 89–98. [CrossRef]
23. Costa, P.F.; Puga, A.M.; Díaz-Gomez, L.; Concheiro, A.; Busch, D.H.; Alvarez-Lorenzo, C. Additive manufacturing of scaffolds with dexamethasone controlled release for enhanced bone regeneration. *Int. J. Pharm.* **2015**, *496*, 541–550. [CrossRef] [PubMed]
24. Langenbach, F.; Handsche, J. Effects of dexamethasone, ascorbic acid and β-glycerophosphate on the osteogenic differentiation of stem cells in vitro. *Stem Cell Res. Ther.* **2013**, *4*, 423–430. [CrossRef] [PubMed]
25. Helledie, T.; Dombrowski, C.; Rai, B.; Lim, Z.X.H.; Hin, I.L.H.; Rider, D.A.; Stein, G.S.; Hong, W.; van Wijnen, A.J.; Hui, J.H.; et al. Heparan sulfate enhances the self-renewal and therapeutic potential of mesenchymal stem cells from human adult bone marrow. *Stem Cells Dev.* **2012**, *21*, 1897–1910. [CrossRef] [PubMed]
26. Martins, A.; Duarte, A.R.C.; Faria, S.; Marques, A.P.; Reis, R.L.; Neves, N.M. Osteogenic induction of hBMSCs by electrospun scaffolds with dexamethasone release functionality. *Biomaterials* **2010**, *31*, 5875–5885. [CrossRef] [PubMed]
27. Goimil, L.; Santos-Rosales, V.; Delgado, A.; Évora, C.; Reyes, R.; Lozano-Pérez, A.A.; Aznar-Cervantes, S.D.; Cenis, J.L.; Gómez-Amoza, J.L.; Concheiro, A.; et al. ScCO2-foamed silk fibroin aerogel/poly(ε-caprolactone) scaffolds containing dexamethasone for bone regeneration. *J. CO2 Util.* **2019**, *31*, 51–64. [CrossRef]
28. Chu, C.C.; Hsing, C.H.; Shieh, J.P.; Chien, C.C.; Ho, C.M.; Wang, J.J. The cellular mechanisms of the antiemetic action of dexamethasone and related glucocorticoids against vomiting. *Eur. J. Pharmacol.* **2014**, *722*, 48–54. [CrossRef]
29. Zamora-Sequeira, R.; Ardao, I.; Starbird, R.; García-González, C.A. Conductive nanostructured materials based on poly-(3,4-ethylenedioxythiophene) (PEDOT) and starch/κ-carrageenan for biomedical applications. *Carbohydr. Polym.* **2018**, *189*, 304–312. [CrossRef]

30. Hernández-Suarez, P.; Ramírez, K.; Alvarado, F.; Avendaño, E.; Starbird, R. Electrochemical characterization of poly(3,4-ethylenedioxythiophene)/κ-carrageenan as a biocompatible conductive coat for biologic applications. *MRS Commun.* **2018**, 1–6. [CrossRef]
31. Pourjavadi, A.; Harzandi, A.M.; Hosseinzadeh, H. Modified carrageenan 3. Synthesis of a novel polysaccharide-based superabsorbent hydrogel via graft copolymerization of acrylic acid onto kappa-carrageenan in air. *Eur. Polym. J.* **2004**, *40*, 1363–1370. [CrossRef]
32. Hunter, R. *Zeta Potential in Colloid Science: Principles and Applications*; Academic Press: Cambridge, MA, USA, 2013; pp. 6–7.
33. Lowry, G.V.; Hill, R.J.; Harper, S.; Rawle, A.F.; Hendren, C.O.; Klaessig, F.; Nobbmann, U.; Sayre, P.; Rumble, J. Guidance to improve the scientific value of zeta-potential measurements in nanoEHS. *Environ. Sci. Nano* **2016**, *3*, 953–965. [CrossRef]
34. Ali, H.; Kalashnikova, I.; White, M.A.; Sherman, M.; Rytting, E. Preparation, characterization, and transport of dexamethasone-loaded polymeric nanoparticles across a human placental in vitro model. *Int. J. Pharm.* **2013**, *454*, 149–157. [CrossRef]
35. Pargaonkar, N.; Lvov, Y.M.; Li, N.; Steenekamp, J.H.; De Villiers, M.M. Controlled release of dexamethasone from microcapsules produced by polyelectrolyte layer-by-layer nanoassembly. *Pharm. Res.* **2005**, *22*, 826–835. [CrossRef]
36. Sagbas, S.; Butun, S.; Sahiner, N. Modifiable chemically crosslinked poli(κ-carrageenan) particles. *Carbohydr. Polym.* **2012**, *87*, 2718–2724. [CrossRef]
37. Antonov, Y.A.; Zhuravleva, I.L.; Cardinaels, R.; Moldenaers, P. Macromolecular complexes of lysozyme with kappa carrageenan. *Food Hydrocoll.* **2018**, *74*, 227–238. [CrossRef]
38. Zhang, Z.; Grijpma, D.W.; Feijen, J. Poly(trimethylene carbonate) and monomethoxy poly(ethylene glycol)-block-poly(trimethylene carbonate) nanoparticles for the controlled release of dexamethasone. *J. Control. Release* **2006**, *111*, 263–270. [CrossRef]
39. Walsh, F.C.; Ponce De Leon, C. A review of the electrodeposition of metal matrix composite coatings by inclusion of particles in a metal layer: An established and diversifying technology. *Trans. Inst. Met. Finish.* **2014**, *92*, 83–98. [CrossRef]
40. Deligianni, D.D.; Katsala, N.D.; Koutsoukos, P.G.; Missirlis, Y.F. Effect of surface roughness of hydroxyapatite on human bone marrow cell adhesion, proliferation, differentiation and detachment strength. *Biomaterials* **2000**, *22*, 87–96. [CrossRef]
41. Kokkinos, P.A.; Koutsoukos, P.G.; Deligianni, D.D. Detachment strength of human osteoblasts cultured on hydroxyapatite with various surface roughness. Contribution of integrin subunits. *J. Mater. Sci. Mater. Med.* **2012**, *23*, 1489–1498. [CrossRef]
42. Hotchkiss, K.M.; Reddy, G.B.; Hyzy, S.L.; Schwartz, Z.; Boyan, B.D.; Olivares-Navarrete, R. Titanium surface characteristics, including topography and wettability, alter macrophage activation. *Acta Biomater.* **2016**, *31*, 425–434. [CrossRef]
43. Tran-Van, F.; Garreau, S.; Louarn, G.; Froyer, G.; Chevrot, C. Fully undoped and soluble oligo(3,4-ethylenedioxythiophene)s: Spectroscopic study and electrochemical characterization. *J. Mater. Chem.* **2001**, *11*, 1378–1382. [CrossRef]
44. Stevenson, G.; Moulton, S.E.; Innis, P.C.; Wallace, G.G. Polyterthiophene as an electrostimulated controlled drug release material of therapeutic levels of dexamethasone. *Synth. Met.* **2010**, *160*, 1107–1114. [CrossRef]
45. Leprince, L.; Dogimont, A.; Magnin, D.; Demoustier-Champagne, S. Dexamethasone electrically controlled release from polypyrrole-coated nanostructured electrodes. *J. Mater. Sci. Mater. Med.* **2010**, *21*, 925–930. [CrossRef]
46. Balint, R.; Cassidy, N.J.; Cartmell, S.H. conductive polymers: Towards a smart biomaterial for tissue engineering. *Acta Biomater.* **2014**, *10*, 2341–2353. [CrossRef]
47. Bredas, J.; Street, B. Polarons, bipolarons, and solitons in conducting polymers. *Acc. Chem. Res.* **1985**, *18*, 309–315. [CrossRef]
48. Ritger, P.L.; Peppas, N.A. A simple equation for description of solute release II. Fickian and anomalous release from swellable devices. *J. Control. Release* **1987**, *5*, 37–42. [CrossRef]
49. Thomas, D.; Nair, V.V.; Latha, M.S.; Thomas, K.K. Theoretical and experimental studies on theophylline release from hydrophilic alginate nanoparticles. *Futur. J. Pharm. Sci.* **2019**, *5*, 2. [CrossRef]

50. Siepmann, J.; Peppas, N.A. Higuchi equation: Derivation, applications, use and misuse. *Int. J. Pharm.* **2011**, *418*, 6–12. [CrossRef]
51. Kleber, C.; Lienkamp, K.; Rühe, J.; Asplund, M. Electrochemically controlled drug release from a conducting polymer hydrogel (PDMAAp/PEDOT) for local therapy and bioelectronics. *Adv. Healthc. Mater.* **2019**, *8*, 1–11. [CrossRef]
52. Hong, D.; Chen, H.X.; Xue, Y.; Li, D.M.; Wan, X.C.; Ge, R.; Li, J.C. Osteoblastogenic effects of dexamethasone through upregulation of TAZ expression in rat mesenchymal stem cells. *J. Steroid Biochem. Mol. Biol.* **2009**, *116*, 86–92. [CrossRef]
53. Simann, M.; Schneider, V.; Le Blanc, S.; Dotterweich, J.; Zehe, V.; Krug, M.; Jakob, F.; Schilling, T.; Schütze, N. Heparin affects human bone marrow stromal cell fate: Promoting osteogenic and reducing adipogenic differentiation and conversion. *Bone* **2015**, *78*, 102–113. [CrossRef] [PubMed]
54. Spataro, L.; Dilgen, J.; Retterer, S.; Spence, A.J.; Isaacson, M.; Turner, J.N.; Shain, W. Dexamethasone treatment reduces astroglia responses to inserted neuroprosthetic devices in rat neocortex. *Exp. Neurol.* **2005**, *194*, 289–300. [CrossRef] [PubMed]
55. Montero-Rodríguez, J.J.; Ramirez-Sanchez, K.; Valladares-Castrillo, G.; Avendano-Soto, E.D.; Starbird-Perez, R. Design and simulation of flexible thin-film electrodes for cell culture stimulation. In Proceedings of the 2020 Latin American Electron Devices Conference (LAEDC), San José, Costa Rica, 25–28 Febuary 2020.
56. Wakkad, E.; Shams, D. The Anodic oxidation of metals at very low current density. Part V.*. *J. Chem. Soc.* **1946**, *1*, 3098–3102.
57. Gómez-Ordóñez, E.; Rupérez, P. FTIR-ATR spectroscopy as a tool for polysaccharide identification in edible brown and red seaweeds. *Food Hydrocoll.* **2011**, *25*, 1514–1520. [CrossRef]
58. Konermann, L. Addressing a common misconception: Ammonium acetate as neutral ph "buffer" for native electrospray mass spectrometry. *J. Am. Soc. Mass Spectrom.* **2017**, *28*, 1827–1835. [CrossRef] [PubMed]
59. Zamora-Sequeira, R.; Alvarado-Hidalgo, F.; Robles-Chaves, D.; Saénz-Arce, G.; Avendaño-Soto, E.; Sànchez-Kooper, A.; Starbird-Pérez, R. Degradation for wastewater treatment using a sensor based on poly (3, 4-ethylenedioxythiophene)(PEDOT) modified with carbon nanotubes and gold nanoparticles. *Polymers (Basel)* **2019**, *11*, 1449. [CrossRef]

Sample Availability: Samples of the compounds are not available from the authors.

© 2020 by the authors. Licensee MDPI, Basel, Switzerland. This article is an open access article distributed under the terms and conditions of the Creative Commons Attribution (CC BY) license (http://creativecommons.org/licenses/by/4.0/).

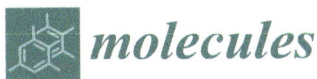

Article

Aerogels from Cellulose Phosphates of Low Degree of Substitution: A TBAF·H₂O/DMSO Based Approach

Christian B. Schimper [1], Paul S. Pachschwoell [1], Hubert Hettegger [1], Marie-Alexandra Neouze [2], Jean-Marie Nedelec [3], Martin Wendland [4], Thomas Rosenau [1,5] and Falk Liebner [1,6,*]

[1] University of Natural Resources and Life Sciences, Vienna (BOKU), Institute for Chemistry of Renewable Resources, Konrad-Lorenz-Straße 24, A-3430 Tulln, Austria; christian.schimper@acticell.at (C.B.S.); paul.pachschwoell@gmail.com (P.S.P.); hubert.hettegger@boku.ac.at (H.H.); thomas.rosenau@boku.ac.at (T.R.)
[2] Vienna University of Technology, Institute of Materials Chemistry, Getreidemarkt 9/165, A-1060 Vienna, Austria; marie-alexandra.neouze@anr.fr
[3] Université Clermont Auvergne, CNRS, SIGMA Clermont, ICCF, F-63000 Clermont-Ferrand, France; jean-marie.nedelec@sigma-clermont.fr
[4] University of Natural Resources and Life Sciences, Vienna (BOKU), Institute for Chemical and Energy Engineering, Muthgasse 107, A-1190 Vienna, Austria; martin.wendland@boku.ac.at
[5] Johan Gadolin Process Chemistry Centre, Åbo Akademi University, Porthansgatan 3, FI-20500 Åbo/Turku, Finland
[6] University Aveiro, Department of Chemistry and CICECO Aveiro Institute of Materials, Campus Universitário de Santiago, 3810-193 Aveiro, Portugal
* Correspondence: falk.liebner@boku.ac.at

Academic Editors: Carlos A. García-González, Pasquale Del Gaudio and Ricardo Starbird
Received: 2 March 2020; Accepted: 5 April 2020; Published: 7 April 2020

Abstract: Biopolymer aerogels of appropriate open-porous morphology, nanotopology, surface chemistry, and mechanical properties can be promising cell scaffolding materials. Here, we report a facile approach towards the preparation of cellulose phosphate aerogels from two types of cellulosic source materials. Since high degrees of phosphorylation would afford water-soluble products inappropriate for cell scaffolding, products of low DS_P (ca. 0.2) were prepared by a heterogeneous approach. Aiming at both i) full preservation of chemical integrity of cellulose during dissolution and ii) utilization of specific phase separation mechanisms upon coagulation of cellulose, TBAF·H₂O/DMSO was employed as a non-derivatizing solvent. Sequential dissolution of cellulose phosphates, casting, coagulation, solvent exchange, and scCO₂ drying afforded lightweight, nano-porous aerogels. Compared to their non-derivatized counterparts, cellulose phosphate aerogels are less sensitive towards shrinking during solvent exchange. This is presumably due to electrostatic repulsion and translates into faster scCO₂ drying. The low DS_P values have no negative impact on pore size distribution, specific surface ($S_{BET} \leq 310$ m² g⁻¹), porosity (Π 95.5–97 vol.%), or stiffness ($E\rho \leq 211$ MPa cm³ g⁻¹). Considering the sterilization capabilities of scCO₂, existing templating opportunities to afford dual-porous scaffolds and the good hemocompatibility of phosphorylated cellulose, TBAF·H₂O/DMSO can be regarded a promising solvent system for the manufacture of cell scaffolding materials.

Keywords: cellulose phosphate; cellulose phosphate aerogel; interconnected porosity; supercritical carbon dioxide; tetrabutylammonium fluoride; TBAF/DMSO

1. Introduction

Amplifying efforts towards a more bio-based economy have recently revived the urge for novel smart processes capable of efficiently transforming biomass or its constituents into functional materials.

Among the broad variety of biopolymers, cellulose is probably the most valuable renewable resource, since it is an abundant unique source of energy, chemicals, and materials. It is easy to access in high purity [1], biocompatible [2,3], and is not a food competitor.

In context with the increasing awareness for a more responsible use of energy and materials in all areas of life, it is easy to understand that research on lightweight, open-porous, and bio-based materials optimized in stiffness-to-weight proportion has greatly advanced in the last decade [4]. This development has been boosted by the nowadays broader availability of supercritical carbon dioxide technologies. The latter allow—besides chemical modification, coating, or foaming—for largely non-destructive drying of biopolymer gels [5]. This gives access to a new family of ultra-lightweight aerogels which would not be accessible with the same features using classical drying techniques [6–8]. Even though not having conquered industrial production yet, cellulose-derived aerogels are promising candidates for a wide range of applications. This includes thermal super-insulation [9], specific sorption of gases or solutes [10], carrier support in catalysis [11], morphological templating [12], energy generation and storage [13], as well as wound dressings [14–16], transdermal drug delivery [17,18], or tissue engineering [19–21].

Depending on the target application, cellulosic aerogels can be required to feature a broad spectrum of specific properties. The demands are rather simple for thermal superinsulation panels. The latter would require low apparent density, narrow mesopore distribution, sufficient dimensional stability in humid atmosphere, resistance towards microbial degradation, and facile processability [22]. Cell scaffolding materials, however, have to meet complex requirements [19,23,24]. Dual-porosity, i.e., interconnected micron-size pores accommodated in networks of nanoporous struts, and biocompatibility for example are key features. While biocompatibility is inherent to cellulose, dual-porosity can be provided, such as using temporary scaffolds of packed beds of porogens [25]. Besides dual-porous architecture, appropriate nanotopology, surface chemistry, electrical charge density, mechanical properties, or availability of growth factors are further important prerequisites [26]. This is complemented by purity and preservation of chemical integrity of cellulose throughout processing into the desired cell scaffolding materials.

Solution casting and subsequent coagulation of cellulose by an antisolvent is one of the most facile and efficient approaches towards shaped open-porous materials [27,28]. However, the choice of solvents able to solubilize cellulose is rather limited [7]. The complex requirements of cell scaffolding materials in terms of purity, morphology, or surface properties further narrow the range of potentially applicable solvents. Reasons include potential derivatization as demonstrated for common ionic liquids [29], hydrolytic cleavage [30], and formation of undesired by-products [31].

Recently we reported about the impact of different cellulose solvents and antisolvents on nanomorphological and -topological features (e.g., crystallinity, size and shape of pores, dimension, organization, and surface roughness of network building nanoparticles) of cellulose II aerogels [32]. Both nanomorphology and nanotopography play a crucial role in tissue engineering. This has been recently demonstrated for neurite extension by neuronal PC12 cells grown on collagen-coated mesoporous silica aerogels [33,34] and on electrically conductive carbon aerogels [35]. Based on the finding that the non-derivatizing solvent system tetrabutylammonium fluoride / dimethylsulfoxide (TBAF/DMSO) affords the formation of particularly small particles, and hence, finely substructured cellulose II networks [32], we extended the exploration of this solvent for processing different types of pulp into cellulose aerogels [36]. Simultaneously we were aiming to improve the dissolution performance of TBAF·xH$_2$O/DMSO. Optimization of the water-to-fluoride ratio was one target, since the latter is a sensitive parameter governing dissolution kinetics. It turned out that the optimum of cellulose dissolution is reached at water-to-fluoride molar ratios of ($0.8 \leq \chi_{wf} \leq 2$). Water contents outside this range impede cellulose dissolution either by E2-type Hofmann decomposition of TBAF into but-1-ene, tributylamine and thermodynamically stable HF$_2^-$ ions ($\chi_{wf} \leq 0.8$) [37] or simply by insufficient rearrangement capabilities for the hydrogen bonding network in cellulose ($\chi_{wf} \geq 2$) [38].

This study investigates the utilization of TBAF·xH$_2$O/DMSO for the preparation of cellulose phosphate aerogels since the latter have shown promise as cell scaffolding materials. Recently, cross-linked aerogels obtained from cellulose nanocrystals carrying a low count of phosphate halfester groups on their surface were reported to fulfil many requirements of viable bone tissue scaffolds [21]. This complements the results of earlier attempts aiming at the preparation of cellulose II phosphate aerogels via shaping and coagulation of cellulose phosphates from *Lyocell* dopes, i.e., using the solvent system *N*-methylmorpholine-*N*-oxide (NMMO)/water. Already at low degrees of phosphorylation (DS$_P$ ca. 0.2), biomineralization and good hemocompatibility in terms of hemostasis and inflammatory response were observed [39]. However, some shortcomings of NMMO related to its elevated melting point, its proneness towards autocatalytic degradation (in the presence of acidic phosphate groups) and the specific solidification behavior of cooling dopes were reasons enough to look for alternatives.

This study investigates the preparation of cellulose phosphate aerogels using TBAF·xH$_2$O/DMSO as a non-derivatizing solvent for the preparation of cellulose phosphate aerogels of low degree of phosphorylation. It has been tested with the example of two representative cellulosic source materials. The exploratory work was expected to provide data for developing a cellulose phosphate 3D printing approach for cell scaffolding materials.

2. Results and Discussion

2.1. Phosphorylation

Phosphorylation of the two selected cellulosic source materials of this study—cotton linters (CL) and eucalyptus prehydrolysis kraft pulp (hwPHK)—was accomplished using concentrated phosphoric acid. Triethyl phosphate was used as solvent and phosphorus pentoxide served as a reactive binder for water released during esterification. Microwave-assisted pressure digestion in HNO$_3$/H$_2$O$_2$ and subsequent ICP-OES analyses confirmed that the desired low degrees of phosphorylation were obtained. While the degree of substitution by phosphate moieties (DS$_P$) was 0.18 for the cotton linters sample (corresponding to a phosphorous content of 33.4 g kg^{-1}; Table 1), it was 0.24 for hwPHK (49.1 g kg^{-1}). At this low degree of phosphorylation, the cellulose derivatives were proven not to be water-soluble yet. This is a prerequisite for cellulose coagulation from solution state, such as in NMMO/H$_2$O or TBAF/DMSO, triggered by the addition of the anti-solvent water. Dissolution in aqueous media is also not desired for any use as cell scaffolding material. ^{31}P NMR as exemplarily conducted for the hwPHK sample confirmed the expected selective substitution of the primary alcohol groups in C6 position of the anhydroglucose units (data not shown).

Table 1. Phosphorous contents, DS$_P$ values (degree of phosphorylation), and selected properties of 3% cellulose phosphate lyogels and aerogels compared to the non-derivatized starting materials. The range of variation represents the 95% confidence interval.

| Sample | P Content [wt.%] | DS$_P$ | Shrinking (−) / Swelling (+) | | Apparent Density [mg cm^{-3}] |
			Regeneration (EtOH, before Drying) [%]	After scCO$_2$ Drying [%]	
hwPHK	-	-	−16.2 ± 4.9	−39.1 ± 5.5	58.1 ± 3.5
hwPHK-P	4.91	0.24	+4.0 ± 2.5	−28.3 ± 6.8	47.0 ± 5.8
CL	-	-	−17.8 ± 4.5	−45.7 ± 6.8	71.2 ± 5.0
CL-P	3.34	0.18	−2.4 ± 2.8	−31.4 ± 6.7	50.0 ± 4.0

Previously, we have shown that a wide range of cellulosic source materials can be dissolved up to 3 wt.% cellulose content within comparatively short dissolution time [36]. Optically clear solutions of sufficiently low viscosity, and hence, good workability, were obtained. Targeting solution casting, a solid content of 3 wt.% was envisaged for the cellulose phosphates of this study, too.

Like their non-derivatized counterparts, the two types of cellulose phosphates could be easily dissolved at the target concentration of 3 wt.% in DMSO that contained 16.6 wt.% TBAF and 0.95 wt.% H_2O. Visually and microscopically clear solutions were obtained within 4 h of dissolution at 60 °C. Solution casting of the comparatively low-viscous solutions and subsequent submersion of the molds in water afforded self-standing transparent hydrogels. According to common practice, the hydrogels were subjected to a series of solvent exchange steps aiming to incrementally increase the ethanol content up to 100% to prepare the gels for supercritical carbon dioxide ($scCO_2$) drying. Since dimensional stability is a key property for many applications, and particularly challenging to achieve for ultra-lightweight biopolymer-derived polysaccharide materials, possible swelling and shrinking throughout all steps of the aerogel preparation procedure were assessed. It was shown that coagulation and hydrogel formation, respectively, occurred across the entire cast solution as evident from the shape and dimensions of the free-standing hydrogels obtained. However, slight shrinkage by syneresis was observed when the gels were left in the PTFE molds, such as for 72 h. Interestingly, this was not the case when cardboard molds were used [40]. Immersion of the CL and hwPHK hydrogel samples in water of incrementally increasing ethanol content (50%, 75%, 96%, and 100%) caused the gels to shrink by up to 18 vol.% (Figure 1, Table 1). This is in agreement with previous work [36] and has been observed for other cellulose II gels too. Examples include gels formed by water-induced coagulation of cellulose from solvent systems like $NMMO \cdot H_2O$, [EMIm][OAc]/DMSO, or $Ca(SCN)_2 \cdot 8H_2O/LiCl$ [32].

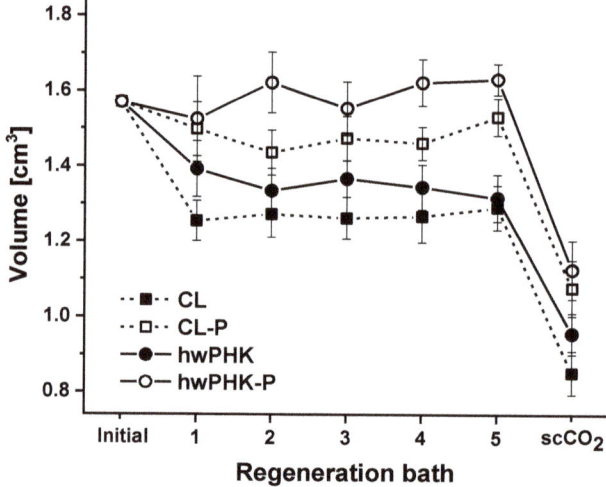

Figure 1. Change in volume of the gels during regeneration in ethanol followed by supercritical carbon dioxide ($scCO_2$) drying (-P indicates phosphorylated samples). Error bars indicate the 95% confidence interval.

Interestingly, both types of hydrogels prepared from the respective phosphorylated cellulosic materials suffered from less shrinkage during the solvent exchange sequence than their P-free counterparts (Figure 1). This is presumably due to the presence of negatively charged phosphate groups on the surface of cellulose II nanoparticles that form and aggregate spontaneously during coagulation to afford three-dimensional networks [7]. Repulsive forces and possibly steric hindrance can partially impede supramolecular arrangement of cellulose chains. This could explain why virtually no shrinkage—in case of hwPHK-P even minimal swelling—was observed after completing the solvent exchange (Table 1). Significant shrinkage of all gels, however, was caused by the final $scCO_2$ drying step. In sum of the entire solvent exchange and $scCO_2$ drying process, the volume loss for the resulting aerogels was about 39–46% for the non-derivatized cellulosic materials and 28–31% for their phosphorylated counterparts. A similar extent of shrinkage (29 vol.%)—occurring mostly during the final scCO$_2$ drying step—has been recently reported for anisotropic cellulose II gels. The latter were obtained by self-assembly of cellulose (3 wt.%) in super-cooled 1,1,3,3-tetramethylguanidinium acetate under the impact of decelerated antisolvent infusion [28]. As discussed earlier [12], shrinkage is governed by solvent-polymer as well as polymer-polymer interactions. They can be quantified by cohesive energy E_{coh} or cohesive energy density e_{coh} when E_{coh} is related to unit volume. The square root of e_{coh} and Hildebrand solubility parameter δ_H, respectively, is frequently used to predict solvent–polymer interactions. Since E_{coh} represents the sum of contributions by dispersion forces, permanent dipol-dipol forces, and hydrogen bonding, any variation of polymer-solvent composition potentially impacts these interactions. While the changes in composition throughout the lengthy solvent exchange procedure are rather small, scCO$_2$ drying causes rapid changes in composition of the interstitial fluids. This is most pronounced in the initial stage of drying. Molecular dynamics simulations have recently shown that the solubility parameters change significantly with enrichment of scCO$_2$ by co-solvents, such as ethanol. It changes in a reverse way when the volume fraction of co-solvent is reduced [41]. For pure scCO$_2$ (and pure co-solvent), δ_H decreases with temperature and rises with pressure and density. Addition of co-solvents, such as ethanol, increases δ_H significantly, boosting with the amount of added co-solvent. Considering the different stages of scCO$_2$ drying, i.e., i) CO$_2$ pressurization, ii) transition from liquid to supercritical state causing considerable changes in density, iii) formation and elution of a scCO$_2$-expanded ethanol phase of rapidly decreasing ethanol content, and iv) final depressurization, it is evident that this part of the aerogel preparation is the most sensitive part with regard to shrinkage, specifically for ultra-lightweight aerogels. Beyond that it is assumed that small quantities of structural water—which acts as a softener for the cellulose II networks—are released towards the end of the drying procedure. This is caused by condensation of labile hydroxyl-groups which seems to start already when the gels are transferred to absolute ethanol since most of the gels stiffened slightly during this stage, comparable to hornification of cellulose at elevated temperature.

According to the different extent of shrinkage throughout the solvent exchange and scCO$_2$ drying procedure, somewhat lower bulk densities were obtained for the cellulose phosphate aerogels. While the values of the latter were largely similar (47 vs. 50 mg cm^{-3}), that of their counterparts from non-derivatized cellulose varied to a larger extent and ranged from 58 (CL) to 71 mg cm^{-3} (hwPHK, Table 1).

2.2. Chemical Integrity of Cellulose Phosphates during Dissolution

In an attempt to verify whether the chemical integrity of the cellulose phosphates was preserved throughout dissolution, both CL-P and hwPHK-P were subjected to elemental analysis prior to and after dissolution in TBAF·H$_2$O/DMSO (20 °C, 16 h). The results revealed a significant loss of phosphate groups for both of the samples. While for CL-P, the DS$_P$ value decreased from 0.18 to 0.13 (−28%) and was more pronounced for hwPHK-P (−55%; DS$_P$ 0.209 vs. 0.095). Kinetic studies, as exemplarily conducted for the hwPHK-P sample, showed that the losses occur mainly in the initial stage of dissolution since the DS$_P$ values remained largely constant after two hours of dissolution time (Table 2).

Table 2. DS_P values of hwPHK-P (initial DS_P = 0.209) after extraction with DMSO or a solution of 16.6 wt.% TBAF in DMSO having a water content of 0.95 wt.% (labeled TBAF/DMSO) at room temperature and for different time periods. The range of variation indicates the 95% confidence interval (n = 3).

Extraction Medium	Extraction Time [h]	Final DS_P	[%] of Initial DS_P	
DMSO (control)	4	0.149	71	±0.0
TBAF/DMSO	2	0.094	45	±1.9
	4	0.093	44	±1.2
	8	0.096	46	±0.0
	8 (60 °C)	0.096	46	±0.0
	16	0.093	44	±0.5

This suggests that for hwPHK about 55% of the presumably introduced phosphates were not covalently bonded but resisted being trapped in the phosphorylated cellulose. Even if released during dissolution in TBAF/DMSO, it was trapped again upon water-induced coagulation, but was then largely removed during the various solvent exchange steps. This conclusion is supported by the fact that identical final DS_P values (0.096) were obtained after 8 h of dissolution time at both room temperature and 60 °C. Aiming to exclude interference of TBAF, the hwPHK-P dissolution experiment was repeated, however, using DMSO as solvent only (4 h, room temperature). Following repeated washings with ethanol and vacuum drying, a remaining P content of 71% was found. Altogether, this implies that the used washing procedure after phosphorylation (*n*-hexanol, ethanol, water) as proposed elsewhere [42] is not efficient enough. The results were also a motivation to re-check similar hwPHK-P retention samples of a previous study for any possible reduction of DS_P. These samples had been used for preparation of potential cell scaffolding materials via the *Lyocell* route [39]. Cellulose was here dissolved in molten *N*-methylmorpholine-*N*-oxide monohydrate (NMMO·H_2O) at 100 °C using propyl gallate and *N*-benzylmorpholine-*N*-oxide (NBnMO) as stabilizers. Repeating dissolution of the hwPHK-P retention samples (DS_P = 0.25) in NMMO·H_2O at 110 °C, subsequent coagulation by ethanol and final scCO_2 drying revealed that also in this dissolution/coagulation approach the DS_P decreased; however to a lesser extent (33%, DS_P = 0.17). A DS_P value of 0.22 was obtained (13% loss) when the hwPHK-P sample was extracted with ethanol only at room temperature.

2.3. TBAF Content of Cellulose Phosphate Aerogels

Even though TBAF/DMSO is considered a direct, non-derivatizing cellulose solvent, selected aerogel samples were subjected to nitrogen and fluorine analysis by energy-dispersive X-ray spectroscopy (EDAX). While for CL and hwPHK aerogels low nitrogen (and fluorine) contents close to the detection limit were determined (0.05% N, data not shown), the latter were significantly higher for their phosphorylated counterparts (Figure 2A). Independent of the cellulosic source material and degree of phosphorylation (CL-P DS_P = 0.18; hwPHK-P DS_P = 0.24), respectively, significantly higher values of 0.74% N were obtained. Considering both the nominal DS_P values of the two phosphorylated cellulosic source materials (DS_P = 0.2 on rough estimate) and the real DS_P ones (DS_P = 0.09 = 45% of the nominal DS_P), it can be concluded that about all covalently introduced phosphate moieties carry one ammonium counter ion. The over-proportional residual content of fluoride ions is difficult to explain. Likely reasons could be remnants of phosphoric acid competing with fluorine for TBA cations or partial degradation of TBAF (triggering release of tributylamine, but-1-ene and the thermodynamically stable HF_2^- ions; cf. above) and preferred removal of the nitrogenous compounds during solvent exchange and scCO_2 drying.

Covalent immobilization of both nitrogen and fluorine, however, can be ruled out since repeated washing of the samples with deionized water (3×) afforded EDAX spectra free of any N and F signals (Figure 2B).

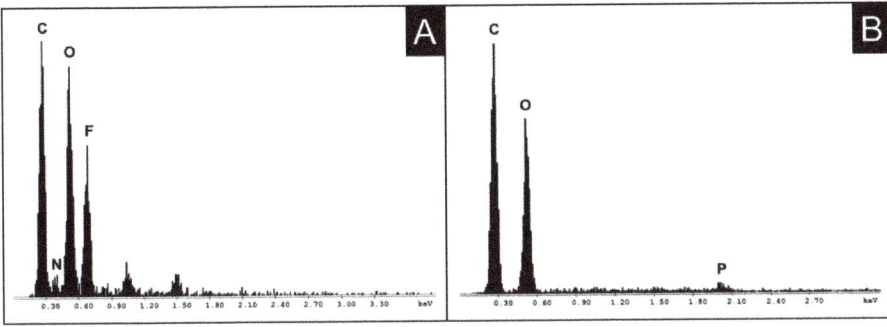

Figure 2. EDAX spectra of aerogels obtained without (**A**, non-derivatized CL) and after (**B**, phosphorylated CL) implementing a H_2O washing step prior solvent exchange and scCO$_2$ drying.

2.4. Aerogel Morphology

Selected aerogel samples were split open by gently pulling apart the two halves of the cylindrical specimen using a small fork with narrow teeth. Scanning electron microscopy (SEM) of the interior of these aerogels revealed the presence of an isotropic network largely composed of interconnected spherical particles (Figure 3). Its appearance resembles that of other cellulose gels formed by spinodal decomposition, such as from cellulose solutions in ionic liquids (e.g., [EMIm][OAc]) or molten NMMO·H_2O) [43,44]. The isotropic networks are formed from (partially elongated) single-digit micron-sized clusters of cellulosic spheres being a few hundred nanometers in diameter. The voids in between the clusters are interconnected and of similar spatial shape and dimension (diameter 2–4 µm, partially elongated). A closer look revealed the coexistence of a further substructure for all of the studied aerogels. In particular, the micrograph of Figure 3E suggests that the spherical submicron particles are composed of finer fibrils, which is in agreement with previous studies [32,36]. Phosphorylation at the low degrees of substitution envisaged in this study had, however, virtually no impact on microscale morphology (*cf.* Figure 3A vs. Figures 3C and 3E vs. Figure 3G).

SEM micrographs of the cutting edges close to the exterior surface revealed that a comparably dense skin had formed in case of the aerogels from the non-derivatized cellulosic materials. It has an average thickness of 10–50 µm and is deficient in micron-size pores (Figures 3B and 3F). Skin formation is evidently less pronounced in the cellulose phosphate aerogels. In particular, the hwPHK-P sample features a largely skin-free open-porous flaky structure (Figure 3H). Skin formation is a well-known phenomenon occurring during cellulose processing from solution state, such as in the course of wet spinning of *Lyocell* dopes. Different coagulation kinetics across the diameter of the extruded dope strands result in significant morphological variation, typically comprising of a compact fiber core, a porous middle zone, and a semipermeable fiber skin [45].

Although relying on different coagulation mechanisms, also membranes prepared from cellulose solutions in mixtures of sodium hydroxide and urea exhibited morphological differences between surface and core of the respective materials. Their extent differed with the type of antisolvent used for cellulose coagulation and was most pronounced for ethanol [46]. Formation of a layered structure comprising of denser outer and looser inner zones has been shown also for cellophane films (sheet-extruded viscose rayon; [47]). Anisotropic cellulose II aerogels (Hermans orientation factor 0.46) obtained by self-assembly of cellulose in super-cooled ionic liquid under the impact of decelerated antisolvent infusion [28] feature skin formation too.

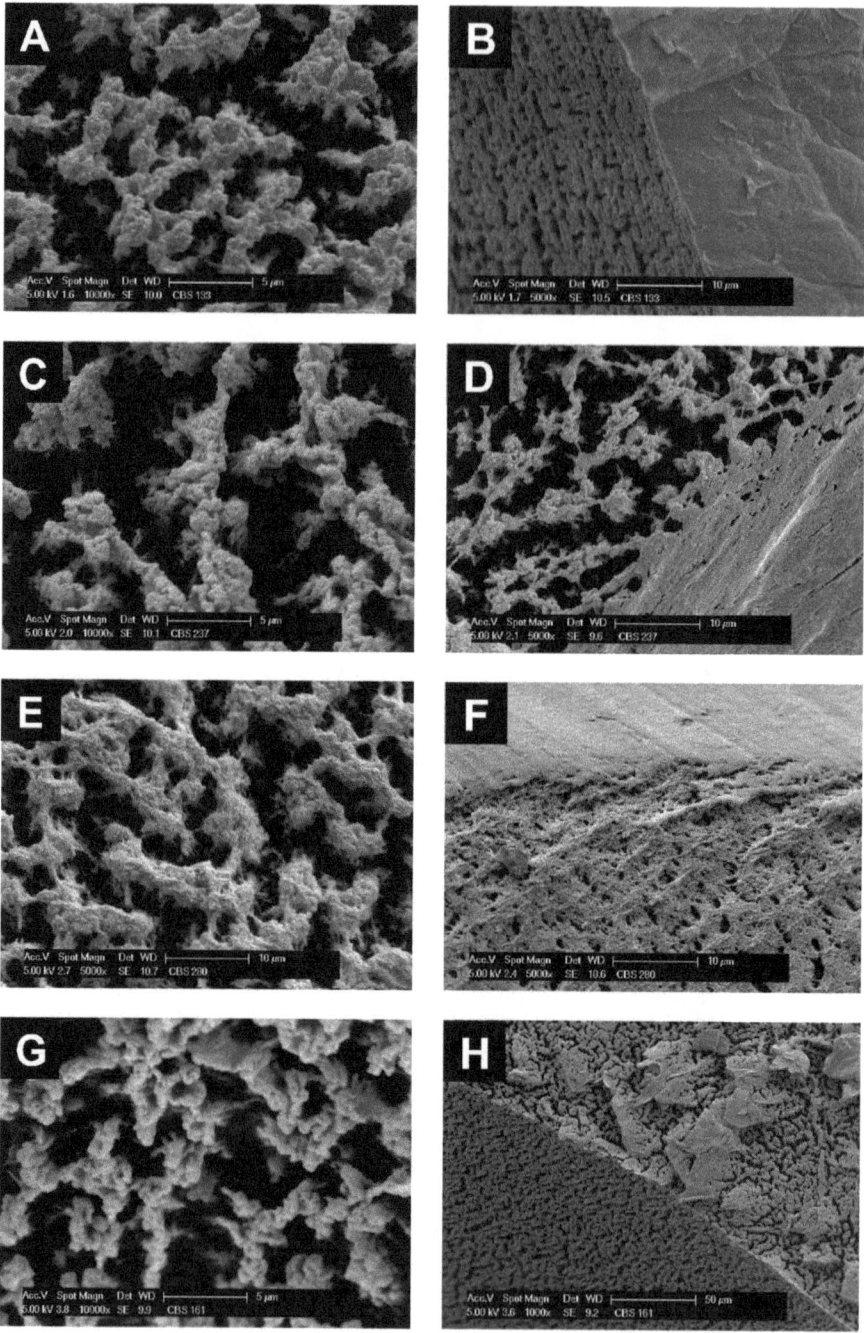

Figure 3. SEM micrographs of the interior (**A**, **C**, **E**, **G**) and near-surface breaking edge (**B**, **D**, **F**, **H**) of aerogels from non-derivatized cellulose (CL: **A**, **B**; hwPHK: **E**, **F**) and their phosphorylated counterparts (CL-P: **C**, **D**; hwPHK-P: **G**, **H**) at different magnification.

2.5. Compression Testing

Uniaxial compression testing and evaluation of the respective stress–strain relationships confirmed the typical compression behavior of lightweight cellulose II aerogels as discussed elsewhere [32]. Besides ductility, low rigidity as expressed by Young's modulus ($E \leq 14.5$ MPa), and absence of sample buckling (zero Poisson ratio), the stress-strain curves exhibit a pronounced plateau region (10–50% strain). In this region, compression energy is dissipated by gradual collapsing of the cellular structure. Beyond that plateau, strain hardening sets in. Recently, it has been shown for aerogels from nanofibrillated 2,3-dicarboxyl cellulose that strain hardening can coincide with pore size harmonization in favor of mesopores giving access towards superinsulating aerogels [9]. Interestingly, both Young's modulus and density-normalized specific Young's modulus of the CL aerogel were higher than that of comparable CL aerogels obtained using NMMO·H$_2$O or [EMIm][OAc]/DMSO as cellulose solvent (Table 3; [32]). Phosphorylation, at least at the envisaged low degrees of substitution, had no clear impact on the anyway low values of Young's modulus E, yield stress (σ_y) and yield strain (ε_y). While E_ρ and ε_y slightly increased with phosphorylation for the aerogels derived from cotton linters, it was the reverse for the hwPHK samples.

Table 3. Young's modulus (E), specific modulus (E_ρ), yield strength (σ_y), and yield stress (ε_y) as obtained from uniaxial compression testing of the prepared aerogels.

Sample	E [MPa]	E_ρ [MPa cm^3 g^{-1}]	σ_y [MPa]	ε_y [%]
CL (TBAF/DMSO)	11.9	167	5.3	3.4
([EMIM][OAc]/DMSO) [a]	1.121 [a]	20 [a]	2.1 [a]	n.d. [b]
NMMO·H$_2$O [a]	4.26 [a]	68 [a]	2.9 [a]	n.d. [b]
CL-P	10.8	216	3.6	5.1
hwPHK	5.9	102	5.7	7.6
hwPHK-P	3.2	68	1.9	3.4

[a] data taken from [15], [b] not determined.

Based on the apparent density (ρ_A) of the aerogels and assuming a skeletal cellulose density of $\rho_S = 1.56$ g cm^{-3}, porosity (Π) values ranging between 95.46 and 96.99% were calculated using the following equation: Π (%) = $1 - \rho_A / \rho_S$ (Table 4). At a first glance, these values combined with the information of the SEM pictures (Figure 3) could be perceived as indicative for the presence of very low specific surfaces only in all prepared aerogels. However, nitrogen sorption experiments at 77 K provided a different picture. Evaluation of the isotherms in the low relative pressure range ($p/p^0 = 0.05$–0.2) of the adsorption branches using the Brunauer–Emmett–Teller (BET) approach revealed a considerable monolayer nitrogen adsorption. It corresponds to about 350–370 m^2 g^{-1} which is almost as high as reported for anisotropic mesoporous aerogels of narrow size distribution [9]. These relatively high values are indicative of the presence of a well-developed nanoporous substructure not visible in the micrographs of Figure 3. Somewhat lower specific surface values were calculated for both types of phosphorylated cellulose aerogels (Table 4). However, these results require careful treatment since gas sorption in aerogels of multiscale porosity depends on many factors. It also includes the C factor of the BET equation. Its significance is low since the C factor—in the strict sense—is a measure of interaction between a non-porous surface and adsorbent molecules [48]. Assuming largely similar morphology, however, the significantly lower C values obtained for the phosphorylated samples can be interpreted as a considerable drop in interaction due to the introduction of the polar phosphate moieties.

Table 4. Calculated porosity, results of nitrogen sorption experiments and pore characteristics derived from thermoporosimetry. Numbers in brackets indicate the 95% confidence interval ($n = 3$).

Sample	Calculated Porosity [%]	Nitrogen Sorption Experiments			Thermoporosimetry	
		Specific Surface [$m^2\ g^{-1}$]	Sorbed Volume [$cm^3\ g^{-1}$]	C Constant	V_p PSD [$cm^3\ g^{-1}$]	R_p [nm] max PSD
CL	96.28	355 (43)	0.80 (0.20)	101 (1.0)	6.06	19.19
CL-P	96.99	311 (6.9)	0.55 (0.10)	48 (2.0)	9.27	21.23
hwPHK	95.46	366 (2.0)	0.7 (0)	104 (2.0)	7.32	19.74
hwPHK-P	96.80	270 (20)	0.5 (0)	45 (5.9)	10.60	24.49

All sorption isotherms confirmed the presence of a considerable volume fraction of mesopores as strongly evident from their IUPAC type IV shape [49]. The latter is characterized by slow monolayer adsorption at relatively low relative pressure ($p/p^0 \leq 60$ kPa), but higher ad- and desorption rates beyond that ($0.07 \leq p/p^0 \leq 0.1$ MPa).

Due to the fragility of lightweight cellulosic aerogels, pore size distributions representing the true porosity are methodologically difficult to obtain, in particular for aerogels of multiscale pore size distribution. While mercury intrusion is not applicable (the high specific density causes pore collapsing), other methods are limited to a certain range of pore size. Evaluation of data points taken from the desorption branches of the nitrogen sorption isotherms using the Barrett–Joyner–Halenda model (BJH) suggested the presence of mesoporous domains. The latter are characterized by a narrow pore size distribution peaking at around 9–11 nm. They seem to exist in all studied materials. The results of the BJH calculations, however, also indicate the presence of larger pores. This is in agreement with the transition of the two branches of the adsorption isotherms at $p/p^0 = 0.1$ MPa and the SEM micrographs. Thermoporosimetry studies confirmed both the presence of mesopores and coexistence of significantly larger pores (Figure 4). All pore-size distributions have their maximum at about 50 nm diameter. The results of the nitrogen sorption experiments, thermoporosimetry data, and SEM micrographs suggest that phosphorylation at the studied low DS_P values has only a marginal impact on morphological features. This includes specific surface and pore-size distribution.

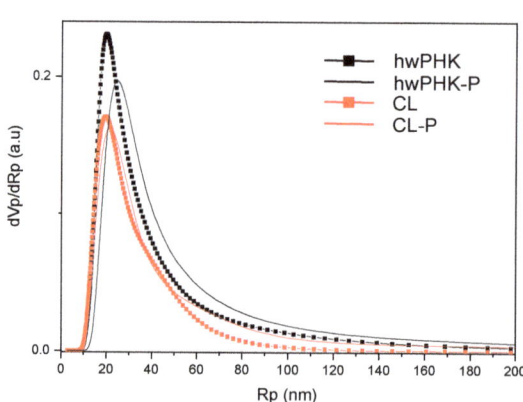

Figure 4. Normalized pore-size distributions as obtained by thermoporosimetry.

2.6. Aerogel Stability and Moisture Sorption during Storage

The abundance of hydroxyl groups renders cellulosic surfaces very sensitive towards moisture sorption. While this feature is highly desired in some applications like wound dressings [15], it is the opposite for lightweight cellulose aerogels. Their high volume fractions of interconnected nanopores exceeding sometimes 99 vol.% render them very fragile, in particular in moist environments. Capillary condensation is a phenomenon that occurs in hydrophobic materials as well, but is amplified by huge internal surfaces of high hydrophilicity. Water condensation in capillaries give rise to the formation of strong inward forces alongside a capillary gradient adjacent to the water menisci formed. These forces are caused by differences in specific energies of the involved phases. Their strength is reversely correlated with pore radii, which renders open-nanoporous, hydrophilic and soft materials particularly sensitive towards shrinkage. Considering both the anhydrous conditions in the last stages of solvent exchange and scCO$_2$ drying, as well as the hydrophilicity of the studied cellulosic materials, it was assumed that the aerogels would gain weight immediately once exposed to air. However, this was not the case. It turned out that the aerogels prepared from the non-derivatized source materials lost about 5–7 wt.% instead within 60 min after scCO$_2$ drying (Figure 5). This is surprising at a first glance and needed a more thorough investigation since this weight loss could be explained solely by degassing of CO$_2$ and replacement by air. Considering a bulk density of 71.2 mg cm^{-3} for the CL aerogels for example and a cellulose skeletal density of 1.56 g cm^{-3}, the corresponding pore volume would be about 0.95 cm^{-3}. Assuming ideal gas behavior, standard conditions and occupation of the entire pore volume by CO$_2$, its quantitative replacement by dry air (80% N$_2$ and 20% O$_2$) would cause a weight loss of ca. 1.22 mg. This would be equivalent to 1.7% loss related to the bulk density calculated from weight and spatial dimensions shortly after scCO$_2$ drying. Even if water sorption would have caused the difference between measured bulk density (71.2 mg cm^{-3}) and theoretical density (55.25 mg cm^{-3})—calculated from the original cellulose content of the CL gel (3 wt.%) and the volume loss throughout aerogel preparation (45.7 vol.%)—the maximum possible weight loss would be 2.21 wt.% only. Therefore, it is reasonable to conclude that small quantities of ethanol were still present in the scCO$_2$ dried aerogels, which is in agreement with olfactory impressions. Headspace-GC/MS investigations confirmed this assumption. They revealed that—depending on the cellulosic material processed into aerogels—considerable amounts of ethanol can remain after scCO$_2$ drying. While scCO$_2$ extracted virtually all ethanol from the pores of bacterial cellulose aerogels of similar sample size and shape within one hour drying time, more than the ten-fold amount of ethanol remained for the significantly denser CL aerogels. Phosphorylation, even at low degree of substitution, seems to disfavor ethanol sorption as evident from the slight weight losses after scCO$_2$ drying.

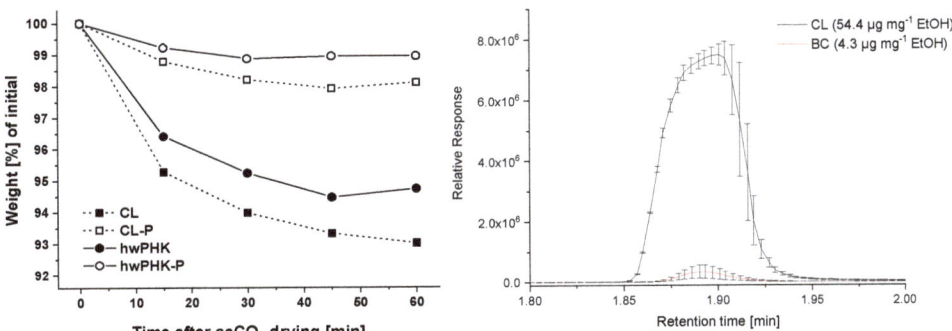

Figure 5. Weight [%] of the materials recorded over 60 min after scCO$_2$ drying (left). Release of ethanol from freshly scCO$_2$ dried cotton linters aerogels (CL) and bacterial cellulose aerogels (BC) under headspace (80 °C) GC-MS conditions (right).

Long-term dimensional stability and moisture sorption of all aerogels were studied for a time period of 84 days and controlled levels of relative humidity. Weight gain and shrinkage values revealed that moisture uptake occurs for all studied aerogels mainly during the first 24 h (data not shown) and is largely completed after 48 h. This was independent of cellulose type, degree of phosphorylation, and relative humidity (Table 5) except for the highest value of 98%RH. Here, water sorption increased by 2.2 wt.% for the CL sample from 23.6% after 2 days to 25.8% after 84 days. The amount of water adsorbed was confirmed to depend on the air moisture content. While at 30% RH, water uptake was negligible for all samples, it was moderate at 65% RH (5.0–6.6%) but strong at 98% RH (23.6–24.2%). Corresponding to the amounts of adsorbed water, all samples suffered from significant shrinkage, specifically within the first two days of storage. Here, the extent of shrinkage increased strongly in the order 30%RH (24–28%) < 65%RH (64–73%) < 98%RH (90–93%). Storage in anhydrous environment as accomplished by placing the samples in a closed compartment over P_4O_{10} is not recommended. Removal of structural water and hornification cause the aerogels to shrink at an extent comparable to that observed for 30% RH.

Table 5. Volume and weight changes of studied aerogels in dependence on relative humidity and storage time (% of initial mass and volume right after $scCO_2$ drying). Numbers in brackets indicate the 95% confidence interval ($n = 4$).

Sample	Conditioning [% RH]	2 d		84 d	
		Volume [%]	Weight [%]	Volume [%]	Weight [%]
CL	0	78.7 (1.3)	−4.2 (0.48)	68.0 (1.6)	−6.7 (0.25)
	30	72.0 (4.8)	−1.4 (0.06)	62.6 (5.2)	−1.5 (0.29)
	65	30.5 (3.0)	5.0 (1.0)	24.7 (2.9)	5.2 (0.63)
	98	10.0 (3.0)	23.6 (0.53)	10.4 (5.5)	25.8 (0.05)
CL-P	0	88.6 (1,4)	−1.7 (0.04)	78.9 (5.1)	−3.1 (0.13)
	65	27.4 (1.1)	6.6 (0.39)	19.7 (1.7)	5.8 (0.21)
hwPHK	0	85.6 (11)	−4.8 (0.37)	76.9 (8.4)	−4.9 (0.36)
	30	76.0 (6.5)	−0.3 (0.02)	68.7 (6.2)	−0.7 (0.13)
	65	36.3 (0.48)	5.5 (0.54)	27.2 (0.13)	5.4 (0.81)
	98	7.1 (0.72)	24.2 (0.01)	6.5 (0.08)	25.0 (0.07)
hwPHK-P	0	95.6 (5.2)	−0.6 (0.01)	87.6 (4.9)	−1.8 (0.01)
	65	30.9 (3.3)	6.1 (0.24)	21.4 (3.4)	4.8 (0.17)

As a result of water uptake and shrinkage, the bulk densities of the prepared aerogels increased as well. While it was to a minor extent only when storing them at 0% and 30% RH, three- (65% RH) to 17-fold (98% RH) higher values were obtained for the more humid environments. Phosphorylation rendered the aerogels somewhat more sensitive towards moisture sorption and shrinkage.

2.7. Thermostability

Thermogravimetric analysis (TGA) conducted in helium atmosphere revealed some interesting differences between the different sets of samples. This applies not only to the cellulosic source materials and the aerogels obtained thereof. It refers also to the comparison between aerogels prepared from non-derivatized cellulose and their phosphorylated analogues (*cf.* Figure 6, right). The two non-processed CL and hwPHK samples were virtually fully stable up to about 325 °C. Here, prominent polymer degradation sets in, exactly as reported for cotton linters before [50]. Thermal degradation is largely completed at 350 °C already when about 90% of the initial weight has been released as volatiles. Continued pyrolysis and carbonization up to 950 °C caused a further 50% reduction of the remaining mass.

Processing of the cellulosic source materials into lightweight open-porous aerogels gives rise to a series of differences in material properties. Compared to the cellulosic fibers of the source materials, the diameters of the aerogel network forming fibrils is much smaller [36] and the degree of crystallinity lower [32]. This translated into much higher specific surface areas and moisture sensitivity. Nanostructuration furthermore imparts thermal insulation properties to aerogels presumably considerably retarding heat-transfer. These properties are assumed to increase the sensitivity of respective aerogels towards temperature alterations and may promote kinetically less favored side reactions. This is supported by the following observations: (i) the above-described humidity-dependent adsorption of water is well reflected by smaller weight losses (ca. 2–4 wt.%) in the temperature range ≤ 150 °C; (ii) intra- and intermolecular condensation occurring between 150 and

240 °C [51] give rise to further weight loss of 1–2 wt.%; (iii) depolymerization starts at 300 °C already likely due to reduced crystallinity, and (iv) the mass remaining at 350 °C (36–37 wt.%) and 950 °C (24–25 wt.%) was much higher compared to the non-processed cellulosic source materials. The latter might be a result of stabilization by cross-linking and hornification.

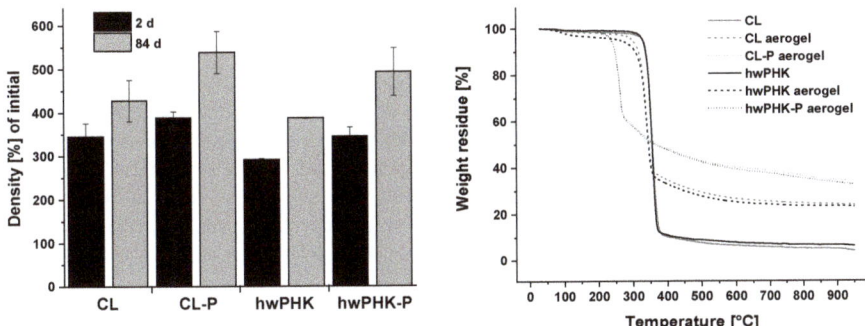

Figure 6. Bulk density [%] of phosphorylated and non-derivatized aerogels after two and 84 days during conditioning at 65% RH (left). Thermogravimetric analysis of cellulose II aerogels from non-derivatized and slightly phosphorylated cotton linters (CL, CL-P) and hardwood prehydrolysis kraft pulp (hwPHK, hwPHK-P). TGA profiles of the unprocessed source materials were recorded for reference purposes (right).

The TGA profiles of the CL-P and hwPHK-P aerogels differed strongly from that of their non-derivatized analogues despite the low degrees of phosphorylation. While desorption of physically bonded water was negligible for the CL-P and hwPHK-P samples, prominent weight reduction started at 235 °C already. However, only about 36% of the initial weight was lost in this step, which is much lower compared to the cellulosic source materials (90 wt.%). Formation of volatiles continued at significantly lower rates until the final temperature of 950 °C and a residual weight of about 40% relative to the initial weight of the samples was reached. It is assumed that acidic phosphate groups as present in CL-P and hwPHK-P are capable to boost formation of low-molecular compounds. This includes levoglucosan, which has been shown to be involved in re-polymerization of volatile cellulose pyrolysis products and secondary char formation (*cf.* [52,53]). The latter could give rise to the formation of thin, heat-shielding char layers efficiently preserving a reasonably large weight fraction under enhanced pyrolytic conditions.

3. Experimental Section

Phosphoric acid (99%), phosphorus pentoxide (98.5%), triethyl phosphate (99.8%, all Sigma-Aldrich, Schnelldorf, Germany), *n*-hexanol (98%, Acros Organics, Geel, Belgium), tetra-*n*-butylammonium fluoride (TBAF) trihydrate (≥97%, Sigma-Aldrich, Schnelldorf, Germany), dimethyl sulfoxide (DMSO, ≥99.9%, Merck, Darmstadt, Germany), molecular sieves 4 Å (Roth, Karlsruhe, Germany), and ethanol (96 vol.% and absolute, Merck, Darmstadt, Germany) were of highest available grade.

Cotton linters (CL) and total chlorine-free bleached hardwood (eucalyptus) pre-hydrolysis kraft pulp (hwPHK) were provided by collaboration partners of the COST E41 action. Their weight average molecular weight (M_W) as well contents of carbonyl group were determined as detailed elsewhere [36,54]:

- CL: M_W 143.2 kg mol^{-1}, 4.4 mmol g^{-1} C=O (fluorescence labelling of cellulose using carbazole-9-carbonyl-oxy-amine, CCOA;
- hwPHK: M_W 154.8 kg mol^{-1}, 8.1 mmol g^{-1} C=O;

Prior to dissolution or phosphorylation, the cellulosic source materials were activated by disintegration in water (solid-to-liquid ratio 1:400, wt./wt.). The obtained slurry was freeze-dried and stored at +4 °C until further processing.

3.1. Phosphorylation of Cellulose

Phosphorylation was accomplished as described elsewhere [39,42,55]. In brief, 250 g of phosphorus pentoxide was placed under argon atmosphere protection in a 1 L 3-necked round-bottom flask equipped with air-tight mechanical stirrer, condenser, and dropping funnel. Phosphoric acid (354 g) was added portion-wise under external ice-cooling. Triethyl phosphate (185 mL) was added slowly within 6 h. A clear, highly viscous solution was obtained after about 48 h of continued stirring. The thus prepared phosphorylation reagent (PR) was stored in anhydrous atmosphere at +4 °C until further use. A defined amount of cellulosic source material (typically 1.0 g) was activated for phosphorylation by repeated short-time (10 s) disintegration in a large excess of water (1:400, w/v). This was followed by submersion in consecutive baths of ethanol and n-hexanol (ca. 1:80, w/v; 2 times á 24 h for each of the organic solvents). About 40 mL of the supernatant n-hexanol was then decanted by gentle squeezing and replaced by an equal volume of PR. The flasks containing the reaction mixtures were then mounted onto a heated horizontal shaking device and left at 50 °C for 72 h. After that, phosphorylated cellulose was separated from the liquid phase and consecutively washed twice with n-hexanol, ethanol, and eventually deionized water. The last step was repeated until the filtrates showed a negative molybdenum blue reaction. The degree of phosphorylation (DS_P) was analyzed as suggested previously [56]. An aliquot of the sample (100 mg) was subjected to microwave-assisted pressure digestion in HNO_3/H_2O_2 using the following temperature program: 25 → 85 °C (3 °C min^{-1}), 85 → 145 °C (ca. 1.5 °C min^{-1}), 145 → 200 °C (ca. 1 °C min^{-1}, 12 min hold), cooling to room temperature. The phosphorous content of the obtained digestion liquor was analyzed by ICP-OES and used to calculate the DS_P according to Equation (1) [56].

$$DS_p = \frac{162x}{3100 - 84x} \quad (1)$$

Finally, an aliquot of phosphorylated cellulose was subjected to solid-state ^{31}P and ^{13}C NMR experiments to confirm covalent introduction of monophosphate groups.

3.2. Preparation of the Cellulose Solvent System TBAF (16.6 wt.%) / H_2O (0.95 wt.%) / DMSO

TBAF trihydrate (157.55 g) was dissolved in anhydrous DMSO (342.45 g). Then, 325 g of freshly dried molecular sieves 4 Å (600 °C, 3 h, argon atmosphere) was added portion-wise over a period of 96 h to bind about 50% of the crystal water. When the remaining water content as determined by Karl Fischer titration reached about 1.5 wt.%—coinciding with the onset of a faint yellowish (λ = 420 nm) coloration [36]—the drying agent was filtered off. The solution was stored at +4 °C until further use. Immediately before cellulose dissolution, the above-prepared TBAF/DMSO solution was diluted with anhydrous DMSO as described previously to obtain a final TBAF content of 16.6 wt.%. The final water content was 0.95 wt.% which ensures good dissolution performance and largely avoids decomposition of TBAF [36].

3.3. Cellulose Dissolution, Casting, Coagulation, Solvent Exchange, and $scCO_2$ Drying

The respective non-derivatized and/or phosphorylated cellulosic materials (3 g) were dissolved portion-wise in the pre-heated (60 °C) and continuously stirred solvent system (97 g) to give a 3 wt.% solution. While the obtained cellulose solutions were visually clear after two hours already, optical microscopy (magnification 100×) revealed that full dissolution requires 3–4 h. After four hours, the obtained dopes were cast into molds of cylindrical geometry (Ø = 10 mm, l = 20 mm). The molds were then immersed in 96 vol.% ethanol (EtOH) to initiate cellulose coagulation using a dope-to-ethanol volume ratio of 1:50. After 24 h of residence time, the molds were opened to expose the cylindrical, free-standing lyogels. The latter were transferred into consecutive bathes of 96 vol.% ethanol (3 × 24 h) and absolute ethanol (2 × 24 h) ensuring a gel-to-liquid ratio of 1:20 (v/v). Drying of the transparent gels was performed using supercritical carbon dioxide equipment (scCO$_2$). Samples were loaded in a 500 mL autoclave equipped with two separators for carbon dioxide recycling (Separex SF1, Separex, France). After heating and pressurization to 40 °C and 10.5 MPa, the samples were dried at constant CO$_2$ flow (2.5 kg h^{-1}) for one hour following recommendations of previous studies [57,58]. It has been shown that increasing the pressure beyond 10 MPa slightly reduces the remaining volume [30]. This is similar for increasing the temperature, as hornification and loss of tightly bonded surface water reduce interfibril distances.

Once ethanol was quantitatively extracted from the voids, the system was slowly and isothermally depressurized to prevent pore collapsing and condensation by Joule–Thomson cooling [59]. Both volume (±0.1 mm^3) and weight (±1 mg) of the samples (5 replicates) were recorded after each step of the sequential solvent exchange and after scCO$_2$ drying.

4. Analyses

Scanning electron micrographs of both external and internal aerogel surfaces were taken in different magnification after gold sputtering. A Philips ESEM XL30 or a Quanta 250 FEG with energy dispersive analysis X-ray (EDAX) mapping was used, both operated at an acceleration voltage of 5 kV. Evaluation of the surfaces with regard to remaining traces of TBAF was accomplished by detection of nitrogen and fluorine in EDAX mode.

Nitrogen sorption experiments at 77 K were performed using a Micrometrics ASAP 2020 analyzer. All samples were evacuated overnight at room temperature prior to the measurements. Specific surface areas were calculated according to the Brunauer–Emmett–Teller equation using a set of data points of the respective adsorption branches of the isotherms [60]. Average pore diameters were calculated from data points of the desorption branches using the Barrett–Joyner–Halenda (BJH) approach [61]. Nitrogen sorption experiments were complemented by thermoporosimetry using a Mettler-Toledo DSC 823e differential scanning calorimeter (DSC) equipped with liquid nitrogen module. DSC calibration for both temperature and enthalpy was performed using open-porous metallic standards (In, Pb, Zn). Aerogels were measured by weighing aliquots (ca. 1–5 mg) into 160 µL aluminum pans and submersing the samples in o-xylene. Measurements were carried out in ambient atmosphere using the following temperature program: (i) 0.7 °C min^{-1} from +25 to −70 °C, (ii) 0.7 °C min^{-1} from −70 to −30 °C ≤ T_x ≤ −20 °C, (iii) 0.7 °C min^{-1} from T_x to −70 °C and iv) 0.7 °C min^{-1} from −70 to +25 °C. Three thermograms at least were acquired for each sample. Data processing was accomplished using STARe software.

Moisture sensitivity of the cellulosic aerogels, water uptake at different degrees of relative humidity (RH), and possible triggering of shrinkage of the cellulosic aerogels was studied at ambient temperature (20 ± 2 °C) in RH-controlled environment for a time period of 84 days after scCO$_2$ drying. Desiccators used for these long-term studies were equipped with either phosphorus pentoxide (0% RH) or a saturated aqueous solution of CaCl$_2$ (30% RH), NH$_4$NO$_3$ (65% RH), and K$_2$SO$_4$ (98% RH) to provide different levels of humidity after equilibration. The actual RH inside the desiccators was monitored by digital hygrometers (Voltcraft data logger DL−120TH) and was found to be largely constant (±5% RH). Throughout the entire experiment, weight (±1 mg) and volume (±0.1 mm^3) of the aerogels were recorded periodically.

Uniaxial compression testing in longitudinal direction of the cylindrical aerogels (Ø = 10 mm, l = 20 mm) was performed on a Zwick/Roell Z010 equipment using a feed rate of 2.4 mm min^{-1}. Only samples transferred immediately in argon atmosphere after scCO$_2$ drying were used. Evaluation of the recorded stress strain curves was accomplished using testXpert software. Stiffness of the aerogels as represented by Young's modulus E was determined from the slope of the regression line through the linear elastic region of each stress–strain curve; boundaries were adjusted individually for each curve.

A 0.2% offset yield strength was recorded, i.e., the stress at the intersection of stress-strain curve and regression line through the linear elastic region shifted parallel by 0.2% strain as reported earlier [30].

Thermal analysis was conducted using STA 409 CD Skimmer equipment (Netzsch GmbH, Germany) allowing for simultaneous recording of thermogravimetric (TG) and differential scanning calorimetry (DSC) profiles. Aliquots of the samples (approx. 8–10 mg) were weighed into Al_2O_3 pans and combusted in helium atmosphere (120 mL min^{-1}) using a constant heating rate of 10 °C min^{-1} over the entire temperature range of 30 to 900 °C.

5. Conclusions

Mixtures of tetra-n-butylammonium fluoride, DMSO, and small quantities of water can be used as an efficient, non-derivatizing solvent to prepare sufficiently low viscous dopes of cellulose phosphates (DS_P ca. 0.2) for further processing into lyogels and aerogels. At moderate dissolution conditions (60 °C, 4 h), this solvent system fully preserves the chemical integrity of the processed cellulosic materials. Care should be taken during work-up of the phosphorylated materials to ensure quantitative removal of non-reacted reagent and solvent components. Compared to aerogels from non-derivatized cellulose, cellulose phosphate aerogels suffer considerably less from shrinkage. This is presumably due to repulsive forces being effective throughout the entire solvent exchange procedure except for the last $scCO_2$ drying step. With respect to the latter, it was interesting to observe that cellulose phosphate aerogels require shorter drying time to get rid of adhering ethanol. On the other hand, slightly increased surface polarity of the phosphorylated aerogels gives rise to a somewhat more pronounced sensitivity towards moisture sorption upon long-term storage. However, this drawback would be irrelevant if the materials would be used as lyogels instead. This would bear the advantage of circumventing that fraction of shrinkage that occurs during the $scCO_2$ drying step. On the other hand, this would be at the expense of the better sterilization opportunities for aerogels. It can be summarized that phosphorylation targeting a low degree of substitution has no negative impact on key aerogel properties. This includes bulk density, pore size distribution, specific surface, or pore volume. Skin formation upon cellulose coagulation, on the contrary, is evidently less pronounced for cellulose phosphate aerogels. This would be beneficial for the design of dual-porous cell scaffolding materials, since their nanoporous struts separating interconnected large micron-size voids are supposed to maintain rapid transport of gases, nutrients and metabolic byproducts.

Author Contributions: Conceptualization, F.L.; data curation, C.B.S. and M.-A.N.; funding acquisition, T.R.; investigation, C.B.S., P.S.P., J.-M.N., and M.W.; methodology, C.B.S., M.-A.N. and F.L.; project administration, F.L.; resources, M.-A.N., M.W., and T.R.; supervision, F.L.; visualization, C.B.S. and H.H.; writing—original draft, C.B.S.; writing—review and editing, H.H., T.R., and F.L. All authors have read and agreed to the published version of the manuscript.

Funding: The financial support by the University of Natural Resources and Life Sciences, Vienna (BOKU), through the BOKU DOC Grant 2008 (Funder Id: 10.13039/501100006380) to C.B.S. is gratefully acknowledged.

Acknowledgments: Part of this work was carried out in the frame of the COST-Action "Advanced Engineering of Aerogels for Environment and Life Sciences" (AERoGELS, ref. CA18125) funded by the European Commission. The authors would also like to thank Dr. Sonja Schiehser (Institute for Chemistry of Renewable Resources, BOKU), Johannes Amberger (Institute for Chemical and Energy Engineering, BOKU), and Adeline Hardy-Dessources (Université Clermont Auvergne, CNRS, SIGMA Clermont, ICCF; formerly ENSCCF, France) and Christian Jäger (BAM Bundesanstalt für Materialforschung und -testung) for SEC analyses, lab assistance, thermoporosimetry, and ^{31}P NMR measurements, respectively.

Conflicts of Interest: The authors declare no conflicts of interest.

References

1. Amaral, H.R.; Cipriano, D.F.; Santos, M.S.; Schettino, M.A.; Ferreti, J.V.; Meirelles, C.S.; Pereira, V.S.; Cunha, A.G.; Emmerich, F.G.; Freitas, J.C. Production of high-purity cellulose, cellulose acetate and cellulose-silica composite from babassu coconut shells. *Carbohydr. Polym.* **2019**, *210*, 127–134. [CrossRef] [PubMed]
2. Hickey, R.J.; Pelling, A.E. Cellulose Biomaterials for Tissue Engineering. *Front. Bioeng. Biotechnol.* **2019**, *7*, 45. [CrossRef] [PubMed]
3. Kim, T.; Bao, C.; Hausmann, M.; Siqueira, G.; Zimmermann, T.; Kim, W.S. Electrochemical Sensors: 3D Printed Disposable Wireless Ion Sensors with Biocompatible Cellulose Composites. *Adv. Electron. Mater.* **2019**, *5*, 1800778. [CrossRef]
4. Zhao, S.; Malfait, W.J.; Alburquerque, N.G.; Koebel, M.M.; Nyström, G. Biopolymer Aerogels and Foams: Chemistry, Properties, and Applications. *Angew. Chem. Int. Ed.* **2018**, *57*, 7580–7608. [CrossRef]
5. García-González, C.A.; Alnaief, M.; Smirnova, I. Polysaccharide-based aerogels—Promising biodegradable carriers for drug delivery systems. *Carbohydr. Polym.* **2011**, *86*, 1425–1438. [CrossRef]
6. Cardea, S.; Reverchon, E. Supercritical Fluid Processing of Polymers. *Polymers* **2019**, *11*, 1551. [CrossRef]
7. Liebner, F.; Pircher, N.; Schimper, C.; Haimer, E.; Rosenau, T. Cellulose-based aerogels. In *Encyclopedia of Biomedical Polymers and Polymeric Biomaterials*; CRC Press: New York, NY, USA; Taylor & Francis Group: New York, NY, USA, 2015.
8. Tabernero, A.; Baldino, L.; Cardea, S.; Del Valle, E.M.M.; Reverchon, E. A Phenomenological Approach to Study Mechanical Properties of Polymeric Porous Structures Processed Using Supercritical CO_2. *Polymers* **2019**, *11*, 485. [CrossRef]
9. Plappert, S.; Nedelec, J.-M.; Rennhofer, H.; Lichtenegger, H.; Liebner, F.W. Strain Hardening and Pore Size Harmonization by Uniaxial Densification: A Facile Approach toward Superinsulating Aerogels from Nematic Nanofibrillated 2,3-Dicarboxyl Cellulose. *Chem. Mater.* **2017**, *29*, 6630–6641. [CrossRef]
10. Fauziyah, M.; Widiyastuti, W.; Balgis, R.; Setyawan, H. Production of cellulose aerogels from coir fibers via an alkali–urea method for sorption applications. *Cellulose* **2019**, *26*, 9583–9598. [CrossRef]
11. Kanomata, K.; Tatebayashi, N.; Habaki, X.; Kitaoka, T. Cooperative catalysis of cellulose nanofiber and organocatalyst in direct aldol reactions. *Sci. Rep.* **2018**, *8*, 4098. [CrossRef]
12. Pircher, N.; Veigel, S.; Aigner, N.; Nedelec, J.-M.; Rosenau, T.; Liebner, F.W. Reinforcement of bacterial cellulose aerogels with biocompatible polymers. *Carbohydr. Polym.* **2014**, *111*, 505–513. [CrossRef] [PubMed]
13. Zhuo, H.; Hu, Y.; Chen, Z.; Zhong, L. Cellulose carbon aerogel/PPy composites for high-performance supercapacitor. *Carbohydr. Polym.* **2019**, *215*, 322–329. [CrossRef] [PubMed]
14. Hakkarainen, T.; Koivuniemi, R.; Kosonen, M.; Escobedo-Lucea, C.; Sanz-García, A.; Vuola, J.; Valtonen, J.; Tammela, P.; Mäkitie, A.A.; Luukko, K.; et al. Nanofibrillar cellulose wound dressing in skin graft donor site treatment. *J. Control. Release* **2016**, *244*, 292–301. [CrossRef] [PubMed]
15. Sulaeva, I.; Henniges, U.; Rosenau, T.; Potthast, A. Bacterial cellulose as a material for wound treatment: Properties and modifications. A review. *Biotechnol. Adv.* **2015**, *33*, 1547–1571. [CrossRef]
16. Sulaeva, I.; Hettegger, H.; Bergen, A.; Rohrer, C.; Kostic, M.; Konnerth, J.; Rosenau, T.; Potthast, A. Fabrication of bacterial cellulose-based wound dressings with improved performance by impregnation with alginate. *Mater. Sci. Eng. C* **2020**, *110*, 110619. [CrossRef]
17. Plappert, S.; Liebner, F.W.; Konnerth, J.; Nedelec, J.-M. Anisotropic nanocellulose gel–membranes for drug delivery: Tailoring structure and interface by sequential periodate–chlorite oxidation. *Carbohydr. Polym.* **2019**, *226*, 115306. [CrossRef]
18. Hujaya, S.D.; Lorite, G.S.; Vainio, S.J.; Liimatainen, H. Polyion complex hydrogels from chemically modified cellulose nanofibrils: Structure-function relationship and potential for controlled and pH-responsive release of doxorubicin. *Acta Biomater.* **2018**, *75*, 346–357. [CrossRef]
19. Zaborowska, M.; Bodin, A.; Bäckdahl, H.; Popp, J.; Goldstein, A.; Gatenholm, P. Microporous bacterial cellulose as a potential scaffold for bone regeneration. *Acta Biomater.* **2010**, *6*, 2540–2547. [CrossRef]
20. Bonilla, M.R.; Lopez-Sanchez, P.; Gidley, M.; Stokes, J.R. Micromechanical model of biphasic biomaterials with internal adhesion: Application to nanocellulose hydrogel composites. *Acta Biomater.* **2016**, *29*, 149–160. [CrossRef]

21. Osorio, D.A.; Lee, B.E.J.; Kwiecien, J.M.; Wang, X.; Shahid, I.; Hurley, A.L.; Cranston, E.D.; Grandfield, K. Cross-linked cellulose nanocrystal aerogels as viable bone tissue scaffolds. *Acta Biomater.* **2019**, *87*, 152–165. [CrossRef]
22. Budtova, T. *Bio-based Aerogels: A New Generation of Thermal Superinsulating Materials, In Cellulose Science and Technology: Chemistry, Analysis, and Applications*; John Wiley & Sons: Chichester, UK, 2018; pp. 371–392.
23. Hollister, S. Porous scaffold design for tissue engineering. *Nat. Mater.* **2005**, *4*, 518–524. [CrossRef] [PubMed]
24. Bonfield, W. Designing porous scaffolds for tissue engineering. *Philos. Trans. R. Soc. A Math. Phys. Eng. Sci.* **2005**, *364*, 227–232. [CrossRef] [PubMed]
25. Pircher, N.; Fischhuber, D.; Carbajal, L.; Strauß, C.; Nedelec, J.-M.; Kasper, C.; Rosenau, T.; Liebner, F.W. Preparation and Reinforcement of Dual-Porous Biocompatible Cellulose Scaffolds for Tissue Engineering. *Macromol. Mater. Eng.* **2015**, *300*, 911–924. [CrossRef] [PubMed]
26. Puppi, D.; Chiellini, F.; Piras, A.M.; Chiellini, E. Polymeric materials for bone and cartilage repair. *Prog. Polym. Sci.* **2010**, *35*, 403–440. [CrossRef]
27. Mi, Q.-Y.; Ma, S.-R.; Yu, J.; He, J.-S.; Zhang, J. Flexible and Transparent Cellulose Aerogels with Uniform Nanoporous Structure by a Controlled Regeneration Process. *ACS Sustain. Chem. Eng.* **2016**, *4*, 656–660. [CrossRef]
28. Plappert, S.; Nedelec, J.-M.; Rennhofer, H.; Lichtenegger, H.; Bernstorff, S.; Liebner, F.W. Self-Assembly of Cellulose in Super-Cooled Ionic Liquid under the Impact of Decelerated Antisolvent Infusion: An Approach toward Anisotropic Gels and Aerogels. *Biomacromolecules* **2018**, *19*, 4411–4422. [CrossRef]
29. Ebner, G.; Schiehser, S.; Potthast, A.; Rosenau, T. Side reaction of cellulose with common 1-alkyl-3-methylimidazolium-based ionic liquids. *Tetrahedron Lett.* **2008**, *49*, 7322–7324. [CrossRef]
30. Liebner, F.W.; Haimer, E.; Potthast, A.; Loidl, D.; Tschegg, S.; Neouze, M.-A.; Wendland, M.; Rosenau, T. Cellulosic aerogels as ultra-lightweight materials. Part 2: Synthesis and properties 2nd ICC 2007, Tokyo, Japan, October 25–29, 2007. *Holzforschung* **2009**, *63*, 3–11. [CrossRef]
31. Onwukamike, K.N.; Grelier, S.; Grau, E.; Cramail, H.; Meier, M.A.R. Critical Review on Sustainable Homogeneous Cellulose Modification: Why Renewability Is Not Enough. *ACS Sustain. Chem. Eng.* **2018**, *7*, 1826–1840. [CrossRef]
32. Pircher, N.; Carbajal, L.; Schimper, C.; Bacher, M.; Rennhofer, H.; Nedelec, J.-M.; Lichtenegger, H.; Rosenau, T.; Liebner, F.W. Impact of selected solvent systems on the pore and solid structure of cellulose aerogels. *Cellulose* **2016**, *23*, 1949–1966. [CrossRef]
33. Sala, M.R.; Peng, C.; Skalli, O.; Sabri, F. Tunable neuronal scaffold biomaterials through plasmonic photo-patterning of aerogels. *MRS Commun.* **2019**, *9*, 1249–1255. [CrossRef]
34. Lynch, K.; Skalli, O.; Sabri, F. Growing Neural PC-12 Cell on Crosslinked Silica Aerogels Increases Neurite Extension in the Presence of an Electric Field. *J. Funct. Biomater.* **2018**, *9*, 30. [CrossRef] [PubMed]
35. Sala, M.R.; Lynch, K.; Chandrasekaran, S.; Skalli, O.; Worsley, M.; Sabri, F. PC-12 cells adhesion and differentiation on carbon aerogel scaffolds. *MRS Commun.* **2018**, *8*, 1426–1432. [CrossRef]
36. Schimper, C.B.; Pachschwoell, P.; Wendland, M.; Smid, E.; Neouze, M.-A.; Nedelec, J.-M.; Henniges, U.; Rosenau, T.; Liebner, F.W. Fine-fibrous cellulose II aerogels of high specific surface from pulp solutions in TBAF·H_2O/DMSO. *Holzforschung* **2018**, *73*, 65–81. [CrossRef]
37. Sharma, R.; Fry, J.L. Instability of anhydrous tetra-n-alkylammonium fluorides. *J. Org. Chem.* **1983**, *48*, 2112–2114. [CrossRef]
38. Heinze, T.; Köhler, S. Dimethyl Sulfoxide and Ammonium Fluorides—Novel Cellulose Solvents. In *Chemistry Student Success: A Field-Tested, Evidence-Based Guide*; American Chemical Society: Washington, DC, USA, 2010; Volume 1033, pp. 103–118.
39. Liebner, F.W.; Dunareanu, R.; Opietnik, M.; Haimer, E.; Wendland, M.; Werner, C.; Maitz, M.; Seib, P.; Neouze, M.-A.; Potthast, A.; et al. Shaped hemocompatible aerogels from cellulose phosphates: Preparation and properties. *Holzforschung* **2012**, *66*, 317–321. [CrossRef]
40. Schimper, C.; Haimer, E.; Wendland, M.; Potthast, A.; Rosenau, T.; Liebner, F. The effects of different process parameters on the properties of cellulose aerogels obtained via the Lyocell route. *Lenzing. Ber.* **2011**, *89*, 109–117.
41. Zhang, M.; Dou, M.; Wang, M.; Yu, Y. Study on the solubility parameter of supercritical carbon dioxide system by molecular dynamics simulation. *J. Mol. Liq.* **2017**, *248*, 322–329. [CrossRef]

42. Granja, P.L.; Pouysegu, L.; Petraud, M.; De Jeso, B.; Baquey, C.; Barbosa, M.A. Cellulose phosphates as biomaterials. I. Synthesis and characterisation of highly phosphory-lated cellulose gels. *J. Appl. Polym. Sci.* **2001**, *82*, 3341–3353. [CrossRef]
43. Gavillon, R.; Budtova, T. Aerocellulose: New Highly Porous Cellulose Prepared from Cellulose—NaOH Aqueous Solutions. *Biomacromolecules* **2008**, *9*, 269–277. [CrossRef]
44. Sescousse, R.; Gavillon, R.; Budtova, T. Aerocellulose from cellulose–ionic liquid solutions: Preparation, properties and comparison with cellulose–NaOH and cellulose–NMMO routes. *Carbohydr. Polym.* **2011**, *83*, 1766–1774. [CrossRef]
45. Abu-Rous, M.; Varga, K.; Bechtold, T.; Schuster, K.C. A new method to visualize and characterize the pore structure of TENCEL® (Lyocell) and other man-made cellulosic fibres using a fluorescent dye molecular probe. *J. Appl. Polym. Sci.* **2007**, *106*, 2083–2091. [CrossRef]
46. Mao, Y.; Zhou, J.; Cai, J.; Zhang, L. Effects of coagulants on porous structure of membranes prepared from cellulose in NaOH/urea aqueous solution. *J. Membr. Sci.* **2006**, *279*, 246–255. [CrossRef]
47. Fink, H.-P.; Weigel, P.; Purz, H.; Ganster, J. Structure formation of regenerated cellulose materials from NMMO-solutions. *Prog. Polym. Sci.* **2001**, *26*, 1473–1524. [CrossRef]
48. Ioelovich, M.; Leykin, A. Vapor sorption by cellulose. *BioResources* **2011**, *6*, 178–195.
49. Rouquerol, F.; Rouquerol, J.; King, S. Adsorption by Powders and Porous Solids: Principles. In *Methodology and Applications*, 1st ed.; Academic Press: San Diego, CA, USA, 1999.
50. Lampke, T. Beitrag zur Charakterisierung naturfaserverstärkter Verbundwerkstoffe mit hochpolymerer Matrix, in Fakultät für Maschinenbau und Verfahrenstechnik. Available online: https://monarch.qucosa.de/api/qucosa%3A17757/attachment/ATT-0/ (accessed on 1 March 2020).
51. Tang, M.; Bacon, R. 125. Carbonization of cellulose fibers. I. Low temperature pyrolysis. *Carbon* **1964**, *1*, 390. [CrossRef]
52. Bradbury, A.G.W.; Sakai, Y.; Shafizadeh, F. A kinetic model for pyrolysis of cellulose. *J. Appl. Polym. Sci.* **1979**, *23*, 3271–3280. [CrossRef]
53. Hosoya, T.; Kawamoto, H.; Saka, S. Pyrolysis behaviors of wood and its constituent polymers at gasification temperature. *J. Anal. Appl. Pyrolysis* **2007**, *78*, 328–336. [CrossRef]
54. Röhrling, J.; Potthast, A.; Rosenau, T.; Lange, T.; Ebner, G.; Sixta, H.; Kosma, P. A Novel Method for the Determination of Carbonyl Groups in Cellulosics by Fluorescence Labeling. 1. Method Development. *Biomacromolecules* **2002**, *3*, 959–968. [CrossRef]
55. Patton, H.W.; Touey, G.P. Gas Chromatographic Determination of Some Hydrocarbons in Cigarette Smoke. *Anal. Chem.* **1956**, *28*, 1685–1688. [CrossRef]
56. Suflet, D.M.; Chitanu, G.C.; Popa, V.I. Phosphorylation of polysaccharides: New results on synthesis and characterisation of phosphorylated cellulose. *React. Funct. Polym.* **2006**, *66*, 1240–1249. [CrossRef]
57. Liebner, F.W.; Haimer, E.; Wendland, M.; Neouze, M.-A.; Schlufter, K.; Miethe, P.; Heinze, T.; Potthast, A.; Rosenau, T. Aerogels from Unaltered Bacterial Cellulose: Application of scCO2Drying for the Preparation of Shaped, Ultra-Lightweight Cellulosic Aerogels. *Macromol. Biosci.* **2010**, *10*, 349–352. [CrossRef] [PubMed]
58. Mukhopadhyay, M.; Rao, B.S. Modeling of supercritical drying of ethanol-soaked silica aerogels with carbon dioxide. *J. Chem. Technol. Biotechnol.* **2008**, *83*, 1101–1109. [CrossRef]
59. Fischer, F.; Rigacci, A.; Pirard, R.; Berthon-Fabry, S.; Achard, P. Cellulose-based aerogels. *Polymer* **2006**, *47*, 7636–7645. [CrossRef]
60. International Organization for Standardization. *Determination of the Specific Surface Area of Solids by Gas Adsorption Using the BET Method (ISO Standard No. 9277)*; International Organization for Standardization: Geneva, Switzerland, 2010.
61. Barrett, E.P.; Joyner, L.G.; Halenda, P.P. The determination of pore volume and area distributions in porous substances. I. Computations from nitrogen isotherms. *J. Am. Chem. Soc.* **1951**, *73*, 373–380. [CrossRef]

Sample Availability: Samples of the compounds are not available from the authors.

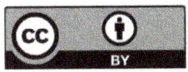

© 2020 by the authors. Licensee MDPI, Basel, Switzerland. This article is an open access article distributed under the terms and conditions of the Creative Commons Attribution (CC BY) license (http://creativecommons.org/licenses/by/4.0/).

MDPI
St. Alban-Anlage 66
4052 Basel
Switzerland
Tel. +41 61 683 77 34
Fax +41 61 302 89 18
www.mdpi.com

Molecules Editorial Office
E-mail: molecules@mdpi.com
www.mdpi.com/journal/molecules

www.ingramcontent.com/pod-product-compliance
Lightning Source LLC
LaVergne TN
LVHW070713100526
838202LV00013B/1088